A Course in Morphometrics for Biologists

This book builds a much-needed bridge between biostatistics and organismal biology by linking the arithmetic of statistical studies of organismal form to the biological inferences that may follow from them. It incorporates a cascade of new explanations of regression, correlation, covariance analysis, and principal components analysis, before applying these techniques to an increasingly common data resource: the description of organismal forms by sets of landmark point configurations. For each data set, multiple analyses are interpreted and compared for insight into the relation between the arithmetic of the measurements and the rhetoric of the subsequent biological explanations. The text includes examples that range broadly over growth, evolution, and disease. For graduate students and researchers alike, this book offers a unique consideration of the scientific context surrounding the analysis of form in today's biosciences.

FRED L. BOOKSTEIN is generally considered the founder of modern morphometrics, an interdisciplinary field bridging computer vision, statistical science, and organismal biology. His most lasting contribution to the field is probably his 1989 invention of the thin-plate spline for depiction and decomposition of changes in landmark configurations, a method that has appeared in countless scientific publications, several courtroom proceedings, and even a dance concert. A Fellow of the Institute of Mathematical Statistics, he was the first winner (2011) of the Rohlf Medal for Excellence in Morphometrics. This is his eighth book.

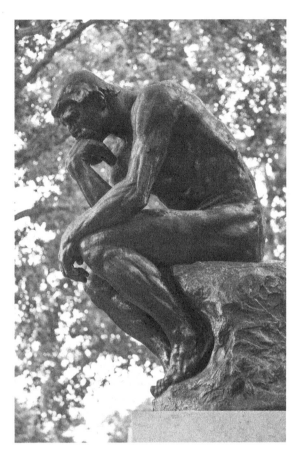

Here, one of the iconic images of Western art, Rodin's *Thinker (Le Penseur)*, is photographed against sunsplashed urban greenery at the Rodin Museum in Philadelphia, Pennsylvania. In its radically different original setting, the same figure, at smaller scale, sits high on the sculptor's *La Porte de l'Enfer* (Gates of Hell), an assemblage of nearly 200 subordinate human forms exemplifying all of the paradoxes of humanity out of Dante's *Inferno*. I take this creation as an emblem of the reflexivity of human biology, humankind studying humankind. There is superb Michelangelesque detail in the heroic musculature here, but it is the pose, not the detail, that lets us infer a specific behavioral/emotional state: meditative study. And even the pedestal on which the creation sits conveys a metaphor for our science, sculpted as it is to project the Thinker off the edge of the secure toward the unknown. We would do well to imitate this level of disinterested engagement in the course of our own studies of this most interesting evolutionary lineage, from the first eukaryotes through the Cambrian explosion of metazoa and so down to our own sudden species.

A Course in Morphometrics for Biologists

Geometry and Statistics for Studies of Organismal Form

FRED L. BOOKSTEIN

University of Washington, Seattle
University of Vienna, Austria

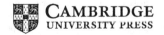

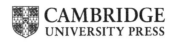

CAMBRIDGE
UNIVERSITY PRESS

Shaftesbury Road, Cambridge CB2 8EA, United Kingdom

One Liberty Plaza, 20th Floor, New York, NY 10006, USA

477 Williamstown Road, Port Melbourne, VIC 3207, Australia

314–321, 3rd Floor, Plot 3, Splendor Forum, Jasola District Centre, New Delhi – 110025, India

103 Penang Road, #05–06/07, Visioncrest Commercial, Singapore 238467

Cambridge University Press is part of Cambridge University Press & Assessment, a department of the University of Cambridge.

We share the University's mission to contribute to society through the pursuit of education, learning and research at the highest international levels of excellence.

www.cambridge.org
Information on this title: www.cambridge.org/9781107190948

DOI: 10.1017/9781108120418

First published 2018

A catalogue record for this publication is available from the British Library

Library of Congress Cataloging-in-Publication data
Names: Bookstein, Fred L., 1947– author.
Title: A course in morphometrics for biologists : Geometry and Statistics for Studies of Organismal Form/ Fred L. Bookstein, University of Washington, Seattle.
Description: Cambridge, United Kingdom ; New York, NY : Cambridge University Press, 2018. | Includes bibliographical references and index.
Identifiers: LCCN 2018012338 | ISBN 9781107190948 (hardback : alk. paper)
Subjects: LCSH: Morphology–Statistical methods. | Morphology–Mathematics. | Organisms–Size–Measurement.
Classification: LCC QH351 .B64 2018 | DDC 571.3–dc23
LC record available at https://lccn.loc.gov/2018012338

ISBN 978-1-107-19094-8 Hardback

....

Epigraphs

When you cannot express it in numbers, your knowledge is of a meagre and unsatisfactory kind.

> Sir William Thompson, Lord Kelvin,
> as quoted in Kuhn, 1961

The most notable achievement of modern science ... so far as its influence on intellectual culture is concerned, is the change that it has brought about in the standard of reasoning, in precision of thought and grasp of fundamental notions; this it has accomplished by creating a new type of rigorous thinking, more accurate and penetrating than the argumentation of an earlier age.

> Edmund Whittaker, 1948

Ah, the nuanced interplay between narrative and number.

> John Allen Paulos, 2015

A large acquaintance with particulars often makes us wiser than the possession of abstract formulas, however deep.

> William James, 1902 (Preface)

Dedication

As ever, I am blessed by the generosity with which my wife Ede and my daughters Victoria Bookstein and Amelia Bookstein Kyazze granted me the solitude needed to construct the arguments here, and revise the text and endlessly redesign all the supporting diagrams, instead of answering their e-mails, admiring the YouTubes of the grandchildren, or participating in the city life of Seattle, Berkeley, or London. To these three Bookstein women, my enduring gratitude, now and forever.

Contents

Appendices to this book, including thirteen of the data sets used for examples, along with Splus code for the main software tools, some useful auxiliary routines, and nearly half of the book's figures, can be found on the book's website, http://www.cambridge.org/9781107190948.

Preface

The book you are holding is the companion to an earlier volume, *Measuring and Reasoning*, concerned with the shared logical structure of numerical inferences over a wide range of basic and applied scientific disciplines. The arguments there are broader than the specific needs of biology or any other single field of study. I needed to complement that treatise with a more accessible offering better suited to my actual teaching assignment, which mainly involved explaining methods for analyzing measurements of shape and form to advanced undergraduates and beginning graduate students in the organismal biosciences at the University of Vienna. Between 2010 and 2015, over a series of drafts and worked examples, a curriculum took shape along these lines. This book assembles the lectures and worked examples from those Vienna courses along with a variety of reflections and extensions.

By "morphometrics," the central noun of this book's title, I do not mean just the subdomain of "geometric morphometrics" that is the concern of most of my scientific papers and essays along with a considerable variety of others' textbooks, software packages, and short courses and workshops these days. Such techniques, specific to the analysis of Cartesian coordinate data from corresponding points or curves of a sample of organisms, are indeed part of our subject, especially in Chapter 5. But in their statistical algebra the analyses driving geometric morphometric studies all rely on a much more fundamental toolkit for the summary of patterns pertaining to one or more numerical measurements per se: patterns that apply to coherently measured suites of variables regardless of their empirical discipline of origin.

A pedagogy for morphometrics must necessarily unify and balance these two source streams, both the "geometry" and the "statistics" of my subtitle. The specifically geometric component of the pedagogy had been laid out recently enough in one of the central chapters of a 2011 textbook with a Vienna colleague, Gerhard Weber, and also in the last two chapters of *Measuring and Reasoning*. But the *bio*metric part, the general language of patterning for studies of evolution or development – explications of the constructs like regressions and principal components that logically precede all the morphometrics – had to be drafted *de novo*. Such a presentation does not go well if it is limited to the standard statistics-textbook terminology of least-squares fits, significance tests, and bell curves. Instead, the pedagogy must anticipate the particular needs of the morphometrics to come – the passage from arithmetic to understanding as it concerns today's best and most carefully collated systems of multiple measurements of biological form. That passage emphasizes some specialized versions of pattern analysis, such as the spatial analysis of multiple measurements, and the corresponding statistical machinery needs to wrestle with models of whole covariance matrices, like the Wishart distribution, not just the simpler, more familiar Gaussian models of observed vector data. Ordinary textbooks of statistics, even advanced texts of multivariate analysis, do not teach the specific pattern languages that today's organismal biologist needs, and so a transition from prediction analysis to pattern analysis is mandatory for this applications domain.

Another central arena for this effort of reimagination was a senior capstone course, Statistics 423, "Regression and allied methods," that I taught at the University of Washington in the winter quarter of 2011. The forty students in that experimental setting were spectators at an improvisation on themes from most of the sample data sets in Chapters 2 and 3, themes that emphasized not the formulas but the justification of the scientific inferences that the formulas sometimes drive. The main examples of these two chapters – didactic data sets from ornithologist Hermon Bumpus and biostatisticians Karl Pearson and Sewall Wright, along with more recent exercises in regression by Secher et al., Tuddenham and Snyder, and Hellung-Larsen – were compiled for that course, and the exegeses here were worked out over the twelve weeks of lectures and student homework assignments in their light.

At the same time, over at the University of Vienna, most of my teaching in the Department of Anthropology was likewise modeled on the content of this accreting manuscript in one way or another. Principles for the appropriate reporting of regressions and correlations in the natural sciences, Chapters 2 and 3, lie at the core of the undergraduate course I taught called Wissenschaftliche Schreiben auf Englisch (Science Writing in English), and the appropriate reporting of covariance structures for shape coordinates, Chapter 5, was the major concern of my graduate course on geometric morphometrics. Five years of these Vienna students struggled through multiple earlier versions of the explanations of eigenanalysis here, and other students and postdocs had to intermittently but repeatedly update their morphometrics dissertations or derived publications whenever I would change the rhetoric of the techniques on which their work had hitherto been based. These stalwart, much-put-upon pioneers include Michael Coquerelle, Sascha Senck, Sonja Windhager, Stefano Benazzi, Jacqueline Domjanić, and Cinzia Fornai. Thanks go to all of you for staying the course. I am particularly grateful to the students in the Introduction to Morphometrics course for the past two years, who, in light of my threat to put any of my figures and any of my equations on the final exam, were obliged to master every detail of Chapters 2 and 3.

For engrossing conversations on these and countless related matters outside the classroom I am grateful to Philipp Mitteroecker (University of Vienna), Verena Winiwarter (University for Natural Resources and Life Sciences, Vienna), Kanti Mardia (University of Leeds), and Joe Felsenstein (University of Washington). Chapter 4, which attempts to ground the study of covariance structures in the classical topic of Wishart distributions, arose from a suggestion Mitteroecker tossed out in connection with the symmetry arguments driving our joint *Evolution* paper of 2009: On a spherical Gaussian hypothesis, why shouldn't the distribution of covariance distance (Figure 5.55) be nearly spherical in the Wishart distribution? (Why not, indeed? According to the elementary sketch of a proof on page 304, it actually is.) All this investment in Viennese pedagogy was under the oversight and continually generous support of Horst Seidler, first as my chairman in the Department of Anthropology and more recently (2008–2014) as Dean of the Faculty of Life Sciences, University of Vienna.

Other audiences for the pre-Broadway tryout period of this pedagogy include those seated for my talks or standing before my posters at the annual conferences of the American Association for Physical Anthropology in Albuquerque, Minneapolis, Portland, Knoxville, Calgary, and St. Louis, between 2010 and 2015; Philipp Gunz and the other thirty-odd predoctoral and postdoctoral fellows of the Marie Curie Labor Mobility Project "EVAN" (European Virtual Anthropology Network), Gerhard Weber (Vienna), director, 2006–2009; and Vienna faculty colleagues Katrin Schaefer, Martin Fieder, Hermann Prossinger, and Karl Grammer. An early formalization of this approach met with some success at a workshop "Measuring Biology" at the Konrad Lorenz Institute for Evolution and Cognition Research, Altenberg, Austria, in September 2008, and a later version at a follow-up conference, "Quality and Quantity," at the same institute (now relocated to Klosterneuburg) in June 2014. The talks at these two meetings were published as Bookstein

(2009a,b) and Bookstein (2015a), respectively. I am grateful to the KLI, to its director Gerd Müller, and to the late Werner Callebaut, its managing intellectual, for their repeated challenge that I turn my intuitions into comprehensible, reviewable presentations in this venue. From 2005 through 2015, the annual meetings of the Leeds Applied Statistics Research (LASR) workshops organized by Mardia and John Kent in Leeds, England, offered a comparable soapbox atop which to promulgate these ideas to a quite different professional audience – applied statisticians. Others who have engaged me at length on these matters include Norm MacLeod, The Natural History Museum, London; Clive Bowman, independent scholar, London; Paul O'Higgins, University of York, England; Daniel Cook, University of Washington; and Benedikt Hallgrimsson, University of Calgary. The specific idea of a relatively basic textbook spanning these topics was hatched over a supper of burgers and beer in 2009 with bioanthropology professor Matt Cartmill (then at Duke, now at Boston University).

The running examples here have several different origins. The Vilmann rodent neurocranial data were originally brought to my attention by the late Melvin Moss more than 35 years ago under a grant supported by the National Institute for Dental Research (a component of the U.S. National Institutes of Health). The data pertaining to fetal alcohol syndrome arose from research projects on adults (1997–2002) and then on newborn infants (2004–2007), led by Ann Streissguth, Fetal Alcohol and Drug Unit, Department of Psychiatry, University of Washington, with support from the National Institute on Alcohol Abuse and Alcoholism (likewise part of NIH). The translation of these studies into the context of discrimination that is their setting in Chapter 3 benefited greatly from conversations with Kathryn Kelly (FADU), William (Billy) Edwards (Office of the Public Defender, Los Angeles), and Arthur Kowell (Neurology, UCLA). Most of the other examples were drawn from one of the two textbooks that I exploited when I taught Statistics 423 in 2011: Per Andersen and Lene Skovgaard, *Regression with Linear Predictors*, 2010, and Sanford Weisberg, *Applied Linear Regression* (I used the 2005 edition). In particular, it was Weisberg who unearthed the Pearson and Tuddenham examples (although the treatment of BMI in Figure 2.40 is new to this volume), and Andersen and Skovgaard who realized the pedagogical value of the *Tetrahymena* and the fetal ultrasound data sets. Some other examples here (Bumpus, Perrin, Hackshaw) are borrowed from my earlier treatise (Bookstein, 2014) but have been rewritten for this disciplinarily focused context. The exemplary data on human skull growth were originally digitized by Philipp Gunz for exploitation in Bookstein, Gunz et al. (2003), with support from a grant to Horst Seidler from the Austrian Ministry of Science, and the Sewall Wright data on leghorn chickens are from the electronic version of Rohlf and Bookstein (1990). Several recent extensions of this work to random walk, to phylogenetic questions, to the assessment of morphological integration, and to aspects of the biomechanical analysis of strain were supported by U.S. National Science Foundation grant DEB–1019583 to Joe Felsenstein and me, as was the pedagogic experiment in expositing the Wishart distribution that concludes Chapter 4.

Since the 1990s I have depended for all my systems programming and computer network support, for the construction of more than a dozen desktop and laptop computer systems, and for two very large bespoke software packages (both named Edgewarp) on Dr. William D. K. Green (wdkg@wdkg.org), nowadays an independent consultant out of Bellingham, Washington, subsequent to intensive productive collaborations with me in Ann Arbor, Seattle, Vienna, and elsewhere. It was Green who guided me through the world of imaging data resources without which geometric morphometrics could not have been brought into the twenty-first century. The adult and baby fetal alcohol brain image data sets could not have been gathered without the Edgewarp program package he designed and wrote, and the dance video (Figure 5.83) fusing grids with the original moving imagery is all his doing. It is also Green who arranges things so that I can carry out computations on computers at three different addresses on two continents without ever needing to know what time zone I am in. Thanks, Bill, for this quarter-century of endlessly patient and creative support.

For their many useful comments I thank Lauren Cowles, my editor at Cambridge University Press, along with several anonymous reviewers. Philipp Mitteroecker and Clive Bowman read every word of an earlier draft in search of unsound generalizations to soften or hopelessly obscure mathematical notation that could be replaced by more accessible visualizations. The errors that remain are not their fault, of course, but mine alone. Please send your comments, complaints, and suggested inserts to flb@stat.washington.edu and fred.bookstein@univie.ac.at (using both addresses will optimize the chances of a comment getting through).

Fred Bookstein
Seattle, Washington, and Vienna, Austria
December, 2017

1

What This Book Is About

1.1 Overview: Where Morphometrics Draws Its Ideas

Morphometrics, the topic of this book, brings together the best modern methods for quantifying the patterns of variation of organismal form that we biologists are most interested in talking about. Sometimes the organisms under study are humans, in which case we usually refer to our work as an aspect of human biology or medicine. Or the research question may be classified under a rubric like zoology, botany, paleontology, or ecology. The objects of study, when they are not actually human subjects, might be living (in which case they may be domesticated, or farmed, or else studied in the wild), but sometimes they are dead or even extinct. They might be observed only once each, or over a short window of time corresponding to some physiological cycle, or perhaps over a substantial fraction of the life cycle or even all of it. Some investigators who make use of our morphometric tools are concerned with the evolutionary, developmental, genetic, or environmental processes that account for those patterns, while others pursue the consequences of those patterns for the biological functions they help govern (physiological energetics, locomotion, predation, reproduction, health), the time course of the organism's life, or the consequences for the ecological system(s) in which the organism can be found. Now a mature scientific interdiscipline, morphometrics combines knowledge bases and expert analytic strategies from geometry, statistics, and classical functional anatomy with the customary investigative styles and question constructions of zoology, paleobiology, medicine, and bioengineering in order to acquire and synthesize the information about organismal form that answers existing questions like those, or to pose new ones.

The underlying intellectual themes on which we draw for the tools and examples this book introduces hence range quite broadly. They are not the property of any single discipline, let alone the discoveries of any single

1

founding father (not even me) or small community of proud progenitors. Rather, they span nearly all the classic branches of the biological sciences and also nearly all of the allied disciplines that build tools for the bioscientist or supply the motivation or the language(s) used for research design, reporting, or dissemination. Here, anticipating nine of the later figures in this book, are some of those components:[1]

- From *comparative anatomy* comes the main thread that links our work to the classic language of organismal form and function:

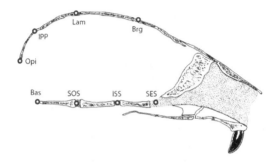

  ⊙ the **homologous anatomical structures** that help us keep track of our place – what we are pointing to – when we talk about variation of complex organismal forms.

- From modern *cognitive psychology* comes our principal diagrammatic device:

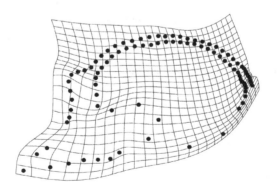

[1] These copy or modify Figures 2.41, 5.2, 5.25, 2.5, 2.10, 2.12, 5.3, 5.55, and 5.83, respectively.

⊙ the **transformation grid** that we use to present an extended comparison of landmark configurations to the intelligent eye.

- From *mathematics* we borrow endlessly, including:

  ⊙ the properties of **derivatives** that let us compute extrema of functions, such as sums of squares or the corresponding likelihoods, when we need those maxima or minima to summarize data;

  ⊙ the theorems of **probability theory**, such as the binomial distributions that summarize tosses of coins, and the rules of **limits** that let us get from there to the bell curve;

  ⊙ the geometry of **quadratic forms** and the ellipses, ellipsoids, parabolas, and the like that illustrate the theorems about them;

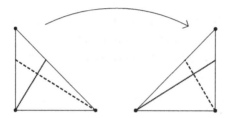

  ⊙ the rules of **tensor algebra**, which authorize us to express shape changes of triangles as ratios along a pair of directions that remain at an invariant angle of 90°;

  ⊙ the related rules of **matrix algebra**, which govern maneuvers such as inversion or eigenanalysis when applied to covariance structures; and

  ⊙ the theorems about **function spaces** that justify the crucial insight that the thin-plate spline interpolant is the "smoothest possible map consistent with the given data," whatever those location data are.

- From *statistics* come these ideas, among many others:

  ⊙ the **least-squares** models that summarize varying empirical data via simple underlying geometrical structures such as lines or planes;

  ⊙ the **covariance coefficient** that summarizes the relationship between two measured quantities – this is the numerator of the usual formula for the slope of the least squares regression line;

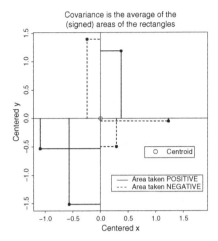

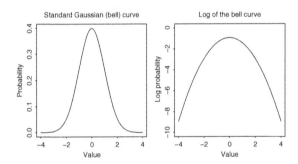

⊙ the **covariance matrices** that summarize the covariances of multiple measurements, all together, in one conceptual object susceptible to the mathematical manipulations of matrix algebra mentioned earlier;

⊙ the Gaussian distribution or "**bell curve**," universal model for disorder in any natural-science system;

⊙ the **Wishart distribution**, equivalent of the bell curve for assessing the disorder in a covariance matrix summarizing some empirical data involving more than one measurement;

⊙ the **information matrix** and its inverse, which summarizes the sampling error variances and covariances of the parameters of any numerical model around their maximum-likelihood estimates;

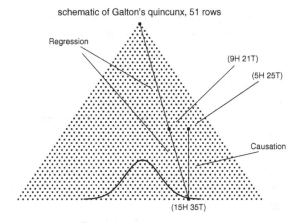

schematic of Galton's quincunx, 51 rows

- ⊙ Francis Galton's **quincunx,** a machine that generates linear regressions as correlated bell curves – straight lines that arise even in the absence of any governing physical theory, and that account for regression to the mean as an intrinsic property of pure noise; and
- ⊙ the algebraic technique of **quadratic discriminant analysis** for classifying organisms among two or more groups that vary in their covariance matrices as well as their group averages.

- From *physics* come three crucial understandings of the disorder through which, under the guise of "variance," we must filter our biological explanations:

  - ⊙ the **Maxwell–Boltzmann distribution**, which accounts for the motion of gas molecules on the Gaussian model;
  - ⊙ the broader notion of **entropy**, in terms of which bell-curve disorder is the universal maximum, and the identification of information (whatever its origin) as the opposite of entropy; and
  - ⊙ the expectation that **mathematics is often unreasonably effective** in summarizing natural variability (as in, for instance, the actual bell-curve formula itself – why on earth should there be a π there?), once the measurement conditions are placed under sufficiently stringent experimental control.

- From the *biological sciences*, broadly considered, come ideas such as

- ⊙ **morphological integration** (substantial but inconstant correlation among most pairs of measurements) as a ubiquitous property of numerical representations for every living system;
- ⊙ the centrality of **measures of extent** – lengths, areas, weight – and **measures of proportion** for summarizing patterns of growth or the relation of biological forms to their causes or effects;
- ⊙ the corresponding centrality of **path coefficients**, slopes of lines, for disentangling genetic or biophysical aspects of the underlying processes we are studying; and
- ⊙ **Brownian motion**, which identifies the disorder of particles in fluid suspension as tracked through a microscope with the disorder of gas molecules and, in a later realization, with the disorder that mathematicians learned to model under the heading of "random walk."

- Finally, from *morphometrics per se,* the literature of tools and expertise for numerical analyses of data on size and shape that this book surveys, we will be systematically reviewing such central strategies as

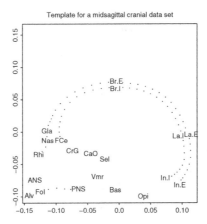

Template for a midsagittal cranial data set

- ⊙ the protocols of **landmarks and semilandmarks** that allow us both to design good measurement schemes based on point, curve, or bounding surface locations and thereafter to report patterns of their differences or covariances by focus and extent;
- ⊙ the **shape coordinates** that convert these multiple point locations into measurement vectors for carefully formulated multivariate statistical analyses;

Example of shape coordinate data

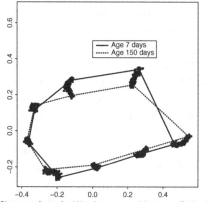

Shape coordinates for 144 rodent neurocranial octagons, Section 5.4

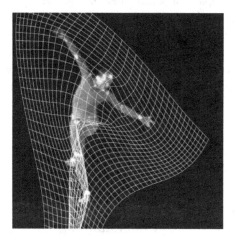

⊙ the **thin-plate spline grids** that convert the customized multivariate
  statistical analyses of those vectors back into the coordinate system of
  the picture of the organism(s) the forms of which we are trying to
  explain; and

⊙ the way that processes of growth or size allometry tend to suit a
  description by the first one or two **principal components** of shape
  coordinates almost as well as they do for multiple measures of extent
  (such as lengths).

The overall development of these ideas across this book falls into two halves with a link. In the first half, Chapters 2 and 3, the classic statistical technology of covariance-based least-squares linear modeling is reviewed as radically rephrased for morphometric studies of physical extents (quantities that add, like length, area, or weight). The second half, Chapter 5, builds on the technologies of the first to fabricate tools specialized for data that come as locations. We extend the covariance methods to incorporate a novel data type, the shape coordinates that convert the Cartesian location data into a format that the covariance-based methods can take hold of and then report using our preferred grid metaphor, the thin-plate spline. In-between these two thrusts is a bridging Chapter 4 that combines the several appearances of the linking statistical theme across the diverse twentieth-century literatures in which they originally appeared: themes as diverse as the Wishart distribution of covariance matrices, the information matrix, the singular-value decomposition, factor analysis, principal component analysis, and the relation of all these to the complexly structured measurement schemes that capture the variations of organismal form study by study. Outside of the morphometric toolkit itself, the shape coordinates and thin-plate splines, hardly any of these tools have the same inventor; it is their combination in dataflows that is crucial, from organismal anatomies through shape coordinates and thin-plate splines and then back to the organisms' picture for interpretation of these patterns as explanations. The reader who perseveres with the technic and the praxis of these preliminary chapters will be richly rewarded with the vistas that their joint application offers across the whole range of pattern studies of organismal form.

1.2 Our Basic Orientation: From Arithmetic to Understanding

Relying on this miscellany of strategies and tactics from so many different disciplines, inside biology or outside it, this book attempts to teach a particular kind of biological explanation, the kind arising from good pattern analyses of good numerical data about organismal form. By "good pattern analyses" I mean the highly structured numerical summaries (often quite clever or detailed) wherein crucial summary quantities match the features that we already know qualitatively to characterize the evolutionary history, life history, physiology, ecology, or pathology of the organisms we are measuring. If a study is about locomotion, energy consumption or transformation, growth, sex dimorphism, predation, reproduction, or selection, then the features of a good pattern analysis should align with those same conceptualizations. By "good numerical data" I mean numbers generated by carefully calibrated machines, operating on physical principles, aggregated over samples whose systematic features correspond to the varieties of "natural kinds" with the aid of which we have some hope of "carving Nature at the joints," as Plato's Socrates famously put it (*Phaedrus* 265e). The word "good" here should be taken in the context of the craft knowledge possessed by the experienced biometrician or human biologist. Or perhaps that should be the phrase "good enough," as in "good enough to convince your colleagues" (for the equivalent in physics, see Krieger, 2012).

The purpose of the book is to sharpen your inferential skills insofar as they pertain to this general bioscientific task of bringing good pattern analyses to bear on good biological data toward our shared goal of heightened bioscientific understanding. Out of the signals detected by the pattern analyses, our aim is to build the explanations that lead to new *questions*, to promising *interventions* (on a human body, a farm, a forest, an ocean, or any other ecosystem), or to deeper academic or public *understanding* of how we became the seven-billion-odd fecund, sentient, frequently rational large mammals who, as I write this, have just outweighed the ants as the most successful eusocial organisms in the history of the planet, at least if success is measured by biomass (E. O. Wilson, 2012).

An especially good pattern analysis will not only meet these criteria but also model the multiple and protean appearances of *noise* in the data. (Here the word "noise" means, roughly, "every aspect of variability that you are uninterested in explaining, at least at this level of measurement.") It is in this way that noise enters into our reasoning here also. If you have taken a statistics class before, you are already acquainted with the commonest quantification of noise in statistical inference, which is the "standard error" of an average or a comparison of averages due to *random sampling*. But this theme, along with its accompanying liturgy of *statistical significance testing*, plays only a very minor role in the explanatory techniques and tools introduced here (see also Mosteller, 1968). We will be much more interested in the ways that measured variables of the same conceptual entity align or misalign, agree or disagree within the same animal or human specimen. And of course the appropriate model for multiple measures of the "same thing" is for them to agree, or, in another jargon, to correlate very highly, not to vary cluelessly with respect to one another. Except in a context of strong and previously confirmed theory, no null hypothesis is likely to play any important role in an organismal study. In fact, the converse is likelier to be true: if the null hypothesis is a serious alternative to the theory in which you are interested as an explanation of the data set you are facing, then you may be reading the wrong book. You should instead be reading the technical manuals that might help you upgrade your instruments, or sharpening your sample descriptions until the appropriate pattern engine can find enough contrast between the signal and the noise to get a numerically reliable grip on the explanatory purpose of your scientific activity. Or maybe you are in the wrong discipline entirely, one that is not so pervasively characterized by systems-level organization and its variation as are the evolved, developed forms of the organisms we study.

This emphasis is different from that of other textbooks in our area, which, when they refer to regression or correlation, typically refer to purposes of "prediction" rather than those of explanation. For instance, in the opening sentence of his textbook on applied regression analysis (a technique that will be of central concern here), Weisberg, 2005) expresses the current conventional wisdom quite clearly without using the word "explanation" even once:

> Regression analysis answers questions about the dependence of a response variable on one or more predictors, including prediction of future values of a response, discovering which predictors are important, and estimating the impact of changing a predictor or a treatment on the value of the response. (p. xiii)

I don't agree – those are not the questions that regression answers, and they are not the biologist's most important questions anyway. In this book, regression analysis will not be argued to be capable of answering questions about "dependence" or "discovery," nor will its "predictions" be of any particular interest or importance in most of the scientific contexts we will be considering. Regression analysis, the way it will be taught here, is only arithmetic, mere numbers. On its own it cannot "predict future values," "discover which predictors are important," or "estimate the impact of changing a predictor or a treatment." Scientific meaning, if any is to obtain, must be based on axioms of causation and control, numerical stability, details of sample design, conditions of observation or intervention, choice(s) of measurements to be made, and, crucially, the route that runs from your data through all your arithmetic to arrive at a *persuasive numerical explanation*, the main scientific goal privileged in this book.

The background I am hoping you bring to the study of this book, then, is not the usual sketchy "introductory statistics" syllabus that focused on elementary probability theory and "significance testing" as part of the customary baccalaureate curriculum in many areas, but instead a background in biometrics or organismal biology that focused on the uses of quantification in the course of pursuing reliable scientific insights pertinent to studies at all levels (not just the molecular or genetic) of the complex systems we call organisms, including the human organism. Much of our expertise about such quantifications is almost independent of the choice of discipline, emphasizing instead the general cognitive role of patterns on paper (or on the computer screen) as a resource for converting numerical regularities into practical understandings or their consequences. A good midcentury overview of most of these themes, though not specific to the biological sciences, is E. B. Wilson, *An Introduction to Scientific Research,* 1952. Among the more recent books along these lines are the gloriously beautiful compendia of scientific information by Georg Glaeser, *Geometry and Its Applications in Arts, Nature, and Technology,* 2012; Philip Ball, *The Self-Made Tapestry: Pattern Formation in Nature,* 1999, and *Patterns in Nature,* 2016; and, for graphical semiotics, S. Rentgen, *Information Graphics,* 2012, and J. Desimini and C. Waldheim, *Cartographic Grounds,* 2016.

The fundamental notion of what, exactly, is being communicated when we report a specifically scientific finding is dealt with in, among other sources, John Ziman, *Reliable Knowledge,* 1978, and James Gleick, *The Information,* 2011. A lengthy but well-written survey of the ways that measured numbers get into biological investigations one by one is implicit in the examples of F. J. Rohlf and R. R. Sokal, *Biometry,* 4th edition, 2012. There is a deeper investigation of the sources of all these ideas in philosophy of science, under the headings of "abduction" and "consilience," in my book-length essay *Measuring and Reasoning: Numerical Inference in the Sciences,* 2014, along with additional commentary on many of these same examples.

This book also differs from most texts in the way its contents are organized. Most books on our topic (retrievable via search keys such as "statistical methods for biologists") begin with formulas, first for particularly simple canonical cases (comparing averages of the same measurement between two groups, fitting a straight line to a point scatter), then for various more complicated settings. The intention is to assure the reader that the tools supply routine arithmetical answers to a wide range of scientific questions. Again I do not agree – if the answer comes from a routinized tool, the question is probably not fundamentally scientific at all, but instead managerial, industrial, opportunistic, fortuitous, or whimsical. So the core of every example described in my pages will be the aspects that are *not* routine, the features that required modification of the standard textbook narrative or rhetoric in order to be of any help in furthering our understanding of the phenomenon under measurement. Note that this word "phenomenon" is in the singular. A good numerical study attempts to account for only one phenomenon, one quantifiable process, no matter the number of different measurements involved.

1.3 The Professional Setting (A Brief Intellectual History)

So why has no book like this been written before? The answer might lie in the unusual intellectual history of morphometrics as an interdiscipline, a history that has always involved a tension between two ways of doing biological science. Indeed, a struggle is under way in the academic halls of organismal bioscience wherever a curriculum committee is meeting to sort out the reasonable requirements that today's specialists in the form, variation, biomechanics, reproduction, development, or evolution of multicellular living creatures should place on tomorrow's. The problem is that we cannot agree on how extensive a familiarity and degree of comfort with applied mathematics and statistics it is sensible to require of our students, first, as prerequisite for studying our subject, and, second, as credential before certifying them as potential colleagues once their studies are completed.

Part of the difficulty is that the committee members themselves likely were taught mutually incommensurate versions of these technologies. Early books on the role of biometrics in evolutionary biology, and also Sewall Wright's late-life masterpiece *Evolution and the Genetics of Populations*, emphasized description and the tie with biological explanation. More recent texts, always excepting the late Richard Reyment's magisterial *Morphometrics* (1971, 1984), *Multidimensional Palaeobiology* (1991), and *Applied Factor Analysis in the Natural Sciences* (1993), have more often been aligned with themes of null-hypothesis statistical significance testing imported (inappropriately, in my opinion – feel free to consult my dissection of the topic in Bookstein, 2014) from other sciences than the biological. The committee's dilemma is not eased by recent progress in bioinformatics, in face recognition technologies, and in genomics, proteomics, etc., all of which, arising as they do in industrial applied biotech, make enormously greater demands on the formal biophysical and probabilistic insights of their practitioners than suit students who are motivated, as you probably are too, more by biophilia than by the more esoteric delights of the exact sciences.

The list in Section 1.1 of the topics we are obliged to "borrow" is, after all, a fairly lengthy one, and parts of it are at a modestly advanced level of mathematical sophistication. Why should we feel obliged to teach our biology students about matrix algebra, for instance, when no actual, measureable organismal quantity manifests itself in the form of a matrix (a rectangular array of numbers)? Yes, a covariance matrix is a familiar information structure (at least to readers who have completed Chapter 4), governed sometimes by a Wishart statistical distribution and thereby useful to us scientific observers of living systems. But we have no real evidence that the organism underlying our data "knows" anything about covariance structures. It is probably not the case that any of the entries in one of these matrices, let alone the corresponding eigenvectors or path coefficients, are encoded in measureable aspects of the individual organism's form, physiology, or bioinformatics per se. And should we be trying to teach the statistics of random walk to students who have not mastered the equations that govern its physical origin (diffusion), or the statistics of uniform deformations to those who have not mastered the corresponding bioengineering of linear strain?

The answer to these and all the parallel rhetorical questions implied in Section 1.1 is the same: to present the essence of the mathematics *in the form that a substantial fraction of the intended audience can master.* The presentations, then, need to rely heavily on analogy, on graphics, and on the student's existing understanding of biological applications that motivate the formalisms. Examples 2.3 and 2.4 in Chapter 2 seem like excellent historical exemplars in this regard: the student already understands enough developmental biology to find Wright's accounting of the correlation pattern sensible, and likewise enough to accept Pearson's certification of those linear regressions in both directions (though not, of course, his eugenics).

It is not obvious how to calibrate this task of comprehension for an audience with the range of mathematical talents that is the reality across today's biological professions. I like to think of the prophylaxis here as a careful balancing among three rhetorical styles: theorems, analogues, and graphical metaphors. At several places in this book I state and prove actual theorems, the kind of communication with which mathematicians (including biomathematicians) are most familiar. These come, generally speaking, in two flavors: statements that a particular formula suits a particular problem setting (the bell curve, the Maxwell–Boltzmann distribution, added-variable plots, two-point shape coordinates) versus statements that a particular formula supplies the optimal quantities for some parameterized explanatory task (least-squares line fitting, Tukey's formula, multiple linear regression, quadratic discrimination, uniform shears, Procrustes shape coordinates as projections). What these more or less fully worked explanations share is a reliance on the simpler parts of college mathematics: exponentials and logarithms, integrals and derivatives, Taylor series, vector algebra. Among the offerings at this level my personal favorite is the demonstration in Section 4.3.3 that the logarithm of Wishart probability in the vicinity of the identity is nearly the same quantity as covariance distance. (However startlingly elementary, this seems to be a new insight.)

The propositions on another list lie deeper: existence and uniqueness of the singular-value decomposition, the Wishart distribution itself, principal components and their biplots, sliding semilandmarks, the information matrix for the variances and covariances of estimated parameters. For these I usually state the general issue, sketch (sometimes algebraically, sometimes diagrammatically) the reason for being concerned, work an example of suitably simple structure or suitably low dimensionality, and then conclude with some version of "So one should be willing to believe that, more generally, ..." followed by that more general version. Among my favorite examples of *these* are two that lie close together in Chapter 4: Pearson's (1898) derivation of the information matrix for the general bivariate Gaussian distribution, and the Fisher–Wishart's (Fisher, 1915; Wishart, 1928) of the elegant and surprisingly terse formula for the sampling distribution of the same multivariate Gaussian. Another is the graphical explanation of the derivation of semilandmarks in Section 5.5.4 via the simplest possible case, just one sliding point.

Finally, there are theorems whose proofs lie so deep that it would be a waste of most readers' time even to sketch them. The most important of these are probably the two involving the formula $r^2 \log r$: the thin-plate spline and its bending energy (Section 5.5) and the self-similarity of the deflated Mardia–Dryden distribution (Section 5.6). To convey these fundamental driving configurations of the morphometric imagination I rely mainly on portfolios of novel graphical metaphors of the underlying mathematical propositions. Figure 5.95, for instance, demonstrates the self-similarity property without hinting in any way about why it holds or how it was discovered. For some readers, this will serve as a provocation to probe the original papers (or the citation chain they launch) in search of the more precise statements and proofs that guarantee the validity of the diagrams. For other readers, probably the majority, the figures will instead serve as the only available anchors for the intuitions that should govern the reasonableness (or not) of particular applications.

This is an appropriate place to note that accompanying this book is an assortment of fragments of **software.** I am not offering any sort of "R library" within which the reader can play *ad libitum.* I am no longer a competent coder, and it would be foolish indeed to compete with the elegance or accuracy of several well-tested packages that are on offer as of this writing (including packages from Ian Dryden, Stanislav Katina, Dean Adams, Chris Klingenberg, and Dennis Slice). What I *can* do is share my own Splus code files (which are easily repunctuated into R) for all the figures in this book that are based on publicly available data sets, along with a personal selection of others that illustrate theorems or simulations. These command files, along with listings of the underlying data or links to such listings, are included in the web resource http://www.cambridge.org/9781107190948 associated with this book. It is divided into one folder for data and another for command files, the latter either numbered figure by figure or corresponding to a few "functions" (subroutines whose names begin with F) called in the course of producing those analyses. These routines are in no way intended as exemplars, merely as conveniences for any reader to exploit or modify.

Over the course of this delicate sorting process of mathematics and graphics I uncovered an unexpected intellectual commonality: the main pedagogical problem is not with the morphometrics, or, more precisely, is not *only* with the morphometrics. Rather, all morphometric detail aside, we professors lack *any* survey of the role of numerical measurements, their variability, and their meaningful patterns suited to the level of the upper undergraduate or introductory graduate curriculum in the biological sciences – any book that fuses even the themes of Section 1.1 that have nothing to do with landmarks or shape. The most recent treatise by a biologist of which I am aware that deals seriously with issues like these (Hogben, 1957) is more than sixty years old. Hogben is very good on the meaning and pitfalls of regression, and also principal components analysis, but he could not critique landmark-based morphometrics because it had not yet been invented.

In short, it is high time for a new essay along these lines, one suited to the quantitative organismal biology of 2017. Hence the notion that I write one of my own. The task is to combine the disciplinary-descriptive and the interdisciplinary-algebraic arithmetic in a series of joint examples that together motivate the tie of the questions to the particular toolkit I am recommending and demonstrating for producing the answers.

The specific fusion that is contemporary geometric morphometrics arose as the vision of several of us, including myself, Kanti Mardia, David Kendall, and Jim Rohlf, that these methods could be extended to govern a previously unformalized realm, the variation of biological form over sampling, growth, and evolution, that had languished over most of the twentieth century pretty much the way pioneers like Rudolf Martin had codified it at the outset. The new tools have been distilled down to an ostensibly routine computational praxis by a wide range of professors and programmers including, among others, William D. K. Green, Dean Adams, Dennis Slice, Jim Rohlf (again), Chris Klingenberg, Ian Dryden, Stan Katina, Paul O'Higgins, and Gerhard Weber.

But in my judgment, this radiation of software contexts has not yet been subjected to sufficiently critical examination as a style of scientific dataflow. Indeed, just as David Freedman's (1991) acid survey of the method of multiple regression finds hardly any sound, arithmetically stable and reliable examples among the myriad of candidate papers, so a survey of the applications of regressions, principal components and like techniques in organismal biology – were anyone so masochistic as to actually carry out such a survey – would likely find few examples that stand up to the degree of skepticism put forward here. An abstract dissection of this general problem can be found in Bookstein (2016b). Meanwhile, this textbook tries to limit itself to a spectrum of unusually sound examples likely to remain persuasive regardless of present and future trends in standards of rigor across my intended range of disciplines.

The approach to the pedagogy of biometrics here differs most from its confrères on the library shelf in its attention to an aspect of biometric structure that transcends the usual emphasis on algebraic manipulations in one particular aspect: the specific concern with *where our variables come from*. In a gentle irony, this was originally the concern of a quite different discipline. Psychometrists like Louis Guttman, Georg Rasch, and Raymond Cattell worked out the appropriate parametric theories of how variables align with factors (e.g., the types of intelligence, as measured by test items having varying degrees of difficulty) long before I finished my own graduate work. Their efforts culminated in books like Lord and Novick (1968) or Cronbach (1972). The creation of the truly *geometric* morphometrics at the core of the "morphometric synthesis" of the late 1990s was the extension of these results to the domain of landmark and semilandmark location data: a newly formalized source of similarly structured measurements that went well beyond the usual approaches of medical image analysis (which originated mainly as imitations of the intuitions of radiologists). These novel techniques, together with the thin-plate spline, quickly proved more fruitful in the context of pattern analysis than of prediction or forecasting – in the contrast of matrix inversion with matrix eigenanalysis (Section 4.1.3), eigenanalysis will always have the upper hand in a morphometric context inasmuch as, if the morphometrics is done correctly, there will always be (indefinitely) many more variables than organisms under analysis.

In an accident that was fortunate for me personally, this aspect of the biometrics of form – its origin in the correspondence of identifiable point-locations – had gone mainly unremarked throughout the mid-twentieth-century ramification that imported nearly all of its main multivariate ideas, such as principal components, principal coordinates, and canonical variate analysis. (There are a few exceptions to this generalization: Jardine [1969], Sneath [1967].) Many of my predecessors were a great deal wiser than I am (e.g., Sewall Wright, Stephen Jay Gould). Nevertheless, the early builders of this bridge between statistical arithmetic and biometrical inference never paid enough attention to this fundamental strategic problem, *the biomathematical rhetoric of anatomical correspondences*. It had been overlooked in all the standard treatises from Martin (1914), shrewd as he was, through Anson (1950) and Yablokov (1974), and on to nearly the turn of the present century before it was foregrounded in my earlier treatise on the topic, Bookstein (1991). The discussion of geometric morphometrics in this book opens (Section 5.1) with this particularly important concern.

To exposit this bridge from "regression of anything on anything" so as to apply coherently to the sciences of organisms, it proved necessary to rebuild the way that regression analysis itself is taught, beginning with the reinterpretation of the regression coefficient in the Pearson context (a scatter, not a law) as a normalized covariance that needs to be un-normalized in order to be meaningful when assembled in the structured collections we now universally refer to as covariance *matrices*. Pearson himself already knew this by 1898, the astonishingly early year in which he introduced the information matrix (which would not be named until 17 years later) and its inverse, which annotates the effect on a calculated likelihood of varying all the parameters of a bivariate Gaussian at the same time, at least in the limit of large samples. Pearson could thereby speak rigorously (and he was the first to do so) of the standard errors of estimate of the correlation coefficients he was mustering as evidence for his dreadful quasi-racialist theories of physical and "psychic" (moral) inheritance. This Pearson approach to whole suites of regressions aligns best not with the regression context of Chapter 2 and Chapter 3, but instead with the Wishart (interdependency) approach discussed later in Chapter 4, and thereafter to the representation of morphogenetic and other comparative morphometric patterns by grids that lies at the core of Chapter 5 and its contemporary extensions.

The translation of least-squares and maximum-likelihood language from the less appropriate context of prediction to this new context of explanatory pattern analysis is probably the greatest achievement of the mathematical statisticians like Kanti Mardia and David Kendall who were present at the birth of modern morphometrics. The emphasis, I repeat, was neither on causation nor on statistical testing; it was on pattern description in our spaces of indefinitely many integrated variables. Here "integrated" means, roughly, "characterized by a pattern of a priori covariances [or correlations] that would make no sense at all if they were near zero, but that when far from zero are expected to make sense in terms of some constitutive theory of ontogenetic or phylogenetic organization." For more on this notion of integration, see Section 5.6.8.

In other domains where statistics is applied within the life sciences there may sometimes be no corresponding challenge. After all, the genome itself is not organized ("integrated") in any equivalently parameterizable way, nor the proteome, nor an ecosystem, nor medicine. Perhaps the specific thrusts of spatial, temporal, and spatiotemporal modeling put forward in this book will have their highest and best application precisely here, in the applied domain of morphometrics. That circumstance would be in keeping with a wide range of other applied statistics approaches emerging earlier – Koch and Link (1971), Riggs (1972), Cressie (1991) – that likewise attempted to constrain statistical methods so as to accommodate the theories governing their intended applications fields rather than, as is most commonly seen in the softer sciences, to use statistical rejections of soft (null) theories as a poor (because noncumulative) substitute for empirical theory instead. This book tries to show how the biology of organismal form can appropriately be brought to dominate the computations and the reasoning processes previously too often ceded to the arithmeticians of "shape data." Our biometric science is a science of patterns and path coefficients, not of p-values, and the pedagogy here will always emphasize patterns of these coefficients in preference to simplistic yes-no statements about "statistical significance" (a concept that is itself of very little practical significance to our community).

1.4 A More Detailed Preview of Coming Attractions

The rest of this book introduces and demonstrates all of the analytic themes that I have just rushed you through too quickly for adequate scrutiny. Chapters 2 through 4 concern a wide range of preliminary themes and anticipations of our overall thrust regarding the art of sound numerical inference from patterns observed in organismal data. The corresponding early examples involve mostly measured "extents" (distances, diameters, areas) or other net measures like weight or strength, with a particular concern for one particular assessment of the relation between two variables, their covariance (numerator of the standard formula for the linear regression coefficient). Chapter 5 weaves all these diverse introductory topics together in a sustained survey of our central domain of rich intended applications, analysis of the highly structured high-dimensional data arising from the labeled point coordinates that we can use to characterize the images by which organisms are viewed in two or three dimensions.

In greater detail: Chapter 2 introduces the fundamental elements of this form of reasoning. We begin (Section 2.1) with some elementary arithmetical properties of averages: their least-squares characterization, their maximum-likelihood property on a Gaussian hypothesis, and the various derived quantities that characterize them, such as variance, standard deviation, and the precision (standard error) of the mean (which decreases as the reciprocal of the square root of the number of observations). Section 2.2 examines the role of straight lines in the formulation of scientific laws, emphasizing the multiple interpretations of least-squares regression slopes (coefficients in laws, covariance divided by variance, weighted averages of observed slopes with respect to a vector mean). At this point the text pauses for two examples. The next section explains everything you need to know about the bell curve of Gaussian distributions, including the many different scientific contexts in which it arises and the quincunx (Francis Galton's wonderful machine) that exploits the Gaussian to produce straight lines as "regressions" for another reason entirely.

Section 2.4 concentrates on another excellent statistical coefficient (this one Karl Pearson's), the correlation, which has nothing to do with causation but which summarizes regressions on the quincunx in a very suggestive way. With its help we interpret examples from classic data sets of Pearson and Sewall Wright, and we explore the deep connection between regression lines and ellipses that justifies our invocation of Gaussian distributions in many inferential contexts. Section 2.5 offers some additional tactics useful in this domain – correlations along causal chains, John Tukey's helpful trick for estimating regression coefficients by hand, and the "hat matrix" that often aids inferences about individual regression residuals. A final section sketches some frequently encountered types of data that do *not* comport with the methods just introduced, in that they do not arise as random samples from a defined population sharing one single distribution, but can be made to suit the preceding formalisms by clever manipulations anyway: data from growth curves, random walks, or phylogenetic schemes, all of which play important roles in parts of organismal biology and bioanthropology.

Where Chapter 2 is concerned with lines as a core component of numerical explanations in the natural sciences, you might say that Chapter 3 is concerned with planes (and their geometric generalizations) as tools toward the same explanatory purpose. We begin with the basic schema of regression on two predictors at the same time, simultaneously introducing the normal equations and the three seemingly incompatible interpretations that apply to their solutions: the counterfactual or interventional version, the multiprocess (path model) version, and the least-squares (optimal prediction) version. To the novice, the fact that all three of these interpretations correspond to the same arithmetic is profoundly disconcerting. The text emphasizes that the choice among these narrative styles must be made on biological, not statistical, grounds. Section 3.2 focuses on one step in the corresponding decision process, the algebra of adding one new predictor to an existing linear scheme. Our example is the prediction of a baby's birthweight from one or two prenatal size measurements. The remainder of this chapter is concerned with three frequently encountered special cases. Section 3.3 shows how analysis of covariance (group differences in regressions) satisfies the same path equations as a fit to a plane and hence can be estimated by the same normal equations. Section 3.4 shows how all this applies to growth series, with implications for the language of persistence versus innovation. The chapter's final concern is the theme of classification and discrimination: Section 3.5 for the conventional linear case, Section 3.6 for the much more common situation where within-class covariance structures are not invariant. The examples here are variously historical (Bumpus's sparrows from 1898) or contemporary (my own research into the fetal alcohol spectrum of brain disorders).

Throughout these two chapters the emphasis is always on just a few variables, often as few as two, and the text is usually focused on accounts of one outcome variable at a time (a predictand, a group identification) that is of particular interest for some applied domain (a baby's birthweight, the slope of the allometric law, the survival of a Rhode Island sparrow, the likelihood of a prenatal alcohol insult to a specific adult brain, the role of height in the prediction of adolescent weight). From these foundations my argument then turns, in Chapter 4, to the more generalized multivariate context in which it is the pattern among our measurements, not any particular singular choice, that is our scientific concern. Correspondingly we will be opening the discussion up to domains offering far more variables than just a few: usually, more variables than we have animals or humans for analysis (what the statistician calls the "$p > n$ problem").

In this context of "indefinitely many variables," still restricting ourselves to discussions that hinge on patterns of covariance, two core formalisms together apply to a great range of questions about organized complex systems like organisms. The chapter begins (Section 4.1.1) with Karl Pearson's classic exposition of the information matrix for a bivariate correlation structure, and goes on in Sections 4.1.2 and 4.1.3 to explain the notion of a square matrix more generally along with its two central derived structures, the matrix inverse and the eigenanalysis, in this explanatory context. We already met the first of these two strategies in connection with the normal equations in Chapter 3. Section 4.2 introduces the second of these, the eigenanalysis, via one of its algorithms, the singular-value decomposition of a data matrix. I then explore its three main variants as used in morphometrics: principal components analysis, Partial Least Squares analyses of cross-covariance patterns, and principal coordinates of distance data. Section 4.3 concludes the chapter with a mostly informal exegesis of the underlying distribution theory for covariance structures like these, the Wishart distribution (an exposition following on one of Fisher's and then on Wishart's own), with applications particularly to the type of descriptions that concerned us in Section 4.2.

By this stage all of the formalisms necessary for a geometric morphometric data analysis are in place. It remains only to introduce them in the context of the several morphometric examples and the numerical inferences about biological process to which they lead. These are the topics of Chapter 5. We begin (Section 5.1) with the notion of a *landmark point*, the formalism that links biometrical shape description to the multivariate analysis that has been our concern hitherto. Section 5.2 shows how a standard maneuver from Chapter 4, the eigenanalysis of a 2×2 matrix, can be converted to specify how landmark data may be reinterpreted as instructions for measurements yet to be made. Section 5.3 switches to another formalism from Chapter 4, the principal coordinates analysis, introducing the celebrated *Procrustes distance* between landmark configurations and the principal coordinates they generate; and Section 5.4 shows another crucial manipulation, John Gower's *Generalized Procrustes Analysis*, that, remarkably enough, lets us install principal components and principal coordinates at the same time. (In other words, GPA supplies the variables for which the principal coordinates of a Procrustes distance analysis are the principal components.) A statistical distribution is introduced, the Mardia–Dryden, that will serve as analogue of the Gaussian in this more complicated context, allowing us to bring concerns of regression and prediction back into the morphometrics of landmark data in parallel to their origins in the data sets of Chapter 2 and 3 involving size measures. But lines and coefficients are not the appropriate formalism for *reporting* these covariance patterns. Section 5.5 introduces a remarkable visualization, the thin-plate spline deformation grid, for this precise purpose. With all these tools in hand, Section 5.6 carries the running morphometric examples of Chapters 2 and 3 to their natural scientific completion, with some surprising implications for other methodological approaches of current interest. Some of the examples are classic. Others pursue current departures from the established tools of Chapter 5 that more closely align arithmetical strategies with the kinds of biological questions that students of organisms are likely to be asking in the coming years, questions typically dealing with the interaction of multiple pattern languages – morphometrics against phylogeny, or biomechanics, or genomics, or medicine.

Some online resources that will help readers make fuller use of this book are collected in the website http://www.cambridge.org/ 9781107190948. These include thirteen of the data sets used for examples, Splus code for the main software tools and some useful auxiliary routines, and complete source code (likewise in Splus) for nearly half of the book's figures.

Throughout this book I deprecate conventional approaches like significance testing and null hypotheses in favor of the much richer scientific possibilities afforded by surprising pattern findings of structured *non*zero covariances, patterns that can potentially be confirmed in new studies, or recreated in reviews of the literature, or elaborated by measurements at other levels of observation or explanation. Keep in mind that organisms hardly ever illustrate null hypotheses or zero covariances. Life and its cycles, after all, are highly organized systems of covariances far from any equilibrium, whether of Gaussian processes (bell-curve noise) or anything analogously disorderly.

By the book's end I hope to have convinced you that the importance of any numerical explanation – any inference from quantitative data – depends less on the correctness of its arithmetic than on the explicit richness of the corresponding sample study design as regards all of the following: the choice of specimens, the carefully controlled conditions of measurement, and the choice of measures taken (single-occasion or repeated, univariate or multivariate). The essence of quantitative reasoning and numerical inference, not only in biometrics but also in all the other natural sciences along with their adjacent interdisciplines like neuropsychology, bioengineering, or cognitive biology, is the transition from arithmetic to understanding: the emphasis on pattern analyses in parallel of all the different channels of synthesis or contrast that a particular scientific measurement strategy affords, and the tight anchoring of the ensuing explanations and interpretations to the content on which these redundant pattern measures agree. The rules taught in this book are the best that I know for making sense of the "blooming, buzzing confusion" that is today's world of quantified organismal forms. They are also, I claim, the best tools for articulating with the domains of evolutionary explanations (such as genomic distances), on the one hand, and developmental, social, or medical applications, on the other. To justify organismal biology as a coherent quantitative discipline, one must demand the richest possible interdisciplinarity of its established explanations – what the myrmecologist and evolutionary biologist E. O. Wilson famously called their *consilience* with the measurements and explanations afforded by all the other sciences, from biophysics or physiology to, say, archaeology or human mating patterns, that communicate across the boundaries dividing the academics and their buildings by reference to the same objects of measurement.

Let us begin, then, in Chapter 2, with the most basic techniques, least-squares fits to individual numbers and to straight lines. Via the role played by computed variances and covariances, these techniques and their formulas lie at the root of every other tool on which we are going to rely.

2

Getting Started: One or Two Measurements Only

Every student of biometrics, even a beginner, already intuits many of the ways that simple arithmetic aids our scientific understanding. Some of these intuitions are valid, and those should survive to the end of our curriculum. Teaching is easier when we can refer to these prior insights wherever they are reasonable – the insights that rely on the geometry of simple linear diagrams or the design and engineering of the elegant machines that provide data matching this simple shared pattern. To the extent that many of our numerical inferences are this straightforward – to the extent we can guess the weight of a baby from its width or an animal's strength or running speed from its body size and shape – we biologists were all born intuitive biometricians anyway.

Chapter 2 is concerned mostly with the algebra that can sometimes sharpen intuitions like these. Its arguments are simpler than the geometries of multiple regression that concern Chapter 3. Chapter 2's arguments emphasize *ties to the logic of the exact sciences,* especially their logic in situations where it is evident what quantities are the essential characteristics of the system under study and what tactics of statistical data collection and analysis can arrive at their values most expeditiously. In other words, this chapter concentrates on applications where theory tells us what number we should expect to get, where it is important to get that correct number or something that is "close enough" to it to be plausible, and where the numerical summary at which we are driving has some of the characteristics of an arithmetical average. This is the role of mathematics in the natural sciences emphasized by such observers of the scientific method as Kuhn (1961) or Wigner (1960): its role in the confirmation or disconfirmation of quantitative theories. We are a long way from the more conventional examples favored in introductory statistics courses, examples driven by qualitative questions like "Do these groups differ?" or "Was this advertisement true?" Part of what makes a natural science numerical is that the answers to its questions are not words like "Yes" or "No" but instead *actual numbers* for which competing theories dictate different values in advance. The most important role that your data can play is to help you decide between theories that were equally reasonable before you started to make your measurements. See also Platt (1964).

The examples to follow will make this point over and over for many different measurement domains. We will see, for instance, how Pearson argued the universality of a relation between measured lengths on parents and their children, although he was totally wrong about what he claimed his findings implied. A famous example from Sewall Wright shows for a data set of measured lengths that the magnitudes of correlations constitute a reasonable guide to the pattern that developmentalists had been calling "morphological integration," commonality of developmental pathways, while a physical argument owing to James Clerk Maxwell shows how the Gaussian distribution beloved of sampling statistics in the hands of humans can be generated just as well in the inanimate world as the natural distribution of the velocities of gas molecules in any direction.

The appropriateness of these relatively simple examples depends not on the discipline generating the data but on the complexity of the contrasts or calibrations that need to be applied to real measurements in order to guarantee that the required summaries and the corresponding tests of positive theory are numerically cogent and clear. In some of the examples, that simplicity will be demonstrated explicitly. In others, it will be just as explicitly contradicted, hence reserving the investigation for the more powerful methods of later chapters.

Within this general framework, our argument here in Chapter 2 has six parts. Section 2.1 reviews something you have probably understood from childhood: the exquisite rationality of averages, their algebraic foundation and their logical import. In a sense, nearly all of statistics reduces to a systematic exploration of the power of averaging quantities, usually many at a time in organized systems of arithmetic. From this topic we turn to an initial algorithmic approach, least-squares linear regression, for which Section 2.2 derives the standard formulas but also shows how they reduce to a straightforward version of weighted averaging. This is particularly convenient inasmuch as of the two terms in the standard formula, covariance divided by variance, there is an intuitive geometry of the denominator (the variance of the predictor) but no equivalently accessible imagery for the numerator. Understanding the biology of covariances will have to wait until whole systems of them can be surveyed in a strict ordering via the matrix computations in Chapter 4.

From this construal of regression as the demonstration of a linear scientific law we turn to a seemingly totally different setup, the flipping (tossing) of sets of coins over and over. Mathematicians (and gamblers too) have known for nearly three centuries that as the number of coins increases without limit, these distributions, properly scaled, converge to one shared canonical form, the Gaussian distribution – the celebrated "bell curve." It is only in the presence of a Gaussian distribution that the ordinary average has a rational justification. Helpfully, we have known since about 1860 that one universally encountered physical process, the molecular mixing that homogenizes the air you are breathing as you read this text, is a machine for generating exactly the same bell curves without any need for human interventions like throwing coins or random sampling. Section 2.3 introduces Francis Galton's elegant machine, the *quincunx,* for generating linear regressions in a context of pure disorder like that one yet far from any physical laws about mass or energy. The corresponding geometric descriptors, which can be graphed as ellipses, are an iconography for the sums of squares that actually carry the algebraic load. The central formula for the standardized Gaussian distribution ties all these considerations together.

Either in their original units (millimeters or inches) or after conversion to "z scores" of average zero and variance 1, these tools and visualizations have been used for over a century to convey the essence of many different biological measurement series. Section 2.4 exemplifies this enduring toolkit in two applications, one from Sewall Wright on the relations among multiple measures of length in leghorn chickens, the other from Karl Pearson dealing with similar data across multigenerational British families. The key to good biology in these and all other cases is the multiplicity of available measurements, even if you are only talking about one or two at a time.

The chapter closes with two sections setting out a variety of special formulas for special cases. Section 2.5 introduces various useful ways of combining data that constitute further numerical processing of the weighted averages emphasized thus far – products of correlations, approximations to regression slopes by mean differences (which are so much easier when you don't have a computer handy), assessments of especially large deviations of single points from their ostensible linear summaries. Finally, Section 2.6 introduces three sample designs that fall outside the domain of the "independent identically distributed" kind to which the usual textbook formulas are restricted: random walks, growth series, and branching processes. Discussion of the corresponding enrichment of the dual domain, that of the logical structure of our selected *variables,* is deferred to Chapter 5.

2.1 Elementary Averages from an Intermediate Standpoint[1]

We begin by reviewing a technique that you surely first met in elementary school. Its justification is the key to justifying many more advanced numerical manipulations.

2.1.1 Averages as Least-Squares

Suppose you have N different numerical measurements. Write them down and refer to these inscriptions as the collection x_i of their values, where the subscript i goes from 1 to N. The first number on the list is x_1, the second is x_2, and so on up to the last one, which is x_N. You are a biological scientist, so the numbers stand for measurements of "the same thing" on a sample of organisms, or over a series of times or a range of environments or other perturbations of their lives. In some studies the order of the x's matters (x_1 is for the youngest organism or the oldest ancestor, . . . , x_N for the specimen of greatest age or most recent ancestry) and sometimes it is just the accidental order they were confronted by your ruler. There will be more to say about the consequences of the presence or absence of this ordering in Section 2.6.

Regardless of what the subscript i on the x's stands for, you are certainly already familiar with the notion of their **average**, the total of all their values divided by their count. In the x notation, this is $\bar{x} = (x_1 + x_2 + \cdots + x_N)/N = (\Sigma_{i=1}^{N} x_i)/N$. If you are reading text like this out loud, you usually read the expression $\bar{x}$ as "x-bar," the "bar" part referring to the line ¯ over the x, and the character Σ is the Greek capital S, standing for "sum." (This is the same S that, transformed into the symbol $\int$, is used in calculus to stand for "integral.") If the total count N is already clear from context, equations like this will usually drop the $\substack{N \\ i=1}$ part. A formula like this can be nonsense: for instance, the average number of hockey goals scored per citizen of the United States, or the average number of leaves per North American tree. Or it might seem intuitively to be fairly reasonable, like the average of the heights of the mothers and the daughters in Pearson's family-by-family data (Figure 2.28). Because this is a course in numerical inference within biology, the criteria of "sense" or "nonsense," "meaningfulness" or "meaninglessness" refer not to the data per se, but instead to *inferences* in the intended bioscientific context.

---

[1] This heading is an homage to the German geometer and mathematics pedagogue Felix Klein (1849–1925), whose lectures for mathematics teachers, gathered in two volumes under the title *Elementary Mathematics from an Advanced Standpoint*, were a mainstay of my time as an undergraduate mathematician.

The **sum of squares** of N x's around a value y is straightforwardly written down as the formula $\Sigma(x_i - y)^2$ (which, remember, is short for $\Sigma_{i=1}^{N}(x_i - y)^2$). "As a function of y," meaning, "as you play around with different values of y," this sum of squares is smallest when $y = \bar{x}$: the sum of squares is smallest around the average. This is easy to show by taking derivatives, as long as you remember two formulas for derivatives that you learned in high school: for any function f of y, $\frac{d}{dy}f^2(y) = 2f(y)\frac{df}{dy}$, and if a and b do not depend on y, then $\frac{d}{dy}(ay + b) = a$. Applying these with $f(y) = x_i - y$, so that $a = -1$, one has $\frac{d}{dy}\Sigma(x_i - y)^2 = \Sigma\frac{d}{dy}(x_i - y)^2 = \Sigma 2(x_i - y)(-1) = -2(\Sigma x_i - Ny)$. This expression is zero when $\Sigma x_i = Ny$, which is the case for $y = \bar{x}$. Or, algebraically, we can rearrange the expression of interest as

$$\Sigma(x_i - y)^2 = \Sigma(x_i - \bar{x})^2 + N(\bar{x} - y)^2, \tag{2.1}$$

which, again, is obviously a minimum at $y = \bar{x}$.

This pair of quantities $\bar{x}$ and $\Sigma(x_i - \bar{x})^2$ might be "physical," in this case, **kinematical**, expressions of the geometry of the real physical world. If we imagine a collection of particles of mass 1 located at the position corresponding to each value x_i on a "massless rod" (a rigid armature that doesn't weigh anything), then the value $\bar{x}$ is the point along the rod at which it will balance on a support (such as your finger), and the quantity $\Sigma(x_i - \bar{x})^2$ is proportional to the energy it will take to spin the rod around a vertical axis through that point of support at a fixed rate of turning (say, one revolution every ten seconds).

It will be useful to talk about a second derived quantity, that actual minimizing sum of squares per original item. This is $\left(\Sigma(x_i - \bar{x})^2\right)/N$, the **variance** of the set of N x's, which can be expressed equally well in the alternate formula

$$\mathrm{var}(x) = \overline{x^2} - \bar{x}^2. \tag{2.2}$$

(To get from equation (2.1) to this new equation we relied on the identity $\Sigma(x - \bar{x}) = 0$.) The notation here was cleverly designed (at least from the mathematician's point of view) to use a single symbol twice with two different meanings. The leftmost horizontal line in equation (2.2), the line over the "x^2," means the average of that entire expression – square first, then average. The line over the x at far right, on the other hand, is *only* over the "x" in its expression "$\bar{x}^2$", implying that you average the x's first, then square. In either version, this quantity is also sometimes called the **mean square**, since it likewise takes the form of an average, i.e., a mean.

Please do not confuse this value with the nearly equal value $\left(\Sigma(x_i - \bar{x})^2\right)/$ $(N - 1)$, the same formula except divided by $N - 1$ instead of N. This version of the formula plays a role in likelihood estimates of the variance of a "population" given the variance of a finite sample. For instance, if a sample consists of just two specimens, so that there are only two measurements, x_1 and x_2, then the likeliest estimate of the actual variance of the population from which the pair of specimens was drawn is not $\left(\Sigma(x_i - \bar{x})^2\right)/2$ but twice that value.

A variance comes in different units from the original measurement. If the measurement was in centimeters, then variance is in squared centimeters (area); if the measurement was of area, then the variance is in units of cm^4, whatever those are. Often it is more useful to refer to a quantity that has the same units as the x's that were originally measured. Around 1850, statisticians began to refer to the median of the absolute value of those differences $x_i - \bar{x}$ of individual measures from their average; this quantity was called the *probable error*, as half the deviations were bigger than it and half were less. A better, algebraically more convenient choice, one you have probably heard the name of before, is the *standard deviation* (s.d.), square root of the variance. At the left in Figure 2.1, the average of the six heavy black points is shown as a point above an imagined pivot, an actual balancing point, whereas the variance of the same set of points is the average of the heights achieved (the open circles) by a parabola of formula $y = x^2$ lofted above this same set of points along its axis. (I scaled up the vertical of this parabola by a factor of 4 for legibility.) At the right, we see the same parabolic shape, now shifted vertically, as representing the mean square of the data around every tentative "central tendency": the minimum is indeed to be found right at the ordinary average.

The same "correction," $N - 1$ instead of N, applies to the standard deviation that applied to the variance. For a sample of just two measurements x_1, x_2, the likeliest value of the standard deviation is not the formula $|x_1 - x_2|/2$, the difference of either value from their common mean, but instead $\sqrt{2}$ times that absolute difference. We will not need this maneuver over the course of this book, although it sometimes turns up when data come in the form of paired observations on left and right sides of a single organism. (See, for instance, figure 4 of Bookstein and Domjanić, 2015.)

Suppose we multiply all the x's by some factor. If we are measuring lengths, for instance, and (perhaps thinking about giant sequoias or whales rather than shrews or bats) we switch from centimeters to meters for our ruler, the new x's will be the old ones divided by 100. The average is reduced by the same factor of 100, the variance (because it is an average of squares) by a factor of $100^2 = 10000$. The standard deviation, scaling as the square root of the variance, will be altered by the same factor of 100 as the original data. This is good, because it's supposed to represent a sort of "width" on the physical bar we're talking about. Of course changes of units like this do not alter the biological explanations at which we are trying to arrive.

2.1.2 Precision of Averages

For convenience, let's take a very simple "measurement," the propensity of an ordinary coin to come up Heads, a foraging animal to veer left or right, or some other similarly binary observation. We measure this in the case of the coin by flipping the coin and observing which side ends up facing upward: Heads or Tails,[2] each with probability one-half. In the limit of "a great many" coins, this

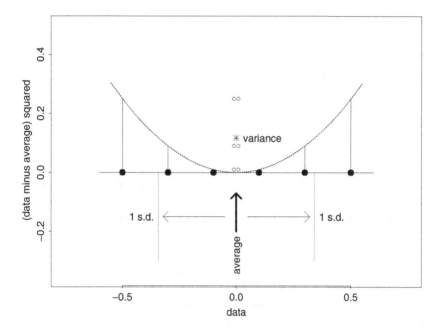

Figure 2.1 Average and variance. Left: definition of the variance as the average squared distance of the data from their average. Dots: six observations of the same measurement x, plotted on an axis. Arrow: their average as a location on the same axis. Vertical: the parabola for squared difference from this position on the horizontal axis. The variance of the set of x-locations is the average height of the six intercepts of the parabola shown; it is proportional to the energy required to spin this particular set of six dots around their average. Right: the same parabola, shifted vertically by the variance, characterizes the mean square of the data around any candidate for the average according to equation (2.3).

---

[2] Other languages have different idioms for these. In the German-speaking world, for instance, the two faces of the coin are *Kopf* and *Zahl*; in French, *face* and *pile*.

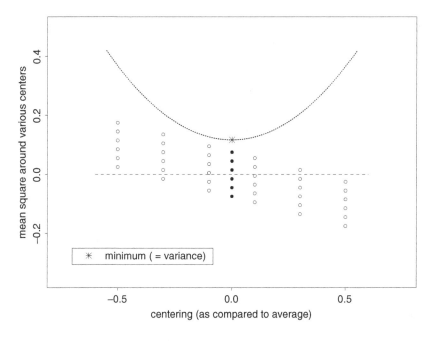

Figure 2.1 *(Cont.)*

example will occupy us extensively later on, in connection with quincunxes and the bell curve. For now, the count of coins might be either small or large, and all we need is the logic of sums of squares, not yet any more abstract style of analysis.

We can imagine assaying the "propensity" of a coin to come up Heads as the average of a large number of coin flips each coded 1 for Heads, 0 for Tails. (There is already a theory here – that the coin *has* a propensity that is a property of the coin rather than, say, the way it is flipped. [For a contrary model, see Diaconis, 2007.] Such theories often arise in genetics, for instance, when we are studying the statistics of two-allele sites or the equivalent for the Y-chromosome that [usually] determines sex.) We want to understand how the variance of this average (or its standard deviation, which encodes the same information) changes as the total number K of coin flips over which we are counting our Heads increases indefinitely.

It is helpful to proceed flip by flip, and we begin as simply as possible, with the flip of just one coin that we consider to be "fair," which means that it has a long-term propensity of producing just 50% Heads. The single flip yields 0 (no Heads) half the time and 1 (one Head) half the time. The average is $\frac{1}{2}$ and the the deviation from the mean is always $\frac{1}{2}$ one way or the other, so that the squared deviation is always $\frac{1}{4}$, and so must average $\frac{1}{4}$ — this, then, is the variance. We can think of this as "two cases," the two outcome possibilities of the one coin.

Flip a second coin. How many Heads did you get? Zero Heads, one-fourth of the time; two Heads, also one-fourth of the time; just one Head, along with one Tail, the other half of the time. The average count of Heads is 1, as it must be (half a Head from the first coin, another half a Head from the second; $\frac{1}{2} + \frac{1}{2} = 1$). What is interesting is the variance of this total. We are 1 away from the average half the time (all Heads or all Tails), and 0 away the other half the time (1 of each), for a total sum of squares around the mean of 2 over our four possible "cases." Divided by $N = 4$, the number of ways you can flip two coins, that gives us a mean-square of $\frac{1}{2}$, which is $\frac{1}{4} + \frac{1}{4}$ — the sum of the variances of the two coins considered separately.

This fact is perfectly general – actually, it is just another version of the Pythagorean theorem: **variances of independent processes add when the scores are totalled.** As a theorem it rests on the definition of "independent," which is an important part of probability theory, more than on the algebra of sums-of-squares. We will note later on that the definition of covariance of any two measurements x and y on the same cases is the difference of the actual variance of $x+y$ from the sum of the variances of x and y separately, divided by 2. Variance and independence thereby have something very fundamental to do with each other, a deep connection that is the topic of courses in mathematical statistics much more advanced than this one.

We can arrive at the same conclusion for K fair coins just as easily from first principles. Write x for the count of Heads for every possible sequence of K coins. We want to know the variance of this collection of x's, which number, in total, $N = 2^K$ — the number of possible outcomes when you have flipped K fair coins is $2 \times 2 \times \ldots \times 2$, a total of K factors of 2. Let's proceed by mathematical induction. Supposing the variance of the count of Heads is $\frac{K}{4}$ for K coins, as we already know to be true for $K = 1$ and $K = 2$, we wish to show that the variance is exactly $\frac{1}{4}$ more for the same computation but with $K + 1$ coins.

If we divide equation (2.1) by N on both sides, we arrive at

$$\Sigma(x_i - y)^2/N = \Sigma(x_i - \bar{x})^2/N + (\bar{x} - y)^2, \tag{2.3}$$

meaning that the mean square of a list of Nx's around any number y is equal to their variance plus the square of the distance from the average to y. Divide the whole series of all 2^{K+1} possible flips of the set that now has $K + 1$ coins into two subsets according to the result on the $(K + 1)^{st}$ flip (the last one): those that ended with a Head, and those that ended with a Tail. In each half there are 2^K different sequences.

For those 2^K sequences that ended with a Head, by the induction assumption, the sum of squares around the mean is $\frac{K}{4}$. The mean around which they have that average, though, is $\frac{K}{2} + 1$. That mean is not the correct mean for the $(K + 1)$-coin problem; we have displaced the correct mean $\frac{K+1}{2}$ by half a Head, and so we need to add the term $(\bar{x} - y)^2$, which is another $(\frac{1}{2})^2 = \frac{1}{4}$, to the mean square, which thereby becomes $\frac{K}{4} + \frac{1}{4} = \frac{K+1}{4}$. Similarly, the sum of squares of the second half of the flips, those that ended in a Tail, is the same $\frac{K}{4}$ we saw before, around a mean that is now unchanged at $\frac{K}{2}$. Again this is the wrong mean, off by $\frac{1}{2}$ from the correct mean (which is still $\frac{K+1}{2}$), so again we add an additional component of $(\frac{1}{2})^2 = \frac{1}{4}$ to the mean-square.

So however the last coin came up, Heads or Tails, its effect on the whole distribution of all the series of flips that preceded is to add just $\frac{1}{4}$ to the expected mean-square: the square of the $\frac{1}{2}$ by which the new coin *must* fail to shift the mean by the precise $\frac{1}{2}$ of the average. The first coin is just like the others in this regard. The net mean-square of the total count is thus $\frac{K+1}{4}$, which is the same as the formula $\frac{K}{4}$ except applied to the next integer, $K + 1$ instead of K, and that's exactly how mathematical induction works.

We've shown, then, that the variance of the total number of Heads in a flip of K fair coins is $\frac{K}{4}$ for *every* K. The average number of Heads is this count divided by K, so the **variance of the average**, the measuring process we're really interested in, is diminished as the *square* of this divisor; it becomes $\frac{K}{4}/K^2$ or $\frac{1}{4K}$. The standard deviation of this average varies as the square root of the variance; that is evidently $\frac{1}{2\sqrt{K}}$. This is a precision of the mean, the plus-or-minus around it for the frequency of Heads. (Often it is called the *standard error of the mean* (s.e.m.), although it does not necessarily have the logical properties you would expect something called an "error" to have.) For 100 flips of a fair coin, for instance, we compute the precision of the fraction of Heads to be $\frac{1}{2\sqrt{100}} = 0.05$; so we write this expected fraction of Heads as $.50 \pm .05$. (The symbol $\pm$ is read "plus or minus"; its counterpart $\mp$ is read, reasonably enough, as "minus or plus.")

The same inverse-root-K formula applies whenever we are averaging independent estimates of the same quantity, whether propensities of Heads or anything else that has a variance. We have in fact shown that **the precision of an average improves (decreases) as the inverse square root of the number of observations that contributed to the average.** We've shown this by an explicit enumeration for coin flips, but it is generally true of averages of any measurement that *has* a variance. (Not every physically realistic process has a variance in this sense: one very simple kinematic system that does not is the location of the spot on an indefinitely long straight wall pointed at by a flashlight spinning around its axis that is sampled at a random moment.) This fact has been known by the cognoscenti, and exploited by gamblers to make a good living, for at least 300 years. For a particularly up-to-date reinterpretation in this specific context, see Nassim Taleb, *The Black Swan,* 2007.

> *Unfair coins.* As one particular example of this general case (or, alternatively, as a particularly simple generalization of the specific distribution of frequency of Heads for a fair coin that we just reviewed), consider the case of an *un*fair coin (in the genetic context, a rare allele). Write the "propensity for Heads" as p, so that the chance of Tails is $1 - p$. The mean count of Heads for the single flip is then, of course, p. To get the variance, we need to average the squared distance from the average. This combines the value of (1 minus the mean) squared — $(1 - p)^2$ — a fraction p of the time with a value of $(0 - p)^2$ a fraction $1 - p$ of the time, for a net sum of squares of $p(1 - p)^2 + p^2(1 - p) = (p + (1 - p))$ $(p(1 - p)) = p(1 - p)$. This is usually written pq where the new letter $q = 1 - p$ stands for the probability of Tails. If pq is the variance of the count of Heads for the flip of *one* unfair coin, the variance for the total Heads after flipping n of them must be npq and the variance of the frequency of Heads thus pq/n. (The square root of this variance, $\sqrt{pq/n}$, is the formula that generates the standard errors following the $\pm$ that reports of public opinion or voter preferences in the United States usually set down.) The formulas for the fair coin are just the special case of these with $p = q = \frac{1}{2}$.

2.1.3 Weighted Averages

Flip a coin 25 times, then 100 more times, then 400 more times: thus a total of 525. Some fraction of Heads will be observed for each set of flips. To pool all these data, evidently you would multiply the 25-flip mean by 25, to turn it back into a total count of Heads; the 100-flip frequency, by 100; the 400-flip frequency, by 400. Add up all the resulting true Head counts, then divide by 525.

The 25-flip mean had a standard error of $1/2\sqrt{25}$, however, the 100-flip mean an s.e. of $1/2\sqrt{100}$, and the 400-flip mean an s.e. of $1/2\sqrt{400}$. So to revert from frequencies to totals, which is the sensible thing to do, is to **multiply by the reciprocals of the variances of the individual estimates,** sum the quotients, then normalize by the sum of those weights.

Again it is easy enough to prove, using only a little more algebra, that this statement is just as true of the general estimate of almost *anything* that arises by combination of independent observations with the same expected value (i.e., "of the same underlying quantity") but different variances. It is enough to talk about combining two different observations of the same underlying physical quantity (though this is itself a supposition worth explicitly checking). Suppose A and B are independent (i.e., physically unlinked) observations of the same mensurand – maybe a measurement twice by the same instrument on different days, or maybe readings by two instruments each calibrated at the factory. Suppose, further, that these observations arrive with squared standard errors V_A and V_B. For instance, A might be an average of $1/V_A$ observations, and B an average of $1/V_B$; or A might be a slope estimate made at a moment $1/\sqrt{V_A}$ units away from the mean predictor value in some regression setup, and B a slope estimate made at a moment $1/\sqrt{V_B}$ units from the mean predictor value.

A weighted average of the measurements A and B is a new quantity $aA + bB$ where $a + b = 1$. Assuming the measurements are independent, the variance of this weighted average is $a^2 V_A + b^2 V_B$. This expression is easy enough to minimize – we have $\frac{d}{da}(a^2 V_A + b^2 V_B) = \frac{d}{da}(a^2 V_A + (1-a)^2 V_B) = 2aV_A - 2(1-a)V_B$, which is zero where $a(V_A + V_B) = V_B$ or $a = V_B/(V_A + V_B)$, whereupon $b = V_A/(V_A + V_B)$ and the minimum value of that variance of the combination $\frac{V_A V_B}{V_A + V_B} = 1/(\frac{1}{V_A} + \frac{1}{V_B})$. Notice that the numerator of each of these ratios is the variance of the *other* component being averaged – the weights are in precisely *inverse* proportion to the variances. That is just the situation we intuited for the coin example preceding. Figure 2.2 sets the weights of the items to be averaged at ratios of 1:4:16, corresponding (if they were sets of coin flips) to sample sizes of 16:4:1. In the left panel, these are drawn in

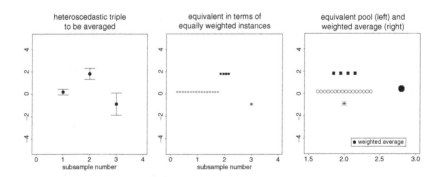

Figure 2.2 Schematic for weighted averages. (left) Three observations, with three different error bars (±1 s.e. ranges), to the same vertical scale. The lengths of the error bars are proportional to 1:2:4. (center) The equivalent layout in terms of equally weighted instances: 16 for the leftmost bar, 4 for the central one, 1 for the rightmost. (right) The equivalent weighted average (big filled circle).

the usual convention, as means with superimposed bars of length 2 s.e.m. In the center is the equivalent construction for the weighted average; the piles of 16 open circles or four closed squares are to be treated as "all at the same height," the height of their separate averages in the left panel. In the right panel we see the construction of the weighted average (big round dot) as, in effect, the average of all 21 replications of one or another of these original scores, where 21 is the sum of the inverses $(1, 4, 16)$ of the squares $(1, \frac{1}{4}, \frac{1}{16})$ of the three original precisions $(1, \frac{1}{2}, \frac{1}{4})$. The weighted average is raised above the value of the most precise original observation (the leftmost) by only a little bit.

In Section 2.2.2 we will see that this formula underlies a particularly congenial reinterpretation of the slope of a fitted line that we are going to concern ourselves with in a moment.

2.1.4 Averages and Likelihoods

We have not yet justified **why** it might be a good idea to use this simple least-squares machinery for thinking of the average independent measurements of the same quantity as a satisfactory "estimate" of its true, underlying value. Any such argument requires a criterion for what it means to behave rationally in estimating values of this kind, and we will need to specify a contingent aspect of the real world in the presence of which the least-squares answer is the correct answer in a specific logical sense.

Let us return to the problem of combining multiple observations of "the same quantity" into an average. It turns out that, just as in the canonical case of the coin's "propensity for Heads," there could have been a hypothesis involved in this maneuver. Specifically, conceive the data x_i we actually measured as having arisen from perturbation of some **true value** μ by independent measurement errors $\Delta_i = x_i - \mu$. (Here μ is the Greek letter "mu," a mnemonic for "mean," and Δ is the Greek capital D that stands for "difference" here.) Suppose, further, we had a function ϕ giving the actual probability distribution of these errors. This means, precisely, that given μ (the *hypothesis*), the probability of a datum in the range $(x_i, x_i + dx)$ will be $\phi(x_i - \mu)dx = \phi(\Delta_i)dx$, *where ϕ is the same distribution for each specimen i.*

We adopt, without any further argument, Laplace's **Principle of Maximum Likelihood.** It can be stated in a variety of ways (see, e.g., Edwards, 1992 or D. R. Anderson, 2008) of which the following construal is probably the simplest. For each parameter that that you might conceivably adopt as your preferred sample summary, compute the probability of generating precisely the data that you did, in fact, encounter.[3] This is called the *likelihood of the data given that specific parameter value*. Then, report the parameter or parameter set for which the data you actually encountered has the maximum of likelihood, which is to say, the highest probability of having been the data you would actually expect to find. (In Chapter 4 we will explore the extension of this method for estimating the standard error of the computed maximum.)

Because we have assumed independence (= multiplication of probabilities) across all the specimens measurement by measurement, the net probability of the whole data set (all the x_i taken as a list) on the hypothesis that the true value is μ must be the product of the ϕ's for each datum separately. By the principle of maximum likelihood, the value of μ we wish to take as our (indirect) measurement of its value – the "most likely" value for μ – is that for which this net probability $\Omega = \phi(\Delta_1)\phi(\Delta_2)\cdots\phi(\Delta_n)$ is a maximum. For given observational data x_i, we could find this maximum as a function of μ, since $\Delta_i = x_i - \mu$, if only we knew the function ϕ.

But, for a great many practical problems, in or out of biometry, *we can know the function* ϕ. Often, as we will see in the next section, it is reasonable to take it as proportional to the initially odd-looking formulation $e^{-\Delta^2/2c}$, a *Gaussian distribution* having some error variance c around the mean μ. Under this seemingly arbitrary (but actually very natural) assumption, we have

$$\begin{aligned}
\Omega &= e^{-\Delta_1^2/2c}\, e^{-\Delta_2^2/2c}\, \cdots\, e^{-\Delta_n^2/2c} \\
&= e^{(-\Sigma_i \Delta_i^2)/2c}.
\end{aligned} \tag{2.4}$$

We maximize Ω by maximizing that exponent. But we *already* know how to maximize it. It is a negative multiple of the sum of squares of the data x_i around μ, so it is guaranteed to be maximized when μ is taken as the average of the data!

Hence:

For data that is known to be distributed around a true mean by "errors" the distribution of which is Gaussian, of any fixed variance, the average of the data is the likeliest candidate for that mean. An easy extension, known already by 1810: if those variances aren't equal, the correct answer is still an average, the one weighted inversely by those error variances, as in the exposition of the section just preceding.

---

[3] The word "parameter" here is a technical term from mathematical statistics that, for the biologist, means roughly "a decimal number that plays some crucial role in the theory you are attempting to show that your data adequately illustrate." If your subject is the comparison of two group averages on one single measurement, probably there is only one parameter, the group mean difference. If your topic is instead the pattern of an extended covariance matrix on p variables, that count is instead $p(p+1)/2$, and so on.

This is the justification of the operation of averaging, and by extension the other least-squares methods, that I have been building up to through this section. Regardless of the variance c, as long as error is Gaussianly distributed the average is the choice of central tendency having the maximum of likelihood for given data. That maximum of likelihood is the justification for choosing it.

This maneuver entails a brilliant notational pun, the interpretation of

$$\Omega = e^{-(x_1-\bar{x})^2/2c} \times e^{-(x_2-\bar{x})^2/2c} \times \cdots \times e^{-(x_n-\bar{x})^2/2c} \tag{2.4a}$$

as the $(1/2c)$th power of

$$e^{-\Sigma_i(x_i-\bar{x})^2} = e^{-\left((x_1-\bar{x})^2+\cdots+(x_n-\bar{x})^2\right)}, \tag{2.4b}$$

the logarithm of which we already know how to maximize (by minimizing the sum of squares that is multiplied by -1 in the exponent). The algebra feels – and is – elegant mainly because the value of c, the precision of the Gaussian distribution involved, is irrelevant to[4] the maximization of likelihood by which we are selecting the best estimate of the true mean, μ. But this double mathematical meaning is combined with the knowledge that such error distributions truly exist in Nature (as Section 2.3 will show) and also can arise from conscientious random sampling. If $\bar{x}$ is known in advance, the likeliest value of c is the same as the formula $\Sigma(x-\bar{x})^2/N$ we are already using for the variance. If instead $\bar{x}$ had to be estimated as part of the same investigation, the formula for c is the same except with the $N-1$ correction.

It is worth pausing here to recount the assumptions that justify the average of a set of data as the likeliest, most reasonable estimate of its central tendency. We must have been persuaded (perhaps by some cogent theory of genomic, biophysical, physiological, or developmental fluctuation) that the measured data arose from a common "true value" by independent Gaussian errors of mean zero and the same variance. Where this compound assumption is *not* reasonable – for instance, where the "true value" is obviously different for different subgroups of the data – the average remains the bare formula it has been all along, the total of the data divided by their count (e.g., the average number of hockey goals per citizen of the United States, or the average number of hairs per North American adult male head). **The meaning of the simplest of all statistics, the ordinary average, is inextricable from the validity of the (equally simple) theories in which its value is implicated.**

When we extend our reasoning to consider the complex organized systems that are the actual organisms we are studying, an additional concern arises, that of *essential heterogeneity.* As the great Austrian-American embryologist Paul

---

[4] This irrelevance, more formally the stochastic *independence* of estimated mean and variance in any sample from a Gaussian distribution, is actually another theorem.

Weiss (1958:140) wryly noted, "Identical twins are more similar than any microscopic sections from corresponding sites you can lay through either of them." What he meant is that identity is a function of the level of measurement under consideration, and for standard deviations to be small and thus standard errors of averages as well, we must be careful to have measured quantities that are under tight control as regards the aspects of their variability that are not the subject of the analysis. Over in the social sciences, "income" is a terrible variable for analysis, especially in America, because it actually has no stable value at all, whether over time or over alternate definitions, at the top end of its distribution. In biology, variables like the "2D-4D ratio" (ratio of lengths of the second and fourth fingers) vary within and across populations by factors of ten more than the size of the effects (sexual dimorphism) by which they are ostensibly interpretable, and thus likewise are unpromising as explananda regardless of the endocrine pathways we can imagine that might have effects on their measured values "other things being equal." Most of the anatomical details of any single human body, for instance the specific course of a secondary cerebral sulcus, cannot easily be converted into quantitative measurements of any sort. This point has been made most earnestly on thermodynamic grounds, by the physicist-turned-biophysicist Walter Elsasser (*The Chief Abstractions of Biology*, 1975). See the discussion in my 2014 treatise.

Gauss's characterization. Exactly the same argument works "in reverse": **if** we want the average to be the likeliest true value, **then** the probability distribution must be a bell curve. This was C. F. Gauss's original argument from around 1800 (see Stigler, 1986), which is why the distribution is named the Gaussian in the first place. It is easy to convey the essence of Gauss's reasoning as follows. Suppose that the average is always the maximum-likelihood estimate of the mean for samples of data from some symmetric distribution. Let $g(u)$ be the logarithm of the symmetric probability density we are looking for, and suppose our sample consists of n values $x_1, x_2, \ldots x_n$ all equal to the same value u, along with one value that is $-nu$ (in order that the set of all $n + 1$ averages zero). Then for 0 to be the maximum of likelihood for the mean of all $n + 1$, the derivative of the log likelihood $\sum g'(\mu - x_i)$ must be zero at $\mu = 0$ – we must have $g'(-nu) = -ng'(u)$. So the derivative of the log of the probability density must be a linear function of u through 0. The exponent must thus be something positive times $-u^2$, in other words, a bell curve.

> *Pearson's astonishing extension.* We will see in Chapter 4 how Karl Pearson found a way to maximize the likelihood of a particularly useful description of the distribution of *two* variables, and, by implication, any number k of variables, at the same time, as long as they were jointly normally distributed. That description is the *multivariate normal model.* For just two measurements, this is the combination of two means, two standard deviations, and a

correlation; for k measurements, $k > 1$, it comprises k means and standard deviations along with $k(k - 1)/2$ correlations. In this way, Pearson, himself a biologist, was responsible for the extension of all these questions from the context of one variable at a time – *univariate* analysis – to the *multivariate* context in which today's quantitative biosciences are almost invariably couched. He was even able to approximate the sampling standard errors of all these quantities, and the covariances of those joint sampling errors. We return to this generalization in Chapter 4 after reviewing a range of simpler questions about the prediction of individual measurements, some dealt with here in Chapter 2 (questions dealing with a single predictor) and others in Chapter 3 (slightly more complicated questions involving multiple predictors).

Summary of Section 2.1

- The ordinary *average* of any set of numbers x_i, $i = 1, \ldots, N$, is at the same time the least-squares estimate of their "common value," where the squared quantity being minimized is $\Sigma_{i=1}^{N}(x_i - \bar{x})^2$, the summed squared arithmetical difference of each observation in turn from the imputed average.
- That minimum sum of squares, divided by the sample size N, is called the *variance* of the x_i, and its square root is the *standard deviation*.
- When observations are independent and of the same variance, the variance of the sum of K of them is K times the variance of any one of them. The variance of the average of K is the variance of any one of them divided by K, and thus the *standard error* of such an average is the standard deviation of any component observation divided by $\sqrt{K}$. In words, the precision of an average increases (its standard deviation decreases) in inverse proportion to the square root of sample size.
- For K flips of a fair coin, the variance of the net count of Heads is $\frac{K}{4}$ around a mean of $\frac{K}{2}$, and so the standard deviation of the frequency of Heads is $\frac{1}{2\sqrt{K}}$ around its mean of $\frac{1}{2}$.
- The optimal weights for averaging estimates of the same quantity having different precisions are proportional to the reciprocals of those precisions. The variance of this weighted sum is the sum of the reciprocals of their precisions, and the precision of that weighted average is the reciprocal of this sum of reciprocals. (For coins, this corresponds to the total of the original coin flips in which the separate estimates presumably originated.)
- When data are distributed around a common true value by normally (Gaussianly) distributed measurement errors of mean zero and the same shared variance – when their probability can be written as $\frac{1}{\sqrt{2\pi}\sigma}e^{-\frac{(x-\mu)^2}{2\sigma^2}}$

for some μ and σ – the best (likeliest) estimate of that true value is the ordinary average of the measured data. And vice versa: if the average truly is the most reasonable way of estimating a true value, the measurement error must have been Gaussian.

2.2 Lines for Laws

2.2.1 Why Organismal Biologists Compute Regressions

So far the discussion has been of only one conceptual entity, one "propensity" or "true value," derived from some collection of closely agreeing separate measurements or averages each of which has some computable precision (standard error of measurement). Such a model suits some standard contexts in the physical sciences, such as estimating a physical constant (the atomic weight of silicon, the speed of light). But estimates of single quantities are not often the subject of investigations in the biosciences – in fact, even in physics these constants are more often the coefficients in equations relating pairs of variables than they are the direct object of unitary measurement themselves. Consider, for example, *Planck's constant h*, the quantum of action. The best classical measurement of its value was that of the physicist Robert Millikan, who, way back in 1916, assessed it via the slope of a linear regression testing Einstein's photoelectric law. Planck's h was equal to the slope of this line divided by the elementary charge e on the electron, a constant that Millikan had also measured. I discussed this example at length in Bookstein (2014), section E4.2.

We are not fully equipped for numerical inferences in any natural science until we extend the methods of the preceding section to *combinations* of measurements, meaning essentially different measurements (for instance, values that come in different units) intended to characterize the same system(s). The simplest such combination is the extension to just *two* measurements, and the rest of this chapter will concentrate mainly on this special case. For Millikan, the horizontal axis of the scatterplot his lines fit was in units of inverse seconds (the frequency of a specific color of light) and the vertical in volts. When we discuss more than two variables, in Chapter 3, we will usually inspect all their pairwise relationships, two at a time, separately, and the best description of the whole system will involve slopes that are analogous to these pairwise formulations but not quite the same.

The units in which a coefficient of biological interest is reported often convey a solid hint about its bivariate origin in a linear fit. A growth rate, for instance, might be reported in units of length divided by time, say, cm/year. It is measured, then, as the slope of a line fitted to a scatter of lengths (along the vertical) by ages (along the horizontal). Many other physiologically crucial coefficients, especially those dealing with energy or its transformations, are computed and then reported in mixed units in just the same way.

Other textbooks often introduce our general topic here, the logical structure of the relation between two variables, by reference to a singular case, the *independence* of the two measures, that is never actually encountered in biometrical practice. Independence (noncorrelation) is purported to be the "null hypothesis" against which we "test" observed pairs of measurements for a "statistically significant association." In general this strategy is hopelessly ineffective as an actual bioscientific research protocol. In the real world of investigations of organisms, whether in the field, the pediatrician's office, or the laboratory, the appropriate reference concept is far more often some approximate *equality* specifying the agreement of two ways of measuring the same underlying thing, or else an (approximate) *linearity*, likewise conveyed by a correlation approaching 1.0, that indicates a system under suitable regulation (the way an elasticity, for example, is measured via the linear part of the relation of strain to applied force). Section 2.2.3 will show one example of each of these where the pair of variables bear the same units. Where units of the two axes of the scatterplot are different, textbooks of physiology, ecology, or theoretical biology might couch the relationship instead via the equations that linearize the expression of one variable as an explicit function of the other one, corresponding to the design of a good experiment in which one variable is explicitly set by the experimenter and then clamped while the complementary value is read off some machine. We are interested, first, in the functional form of this equation; second, in the numerical values of its coefficients; and third, in the magnitude and perhaps other details of the noise *around* this equation. This is the reporting protocol that corresponds, for instance, to the design of the *Tetrahymena* experimental data reported in Section 2.5.

In the simplest setting, the equation under consideration is linear, and the corresponding reference hypothesis entails a correlation that is approximately unity rather than one that is approximately zero as in the conventional null-hypothesis approach. We will shortly see that this scheme permits a nearly verbatim copy of the logic of the preceding section in two separate aspects: a least-squares approach to the estimation problem that is maximum-likelihood in the case of normally (Gaussian) distributed error, and an expression setting out the estimated slope of this best-fitting line as a weighted average of more elementary numbers. The remainder of this subchapter introduces a toy example, derives the so-called "normal equations" and their solution (as expressed in two different formulas), and guides you through two previously published examples.

2.2.2 From Errors-in-Variables to Errors-in-Equations

Suppose, indeed, that we are examining a pair of measurements jointly governed by a "law," which, for the purpose of this exposition, will mean an exact linear equation for the relation between two variables had they been measured "ideally," without error. Such equations are commonly found in physics (consider Newton's *"F = ma"*), in fields like astronomy, that deal with particularly massive physical entities, or in subfields of the biosciences like ecology or physiology (and, nowadays, more and more often, cognitive science), that deal with variation under explicit physical constraints dictated by the laws of thermodynamics, mechanics, or information. In the first example of Section 2.2.3, the equation is a version of Julian Huxley's (1932) "law of relative growth," the approximate linearity of simultaneous variations of common consequences of the same composite genetic cause of form – in this instance, the integration of growth patterns down the length of a single embryonic limb. Linearity here is presumably expressing the relative stability of some biophysical reduction, such as a gradient of some diffusing morphogen. In the second example, the equation is logically an aspect of bioscientific reductionism, a claimed identity between "scaling dimensions" as inferred from fractal geometry and the same quantities as estimated from empirical data on mammals.

To make the algebra as simple as possible, assume that the regularity we are studying takes the mathematical form of an indefinitely extended straight line. Quantitative theories tend to talk about the coefficients in the formulas for these lines – why the slopes have the values they do, why the intercepts are what they are. For now, just consider those "constants" – those slopes or intercepts (and their extensions for more complicated laws, such as planetary orbits) – to be numbers we and our readers are interested in. Can we use the observed data that are supposed to be lawful as if collectively they supplied some sort of measurement of the underlying quantities that theory argues should be seen as the more real?

Yes, we can. Suppose, for instance, a vehicle is moving straight away from you at a constant speed. (How do you know that the speed is constant? What does that mean, anyway?) You have a stopwatch, attached to a loudspeaker, and the car has an odometer, maybe the kind with digital readout. (But how do you know if the readings of the odometer are evenly spaced? What does that mean, anyway?) At some moment when the car is already moving "at constant speed," you start the stopwatch. Then at N different preset times, the speaker sounds a loud click, and when the driver hears this, he calls out the number on the odometer. **How fast is the car traveling?**[5] Notice how those parenthetical phrases seem to pile up after a while. They are all worrying about the "evenness" (really, the lawfulness) of the phenomenon, the linearity of the measuring instruments with respect to one another, and the other real physical factors being treated as "negligible." The question of what to ignore is never closed.

The crucial features of this regression-like measurement scenario setup, then, are the following:

- We can measure distance [position] and time. (In other sciences these might be chemical concentrations, masses, pressures, or other equally fundamental dimensions.) Our machines, or our reports of the readouts of machines, give us these quantities directly. We do not have to know how these machines (odometers, stopwatches) actually work; it is enough that we trust their factory calibrations.
- Our measurements always incorporate small errors. (Which is not to say that we have not striven to make them as small as we possibly can.)
- The laws we seek to support by these data do not use these measurements directly. Raw data depend far too much on accidental factors such as where one happens to be standing or what time of day it is. The truthful, robust, reliable laws are independent of all these arbitrary choices, by specifying constant coefficients ("invariants") for relations among them. For instance, the measurement of age in biology does not designate a calendar date, but a temporal interval elapsed from birth; the height of a standing human child is measured from the floor, not from sea level.
- **The laws are exactly true,** in the sense that **if** the apparent errors could be made as small as we'd like, by incorporating instruments of steadily greater precision or by bringing the whole experiment or measuring session under tighter and tighter experimental control, **then** the resulting measurements would be as enlightening and persuasive as, say, Newton's law of gravitation was (until Einstein corrected it).

As laws go, the one about the motion of this car has unusually small scope. It will be expected to apply only when observers are on the same line as that on which the car is traveling, and only when the whole propulsive mechanism of the car is in a steady state thermodynamically, aerodynamically,

---

[5] You may be amused to learn how different this scenario is from the actual mechanisms by which contemporary cars actually report their speeds. See, for instance, http://www.explainthatstuff.com/how-speedometer-works.html. As the article notes, "it is hard to measure a wheel's speed of rotation." And the mechanism of the policeman's radar gun is different also.

and rheodynamically with respect to its surroundings: level road, warm engine, constant throttle setting, and so forth. This, too, is typical of regression applications in biology: a linearity is observable, and its slope is accessible to a precise computation, only when nearly every other known source of biological or biographical variation has already been controlled.

Returning to the data set at hand, write t_1 for the time the stopwatch emits its first click and s_1 for the first odometer reading called out by the driver. The pair of numbers (t_1, s_1) is the *first pair* of observations. Similarly, (t_2, s_2) is the second pair, (t_i, s_i) the ith pair, and (t_N, s_N) the last pair, Nth of N. In the example shown in Figure 2.3, $N = 10$.

We **know** a priori that these quantities, had they been measured perfectly, would satisfy some equation

$$s_i = s_0 + vt_i,$$

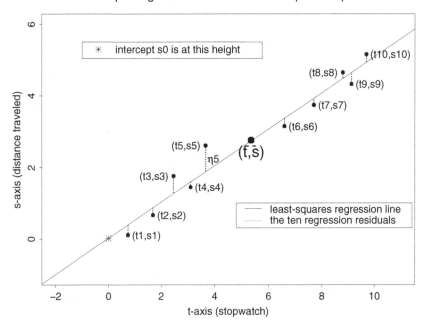

Figure 2.3 Conventional diagram for a least-squares regression line. Dots: ten data pairs (t_i, s_i). The least-squares optimum goes through the centroid $(\bar{t}, \bar{s})$ of all the data with slope equal to the expression in equation (2.7) or equation (2.8a). The star is located where $t = 0$ on the line at height s_0, the *intercept* of the formula. The vertical dotted lines are the ten values of the errors η in the regression equation. (In the figure, only the fifth one is numbered.)

where s_0 is the odometer reading at the moment you started the stopwatch and v (for "velocity") is the actual speed of the car, the number we are seeking. This "knowledge" is what we mean by saying that the car is traveling "at constant speed." We are much more interested in v than in s_0, because although different observers with different stopwatches will have unrelated values for s_0, they ought to arrive at nearly the same values for v. In this respect, at least, our toy example is aligned quite well with the reality of biometrical computations: slopes of regressions are typically a lot more interesting than their intercepts.

Admit, now, that we are measuring with error. There is error in the running of the stopwatch, and in the loudspeaker circuitry; there is error in the mechanism of the odometer, and in the calling out of its values. This means that the "law" really is

$$s_i - \varepsilon_{s_i} = s_0 + v(t_i - \varepsilon_{t_i})$$

where ε_{s_i} is the error of the ith odometer reading and ε_{t_i} that of the ith stopwatch reading. (Here ε is the Greek letter "epsilon.")

Neither the observer nor the statistician can separate the values of the two ε's given only the data of this simplistic measurement scheme. That impasse immediately suggests an improvement in the "experimental design," namely the provenance of additional data (for instance, multiple stopwatches, or a battery of laser-ranging distance measurement devices) that permit better estimates of both quantities. But the car had to be *somewhere* when the stopwatch clicked at "3 seconds," for instance, so we can rewrite the error equation as

$$s_i = s_0 + vt_i - (v\varepsilon_{t_i} - \varepsilon_{s_i})$$
$$= s_0 + vt_i + \eta_i, \text{ say,}$$

where η_i is a new "composite" error – *not* a "measurement error" – referring to the ith equation as a whole. (Here η is the Greek letter "eta") More explicitly, we have

$$\eta_i = s_i - s_0 - vt_i. \tag{2.5}$$

By rearranging terms like this, diverse errors that were once physically distinguishable (here, one error ε_{s_i} of measured position and another error ε_{t_i} of measured time) have been combined into a single term, an "error in the equation." Enormous consequences follow from this tiny rearrangement. Most importantly, while the ε's are functions of one observation at a time, the value of η_i, error in the equation for the ith observation, will turn out to depend on *all* the observations, not just the ith pair. If these errors η are unacceptably large, you can't tell if their magnitude would be more effectively reduced by improvements in the error ε_{s_i} of the odometer, in the error ε_{t_i} of the stopwatch, or in the calibration of the vehicle to constant speed. You must work to ameliorate all these potential flaws simultaneously. When the regression line is computed as the least-squares optimum, these η's are usually called **residuals,** especially if the scientist's intention to interpret at least some of them further (see Section 2.5.3 or Section 3.2).

Whether considered to be measurement errors or instead potentially meaningful "residuals," the η's are the quantities we wish to make small: deviations not in the *data* but in the *law* we are expecting to find. In the usual graphic, a line drawn on the plane of the points (t, s), this "error" looks like the vertical distance of the point from the line of the law. (But there is a better way to understand what is being computed – it is that something reasonable is being averaged, as we will see presently.)

> That we are measuring error around the line by the distance that is vertical in Figure 2.3 breaks what might have seemed to be a symmetry in the formulation of the law before we took measurement error into consideration. In my description of this "experiment" I tacitly led you to imagine that the measurement error of t, electromechanical as it is, is substantially less than the measurement error of s, which, in my little sketch, involved a human observer. Ignoring measurement error, the law written "$s = vt$" could just as well have been written "$t = s/v$," with v estimated as the reciprocal of the slope of a line that fits t as a linear formula in s. By measuring error in the s direction we are implicitly presuming that the error in t is less than the error in s. When no such assumption is plausible, as in the relations among limb lengths of relatives studied by Pearson (see Figure 2.28), one needs to compute both slopes, not just one, and a summary more useful than either slope will be the square root of their product, the *correlation coefficient* explored in Section 2.4, or the covariance coefficient, Chapter 4, that is central to studies involving indefinitely many variables. Both of these coefficients are symmetric in the two variables whose values are combined; that is not the case for the regression slope per se.

One might imagine many criteria for smallness, many desiderata for the η's that would each generate values for s_0 and for v, the speed we wish to have "measured" in this indirect fashion. As you might have guessed from the positioning of this discussion immediately following that in Section 2.1, it turns out to be most useful to measure "smallness" by the mean square of the η's. What makes these so-called *least-squares estimates* of s_0 and v worth considering is that under some circumstances, analogous to those for which the average was the best (likeliest) guess (Section 2.1.4), the particular values of s_0 and v computed in this way are the most *reasonable* estimates of the corresponding "underlying quantities." They are maximum-likelihood (ML) in the same sense that the average was, whenever the probability distribution of η takes the form $e^{-\eta^2/2c}$. And this can happen: certainly, if ε_{s_i} and ε_{t_i} are both

Gaussianly distributed themselves, and if the variance of ε_{t_i} (the "predictor") is substantially less than that of ε_{s_i}, then the errors-in-equation $v\varepsilon_{t_i} - \varepsilon_{s_i} = \eta_i$, their linear combination, will likewise be nearly Gaussian as soon as v has been estimated. When this is the case, the arithmetical values s_0 and v that minimize $\Sigma \eta^2$ are at the same time the most reasonable estimates of those two quantities, the initial odometer reading and the car's speed.

In such circumstances, the actual arithmetic that gives us estimates of that "true speed" v, along with the "true time-zero odometer reading" s_0, comes from straightforward algebra. We want the values of s_0 and v that minimize $\Sigma \eta_i^2 = \Sigma(s_i - s_0 - vt_i)^2$, where the η's, ten in number, are the vertical discrepancies shown by the dashed lines in Figure 2.3. At the minimum, we must have[6]

$$\frac{\partial}{\partial s_0} \Sigma \eta_i^2 = \frac{\partial}{\partial v} \Sigma \eta_i^2 = 0. \tag{2.6}$$

But, from the formula for derivatives of squared binomials and the definition of the η's,

$$\frac{\partial}{\partial s_0} \Sigma \eta_i^2 = 2\Sigma(-1)(s_i - s_0 - vt_i)$$

and

$$\frac{\partial}{\partial v} \Sigma \eta_i^2 = 2\Sigma(-t_i)(s_i - s_0 - vt_i).$$

Notice the pattern that governs these equations. Each one takes the formulas for all the η's at once, multiplies by the coefficient of one of the unknowns (either -1, for s_0, or $-t_i$, for v), and sums all these multiples. In other words, probably we can't make the whole set of all N η's zero at the same time, but we can find values s_0 and r that make both of these partial derivatives zero at the same time. These are called the **normal equations** for the estimation problem; we will see them generalized in Section 3.1.3.

The normal equations are two linear equations in two unknowns; let us solve them. From the first of the equations,

$$\Sigma \eta_i = \Sigma(s_i - s_0 - vt_i) = 0,$$

the η's average zero. Rewrite this as an explicit linear expression in the two unknowns:

$$Ns_0 + (\Sigma t_i)v = \Sigma s_i. \tag{2.6i}$$

---

[6] Perhaps you have not encountered this notation before. The symbol "∂" stands for the *partial derivative*, the derivative of an expression in many variables (here, two of them) that presumes only one of them is changing, the others remaining ostensibly constant. It is not a Greek letter; it is usually read "del."

Dividing by N, this means that our least-squares line must pass precisely through the centroid $(\bar{t}, \bar{s})$ of all the data. (The situation is more symmetric than it looks, since $N = \Sigma 1$, the sum of all the coefficients of s_0.) Likewise, from the second equation,

$$(\Sigma t_i)s_0 + (\Sigma t_i^2)v = \Sigma s_i t_i. \tag{2.6ii}$$

Solving these by the usual rules that you learned when you studied determinants in high school (which reduce to the idea that for either unknown you multiply both equations by the coefficient of that unknown in the *other* equation, then subtract), we get

$$v = \frac{N\Sigma s_i t_i - \Sigma s_i \Sigma t_i}{N\Sigma t_i^2 - (\Sigma t_i)^2} \tag{2.7}$$

after which we simply evaluate s_0 from the simpler equation:

$$s_0 = \frac{\Sigma s_i}{N} - v\frac{\Sigma t_i}{N},$$

so as to guarantee that the errors η in the equations average zero. For the little data set of ten points in Figure 2.3, we have $v = 0.5005$, $s_0 = 0.0775$. Together they specify the equation $y = 0.0775 + 0.5005x$ of the line drawn there.

In this way we have converted raw data – those ten pairs (t_i, s_i) – to a pair of new quantities: an estimate of s_0, which is the location of the car at time $t = 0$ on the stopwatch, and an estimate of the speed v at which the car is moving, the number that is likely to be the main concern of whatever theory lurks behind this particular experiment. I prefer to speak of these quantities, the coefficients in the law $s = s_0 + vt$, as having been **measured**, through this modest extent of algebra, by the application of the **law** (the putative linear relationship) to the data set (t, s). The two parameters s_0 and v of the regression line have in this way been measured *implicitly* at the same time that the separate s's and t's were measured explicitly, as averages of certain modifications of those observations. Their measurement has been **indirect**, mediated via the postulate of that law of constant speed rather than the simpler laws of stopwatches or odometers (or, for that matter, internal-combustion engines) separately. We have, in passing, underlined one of the principal points of Kuhn's (1961) great essay on measurement in the physical sciences: there can be no effective measurement without equivalently effective theory.

After you divide by N^2, the numerator and denominator of equation (2.7) both have names. You recognize the denominator as $\overline{t^2} - \bar{t}^2$, the variance of t. Because $\Sigma(s - \bar{s}) = \Sigma(t - \bar{t}) = 0$ the numerator rearranges as

$$\overline{st} - \overline{\bar{s}\bar{t}} = \overline{(s_i - \bar{s})(t_i - \bar{t})}. \qquad (2.8)$$

This formula specifies the crucial quantity that is called the *covariance* of s and t. (As in equation (2.2), the line over "st" means to take the average of the whole expression under the bar; likewise the line over "$(s_i - \bar{s})(t_i - \bar{t})$".)

We have thus arrived at the **very important equation**

$$v = \frac{\text{cov}(s, t)}{\text{var}(t)}, \qquad (2.8a)$$

which connects the very practical task of estimating the slope v of a line to the two principal descriptors on which multivariate statistical analysis relies throughout. In its denominator, this formula for v invokes the fundamental descriptor of the distribution of one single measured variable, its variance; in its numerator, the same formula invokes this new value, their covariance or *product-moment*. Under either name it is the fundamental descriptor of the relation between two different measurements, As Wright (1968:283) points out, quoting his own earlier work of 1917 (!),

> The product-moment in a heterogeneous population may be analyzed into the sum of the product moment of the weighted means of the subpopulations and the average product moment within these. Because of this additive property, Fisher later renamed this statistic the covariance in analogy with the term variance for the squared standard deviation.

Another useful version of this same sum-of-squares definition is the identity

$$\text{var}(X + Y) = \text{var}(X) + \text{var}(Y) + 2\,\text{cov}(X, Y), \qquad (2.8b)$$

which can be rearranged to characterize the covariance in terms of a multiple of how much "extra" variance it assigns to the sum of X and Y:

$$\text{cov}(X, Y) = (\text{var}(X + Y) - \text{var}(X) - \text{var}(Y))/2. \qquad (2.8c)$$

There will be two more identities of this flavor in Section 5.4.6, in connection with Figure 5.61.

Equation (2.8b) has a simple corollary that is worth keeping in mind. As long as the two measurements or averages X and Y are independent, the variance of their difference is the same as the variance of their sum – just the sum of their separate variances. So the standard error of the difference of means of two groups with the same variance is $\sqrt{2}$ times the standard error of either mean, and the standard error of the difference $x_1 - x_2$ of two samples from the same distribution is $\sqrt{2}$ times the standard deviation of that distribution itself. We encountered this identity already in Section 2.1 – it is a special case of the small-sample formula for maximum-likelihood estimates of variance.

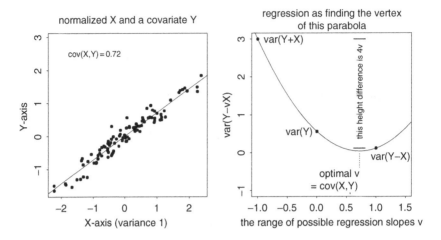

Figure 2.4 The role of the covariance coefficient in regression analysis, via the geometry of parabolas. (left) Scatterplot of two variables X and Y with var$(X) = 1$ and positive covariance between them. (right) In this setting the regression slope for predicting Y from X is the same as the covariance of X and Y, which, in turn, is the same as the horizontal coordinate of the vertex of the parabola diagrammed in this panel. It is an elementary property of parabolas with leading coefficient 1 that this minimum is equal to $\frac{1}{4}$ of the difference in heights of the parabola at ± 1. (If $y = (x - a)^2$, then $a = ((-1 - a)^2 - (1 - a)^2)/4 = (y(-1) - y(1))/4$.) That is, the vertex of the parabola (right) has a horizontal coordinate equal to the covariance of X and Y at left, which, under the assumption var$(X) = 1$, is also the regression slope of Y on X (line at left).

While the covariance $\overline{XY} - \bar{X}\bar{Y}$ thus appears to be a property of the pair of variables (X, Y) independent of any specific applied context, it helps the intuition to keep the least-squares interpretation of regression in mind. Assume without loss of generality that the predictor variable X has variance 1.0. (If not, just divide it by its own standard deviation.) Under that assumption, by equation (2.8a), the covariance of X and Y is equal to the regression slope of Y on X. Remembering that the regression is minimizing something, we can graph the minimand as the variance of $Y - vX$ as a function of v (Figure 2.4). This curve is a parabola, the vertex location of which must necessarily be the same as the value $v = \text{cov}(X, Y)$ in equation (2.7). But also, from the simple algebraic definition in equation 2.8b, we have $\text{cov}(X, Y) = (\text{var}(X + Y) - \text{var}(X - Y))/4$. The equation (2.7) for the optimal v is thus an elementary aspect of the geometry of parabolas.

If var$(X + Y) = \text{var}(X - Y)$, the vertex of the parabola must be at zero, which is $\frac{1}{4}$ of the difference of those two variances. But in this situation, cov(X, Y)

must likewise equal zero: there is no information in either variable that helps us predict the other by a linear formula. If, on the other hand, the height difference of the parabola at $v = -1$ over its height at $v = 1$ is 4, then it must be the case that the vertex is at $v = 1$, implying that the predicted value of Y from X is just X itself, or equivalently, that the covariance of X and Y in this case must be 1.0. (We will see an example of this in the geometry of causation for Galton's quincunx, Section 2.3.2.) The example in Figure 2.4 corresponds to an intermediate case with $v = \frac{1}{\sqrt{2}}$, about 0.7.

The geometry of a variance was displayed in Figure 2.1. We can draw a picture of this new, similarly named quantity, the *covariance*, by diagramming the products we are averaging, each as the area of a rectangle with sides of length x and y, as in the left-hand panel of Figure 2.5. It is a convenience that $\mathrm{cov}(x, y) = \mathrm{cov}\left(x, \left(\frac{\mathrm{cov}(x,y)}{\mathrm{var}(x)}\right) x\right)$ – that is, the covariance of x with y is also the covariance of x with the value of y predicted by the linear regression on x. (The intercept term that this formula ignores makes no difference for the covariance coefficient.) For this reason, we must get the same average area (i.e., the same geometric representation of the covariance coefficient) from the set of similarly shaped rectangles (now with areas all positive) in the right panel as from the dissimilar rectangles, some of negative area, in the left panel. Because the covariance is an average, its variance is just the variance of any individual contribution, the (signed) area of any one of those rectangles in the

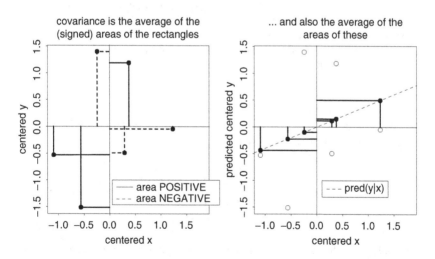

Figure 2.5 Geometry of the covariance coefficient. (left) Average of the observed products xy after mean-centering. (right) Average of the products $x \cdot \left(\frac{\mathrm{cov}(x,y)}{\mathrm{var}(x)}\right) x$. Open circles: original data, copied from the left panel.

figure, divided by n. Here is a handy special case: if x and y have mean zero and are actually independent, then the variance of the sample estimate of that covariance is

$$\text{var}(xy)/n = \left(\overline{(xy)^2} - \overline{(xy)}^2 \right)/n = \overline{(x^2 y^2)}/n - (\overline{x}^2\,\overline{y}^2) = (\overline{x^2}\,\overline{y^2})/n = \sigma_x^2 \sigma_y^2/n,$$
(2.8d)

by two applications each of the definition of the variance and the independence assumption.

> Such diagrams are not innocent of scientific assumptions that it is mandatory to verify; you must think deeply and skeptically before you put any faith in one of them. The preceding figure, for instance, entails a startlingly long list of ancillary assumptions. We tacitly assumed that area has some meaning – that the values of variables x and y can be multiplied (along with their units, whose product needs to make sense, too). Inasmuch as $xy = ((x+y)^2 - (x-y)^2)/4$, it can be seen that what we are really requiring is that our measurements can be added, subtracted, and squared, *all the while remaining meaningful as scientific descriptors*. Geometrically, the construction of the two new numbers $x \pm y$ can be interpreted via one single 45° rotation of the Cartesian plane, and so we can embed this same criterion of meaning within the more general claim that our scatterplot of (x, y) pairs has scientific meaning no matter what direction we inspect it in. This is quite a sweeping assumption – see Figure 5.61. An analogous criterion, applying to arbitrary linear combinations of arbitrarily long lists of measurements, will be an axiom of the more general multivariate approach of Section 4.3. In either of the graphical versions here, the covariance value itself, the numerator of the regression formula (2.7), has no obvious biological meaning. In the more sophisticated point of view of Chapter 4 any single covariance turns out to be best notated as $\text{cov}(X, Y) = r_{XY}\sigma_X\sigma_Y$, the correlation between a pair of variables scaled up by the product of their standard deviations.

2.2.2.1 Edgeworth's Reinterpretation of the Regression Formula

We can go even further in our rearrangement of equation (2.7). In the numerator, multiply and divide by $(t_i - \bar{t})^2$ to arrive at

$$\begin{aligned}
v &= \frac{\Sigma (s_i - \bar{s})(t_i - \bar{t})}{\Sigma (t_i - \bar{t})^2} \\
&= \frac{\Sigma \left(\frac{s_i - \bar{s}}{t_i - \bar{t}} \right)(t_i - \bar{t})^2}{\Sigma (t_i - \bar{t})^2}.
\end{aligned}$$
(2.9)

This takes the form of the weighted average to which you were already introduced in Section 2.1.2. Each raw ratio $\frac{s_i - \bar{s}}{t_i - \bar{t}}$ is multiplied by a factor $(t_i - \bar{t})^2$, the products added up, and their total divided by the sum of those weighting factors. This simple manipulation was apparently first noticed by

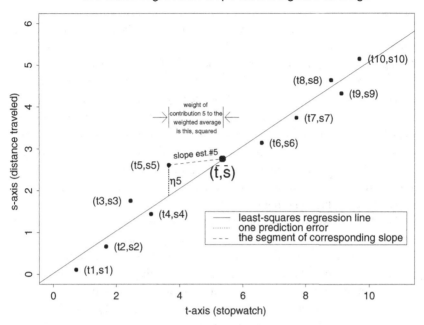

the same regression slope as a weighted average

Figure 2.6 Diagram for the interpretation of a regression coefficient as a weighted average slope. The point $(\bar{t}, \bar{s})$ is, as it was in Figure 2.3, the centroid of the set of ten (t, s) pairs shown. The regression line passes through this point with a slope that is equal to the weighted average value of $(s_i - \bar{s})/(t_i - \bar{t})$, where the weight is the square of the distance $t_i - \bar{t}$ from the average point to the ith point along the horizontal. In the figure this slope and the corresponding weight are shown explicitly for the fifth data pair along with the conventional vertical error term η_5.

F. Y. Edgeworth in 1892, nearly a century after the formula itself was first derived. To interpret it, examine the small print in Figure 2.6, which is an enhancement of the geometry we already inspected in Figure 2.3.

Both of the terms in the bottom line of Edgeworth's equation (2.9), the quantity being averaged and the quantity doing the weighting, are meaningful separately, and add strength to the interpretation of this process of line-fitting as a form of (indirect) measurement. The quantity being averaged, $\frac{s_i - \bar{s}}{t_i - \bar{t}}$, is an elementary slope estimate for v: a distance divided by a time. The distance is distance from the **mean**, however, not from our arbitrary zero, and the time is likewise time from the mean of the stopwatch readings, not from zero.

[If you **knew** the stopwatch was started just as the car ran over it (between the tires, so as not to crush it), you would modify the formula into $v = \Sigma s_i t_i / \Sigma t_i^2$, the same expression "referred to (0,0)." In this form it is clearer that we are averaging separate estimates s_i/t_i of speed using weighting factors t_i^2.]

Supposing that all values of s were measured with the same error variance (an assumption we hadn't explicitly stated before – actually it is embodied in the logic of minimizing the sum of the squares of the η's), then the associated guess $\frac{s_i - \bar{s}}{t_i - \bar{t}}$ for the speed v has the error of s divided by the *absolute value* (not the error ε) of $(t_i - \bar{t})$. The smaller this quantity – the closer t_i is to the mean $\bar{t}$ – the more error-prone is this particular component estimate of the common slope v. The weight of the "observation" $\frac{s_i - \bar{s}}{t_i - \bar{t}}$ of v is the reciprocal of this error variance, and so should be proportional to $(t_i - \bar{t})^2$, just as the formula says. (And so observations at times near the average time $\bar{t}$ do not contribute usefully to the estimation of v, which is why Tukey's formula, Section 2.5.2, does as well as it does while ignoring them entirely.)

We thought we were asking about a least-squares fit of the "law of constant speed" to time, but what we actually got was much more relevant to *measurement* than we expected: a (weighted) least-squares estimate, i.e., an average, of the slope we were really after, the specific object of the indirect measurement. If the car's speed were not known to be constant, this whole procedure would be meaningless. The least-squares logic of kinematics dictates that the line we are looking for has to go through the center of mass of the whole set of data as graphed – the centroid $(\bar{t}, \bar{s})$ of the set of points (t_i, s_i) considered as particles of identical mass on the plane. From the lines through that point we end up selecting the one that has as its slope the weighted least-squares estimate of the average slope over the whole sample of paired observations (t_i, s_i). The effect of one point at separation 2 seconds from the mean observation time $\bar{t}$ would be equivalent to the effect of four points at separation 1 second from that same mean time as read off the stopwatch, except that in this particular setup we don't have access to the requisite number of replicate stopwatches.

Uncertainty of v. The value of v we just computed has an uncertainty of its own with a formula that is so simple it would be churlish of this book to omit it. If $\sigma^2 = \text{var}(y|x)$ is the true error variance of any y-value at every specific x-value, then the variance of the linear estimate of v just printed is $\sigma^2/(n\text{var}(x))$. (The vertical bar in the expression $y|x$ is read "given," so that "$\sigma^2(y|x)$" stands for the variance of the y's associated with a given value of x.) This is easily shown by yet another rearrangement of the same formula (2.9). Assume $\bar{x} = \bar{y} = 0$, by recentering our measurements if necessary, and that the x's have been measured with negligible error. Then we have $v = \frac{\Sigma xy}{\Sigma x^2}$, and (remembering that prediction errors in the individual y's are all independent of one another) we must have

$$\text{var}(v) = \text{var}\left(\frac{\Sigma xy}{\Sigma x^2}\right) = \Sigma \left(\frac{x}{\Sigma x^2}\right)^2 \text{var}(y|x)$$

$$= \text{var}(y|x)\left(\Sigma x^2\right)/\left(\Sigma x^2\right)^2 = \sigma^2/\Sigma x^2 = \sigma^2/\left(n\,\text{var}(x)\right). \qquad (2.10)$$

2.2.3 The Role of Regressions as Lawlike Explanations: Two Examples

As David Freedman said (1991:292), "Regression sometimes works, in the hands of skilled practitioners ... although good examples are quite hard to find." Here are two good examples. (For a third, one that was partly responsible for Robert Millikan's Nobel Prize in Physics in 1923, see the discussion of his paper of 1916 in Bookstein, 2014, chapter E4.2.)

2.2.3.1 Example 2.1: Correlated Length Measurements

In 1932 the American geneticist Sewall Wright (1889–1988) published an extended analysis of six measured lengths on 276 adult leghorn chickens that will concern us when we turn to the topic of factor analysis in Section 4.3.4. Just to exemplify how good a data-based regression in the biosciences actually can be, I call your attention to Figure 2.7, which presents one of the fifteen bivariate scatterplots for this data set: lengths of the humerus and ulna. Data are taken from the tabulation published in Les Marcus's chapter of Rohlf and Bookstein (1990), also included as one of the thirteen data sets set down in the online appendix http://www.cambridge.org/9781107190948 for this book. As the figure shows, one of the points scattered (the one at line 101 of the computer file) is wildly discrepant from the others. Probably it stands for a typing error, 79.7 instead of 69.7, but no scientific insight is lost if I simply delete the point from the data set. There results the very nice scatter of the black dots in the figure, a scatter that is satisfactorily linear (without evident curvature) in accordance with the assumptions. The data really *do* seem to conform to a linear model, either ulna $\sim$ .9164(humerus)+0.476 or humerus $\sim$ 0.9737(ulna)+7.573. (The symbol $\sim$ is read "is distributed as".) As these are all adult chickens, the relation here is what the literature calls *static allometry*, the association of two or more measures of extent (i.e., "size measures") for a conspecific sample of organisms of homogeneous status within a shared life cycle. (Other logical possibilities include *growth allometry*, the form originally studied by Huxley in 1932, and *evolutionary allometry*, the subject of our example in Section 3.3.2.) Following the suggestion from

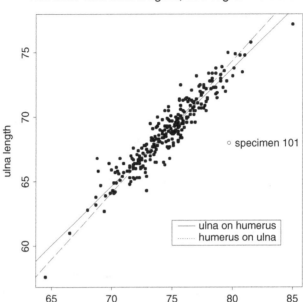

Figure 2.7 Scatter of two measured limb lengths for 276 leghorn chickens, showing both regression lines. Data from Sewall Wright via Marcus (1990). See text.

Karl Pearson that will be reviewed in Section 2.4, it is sufficient to summarize this pair of regressions by the single quantity that is the square root of the product of their slopes, $\sqrt{0.9164 \times 0.9737} = 0.9446$; this is the *correlation* between the two measures. (The square root is taken with the same sign as either of the slopes that it combines; here, that sign is positive.) Its value is larger than the correlation between any other pair of these six length measures, presumably because they share an axis within a single embryonic component (the forelimb).

The result of this fit is to replace the full data set – a total of 2×275 measurements – by a set of five parameters only: the mean and variance of this pair of measurements and either the correlation coefficient of 0.944 or the error variance of either prediction around the regression upon the other. In this form the summary is optimal for serving as a component of a higher-level explanation (see Section 4.1). Our interest was never in the prediction of humerus length from ulna length, or vice versa, but in the pattern of these measured lengths as a whole as an illustration of theories of form-regulation in animal species.

2.2.3.2 Example 2.2: Circulatory and Respiratory Allometries: A Data Set from Geoffrey West

West et al. (1997) report on "a general model for the origin of allometric scaling laws in biology." As we will see when we turn to the topic of brain weight – body weight allometry in Section 3.3.2, the most obvious factor of biological diversity is the variation of body size between and within evolutionary clades, a scaling that presumably affects most biological structures and processes. It is a commonplace that such scaling relationships are often found to be loglinear; it is less common that (particularly when the variables in question are physiologically simplistic in some way, expressive of some energy-minimizing strategy) the corresponding exponents of the dependence on size are often simple proper fractions (ratios of small integers). The West argument, assuming mainly that energy dissipation is minimized and that terminal tubes do not scale with body size, provides predictions of a variety of scaling exponents for mammalian circulatory systems "that are in agreement with data" over the observed size range of approximately three orders of magnitude. A summary table (their page 125) pairs the inferred exponents (fractions) against exponents taken from one of three different monographs. The comparison can be set out in the form of the graphic in Figure 2.8.

This is an unusual scatter in several ways. First, the linear prediction of the observed allometric exponents has a slope differing from the hoped-for value of 1.0 by only 0.63%, and the standard error around this prediction is only 0.025 over a range of 1.75 in value, from $-\frac{3}{4}$ to 1; both of these features are nearly unheard-of in theoretical biology. (The observed correlation, 0.999, is certainly at the high end of correlations between observed and expected quantities encountered anywhere in the biological literature.) Second, the distribution of the variables on either axis is not remotely bell-shaped (Gaussian); rather, it is limited to 0, ±1, and a selection of fractions with denominators 4, 8, or 12. Third, the fractions along the horizontal axis are derived from exact theory, and hence *have* no "measurement error," any more than the number π does. Fourth, the agreement of the observed exponents (themselves regression slopes) with the predictions from the various theories here is remarkable – the line of perfect agreement (dashed) is indistinguishable from the actual regression of observed on predicted slopes. The argument is thereby supported that the form of derivation demonstrated in the article by West et al. is a valid approach to the computation of expected scalings over a wide range of fractal and fractal-like aspects of animal physiology. This, in turn, argues for applications to extinct species, for which physiology is no longer accessible; likewise to comparisons with distribution networks in other taxa, such as insect tracheae; likewise to a wide range of other scaling arguments in biophysics. The regression of

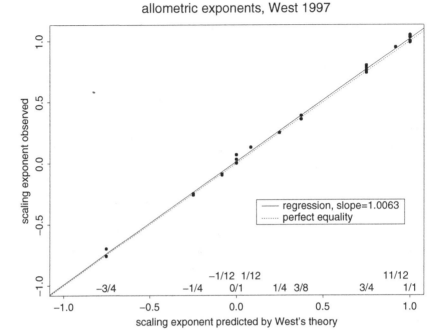

Figure 2.8 Graphical rendering of table 1 of West et al. (1997), showing the remarkable agreement of modeled vs. reported allometric scaling exponents for a variety of aspects of circulatory and respiratory microstructure vis-à-vis body size over the mammals. The regression line is indistinguishable from the line of perfect equality as regards either slope or intercept. The original data for this scatter were selected by West et al. from the tabulations in Peters (1983) and Schmidt-Nielsen (1984).

observed against predicted exponents is evidently much more sharply defined than any of the individual allometric relationships that supply values of the corresponding ordinates. For more on the biophysics of this sort of scaling, see West (2017).

Summary of Section 2.2

- The discussion of the relationship between two separate measurements of an organism (or any other organized system) begins best not with the model of noncorrelation (independence) but with the opposite model, that of a perfect linear relationship (an equation) up to measurement error.

- When the points in a scatterplot of two measured variables x and y lie close to a straight line without curvature, a robust and satisfactory estimate of that line is given by the *normal equations* that minimize the sum of squared distances to it measured perpendicular to the axis of one or the other of the variables.
- The least-squares optimal slope yielded by the normal equations with x as predictor is equal to the ratio $\frac{\text{cov}(x,y)}{\text{var}(x)}$, where "var($x$)" is the variance of the predictor and "cov(x, y)" is the *covariance* of x and y, the average $\Sigma_{i=1}^{N}(x_i - \bar{x})(y_i - \bar{y})/n$ of the product of their deviations from their own averages separately.
- The estimated slope yielded by the normal equations is the same as the weighted average of the slopes from each original paired observation to the point at the grand mean of those pairs of observations, using weights that equal the squared distances of the independent variable from its own mean.
- The square root of the product of the two regression slopes, taken with a minus sign if these are negative, is the *correlation* of the pair of variables under consideration. It is sometimes a useful scale-free summary of their relationship, especially in the context of more than two variables.
- The slope of an estimated regression line is often a biological measurement on its own. As such it has a standard error of estimate that can be computed from the geometry of the least-squares fit that led to it. If σ^2 is the true error variance of the dependent variable around the prediction by the independent variable x, then the variance of the estimated slope is just $\sigma^2/n\text{var}(x)$.

2.3 Gaussian Distributions and Galton's Quincunx

I know of scarcely anything so apt to impress the imagination as the wonderful form of cosmic order expressed by the "Law of Frequency of Error." The law would have been personified by the Greeks and deified, if they had known of it. Whenever a large sample of chaotic elements are taken in hand and marshalled in the order of their magnitude, an unsuspected and most beautiful form of regularity proves to have been latent all along.

(Francis Galton, 1889:66)

The argument in this section, beginning with Pascal's formula for binomial coefficients and ending with the explicit formula $\frac{1}{\sqrt{2\pi}}e^{-x^2/2}$ for the standard Gaussian distribution as applied in both the physical sciences and the biosocial sciences, is one of the all-time classic demonstrations of the power of applied mathematics to make sense of the world. It should be part of the intellectual travel kit of every educated person. So if you have not been shown this derivation before, please take as much time as you need to master this section, rereading it until you can reproduce at least the major steps of either formal argument, Maxwell's or Galton's. It is well worth your while as scientist, scholar, or citizen to understand just *why* the bell curve is the inevitable, universal descriptor of complete quantitative disorder both mathematically and physically. This formula $\frac{1}{\sqrt{2\pi}}e^{-x^2/2}$ is one of the fundamental mathematical insights on which the universe seems to be grounded.

I tell the story of that formula as a sequence of five major milestones in our understanding: the limiting form of the binomial distribution, the working of Galton's quincunx, the linear equation for regression (inference of causes from effects) on the quincunx, the re-expression of all this in the currently standard notation, and the several other origins of this same distribution in alternative models of complete disorder. These are the concerns of Sections 2.3.1 through 2.3.5. A final section returns to the geometry of regression with reference to a different reference structure, the ellipse, in order to clarify the phenomenon usually called "regression to the mean."

2.3.1 Milestone 1: Limits of Binomials

Our **first milestone** is the essentially elementary construction of the master formula as a limiting form of the familiar binomial distribution, the pattern of the coefficients of powers of x in the expansion of $(1 + x)^k$ as k becomes arbitrarily large.[7] We will need two auxiliary formulas. First, one from the ancient Greeks: the sum of the first k odd numbers is k^2. Second, the approximation known as "Stirling's formula," after James Stirling (1730):

$$k! \approx k^k e^{-k}\sqrt{2\pi k} \tag{2.11}$$

Here π is the same constant you have always known as the ratio of the circumference of a circle to its diameter.[8] The expression $k!$, read "k factorial," stands for $1 \times 2 \times \ldots \times k$, the product of all the integers up through k, and you remember from high school that $e \sim 2.71828$ is the basis of the *natural logarithms* used without exception in this book, the value e for which $\int_1^e dx/x$, the area under the curve $y = 1/x$ from 1 to e, is 1. And the symbol $\approx$ means

---

[7] This is not the only role of limiting forms of the binomial distribution in statistics. There is a different limit, where as the number of coins increases indefinitely, the probability of Heads for each in turn drops exactly in proportion. This leads to another famous elementary probability distribution, the *Poisson distribution,* which also has a role to play in physics, for instance in studies of radioactive decay.

[8] This specific notational fact is implicit in the very first argument brought forward by Eugene Wigner (1960) in support of his claim that mathematics is "unreasonably effective" in its applications to the real physical world.

"is approximately equal to," in the sense that as k gets bigger and bigger, the ratio of the left side of equation (2.11) to the right side approaches 1.0 more and more closely.

From Stirling's formula we can proceed to generate useful approximations of Pascal's binomial coefficients $_nC_k = n!/(k!(n-k)!)$, the coefficients of successive powers of x in the expansion of $(1+x)^n$. $_nC_k$ (read this symbol as "enn choose kay") is the count of the ways of choosing k coins out of n to be "Heads-up," and so it is also n times the random variable we are interested in, the frequency of Heads. (There are two common proofs of Pascal's formula, one by mathematical induction via the formula $_nC_k = {}_{n-1}C_k + {}_{n-1}C_{k-1}$ and the other by explicit enumeration of cases – there are n ways of choosing the first coin to come up Heads, times $n-1$ ways of choosing the second, ..., times $n-(k-1)$ ways of choosing the kth – this product is $\frac{n!}{(n-k)!}$ – but we get the same set of Heads whatever the order we decided that one was first, one second, ..., and so we have to divide this ratio by a further factor of $k!$.) Suppose that n is an even number $2m$, for instance, and we want the frequency with which Heads and Tails come out equally in the flip of $2m$ coins. By Pascal's formula, this is $(2m)!/m!\,m!$; by Stirling's formula (2.11), that ratio expands to approximately

$$\frac{(2m)^{2m}e^{-2m}\sqrt{2\pi(2m)}}{(m^m e^{-m}\sqrt{2\pi m})^2} = \frac{2^{2m}m^{2m}e^{-2m}\sqrt{2\pi(2m)}}{m^{2m}e^{-2m}(2\pi m)} = 2^{2m}\sqrt{1/\pi m} \quad (2.12)$$

because all the other terms have cancelled. Dividing by the total count 2^{2m} of sequences of flips, this is just $\sqrt{1/\pi m}$. So, for instance, if you have flipped 100 coins, the chance of counting *exactly* 50 Heads is $1/\sqrt{50\pi} \approx 0.08$.

But it is not only the central probability $((2m)!/m!\,m!)/2^{2m}$ that we can approximate this well; it is also the frequencies $({}_{2m}C_{m\pm l})/2^{2m}$ for the counts of Heads falling off by l to either side of this maximum. The formula for $_{2m}C_{m\pm l}$ changes the formula for $_{2m}C_m$ by dropping factors n, $n-1,\ldots, n-(l-1)$ from the first factorial in the denominator and adding factors $n+1$, $n+2,\ldots, n+l$ to the second factorial in the denominator. We have thus increased the denominator, as a whole, by a factor that we can rearrange helpfully as

$$\frac{m+1}{m} \cdot \frac{m+2}{m-1} \cdots \cdots \frac{m+l}{m-(l-1)}.$$

We need two approximations from elementary calculus: for a, b both small,

$$(1+a)/(1-b) \approx 1 + (a+b) \quad (2.13a)$$

and

$$\log(1+a) \approx a. \quad (2.13b)$$

Apply (2.13a) with $a = 1/m$, $b = 0$, then with $a = 2/m$, $b = 1/n$, ..., up through $a = l/m$, $b = (l-1)/m$. The a's and b's are of the order of $1/\sqrt{m}$ or less, which is small enough for this approximation if m is large, so that our factor by which the denominator of $_{2m}C_{m\pm l}$ has increased over the denominator of $_{2m}C_m$ becomes, approximately,

$$\left(1 + \frac{1}{m}\right) \cdot \left(1 + \frac{3}{m}\right) \cdot \cdots \cdot \left(1 + \frac{2l-1}{m}\right).$$

The logarithm of this product is the sum of the logs of the factors, each of which is approximated with the aid of (2.13b): $\log (_{2m}C_{m\pm l}/_{2m}C_m)$ is thereby very nearly $(1/m) + (3/m) + (5/m) + \cdots + (2l-1)/m$. But from the ancient formula, that is just l^2/m.

By undoing the logging, and keeping in mind that we were working in the *denominator* of the formula for $_{2m}C_{m\pm l}$, it turns out we have shown that **the terms $_{2m}C_{m\pm l}$ fall off from their maximum $_{2m}C_m$ approximately as** $e^{-l^2/m}$. As we already saw for the precision of the average, Section 2.1.2, this is an inverse square-root scaling. For equal ratios l^2/m, quadrupling m only doubles the value of l for which the fall-off achieves any particular threshold of negligibility, say, one chance in a thousand or so.

If we rewrite to refer to the flip of n coins instead of $2m$, the exponent becomes $-l^2/(n/2)$, or $-2l^2/n$. So for a count of Heads $n/2 \pm l$ that differs by l from the maximum ($n/2$ Heads) in either direction, the peak frequency is multiplied by $e^{-2l^2/n}$. It is worth setting this down as an equation we can crossreference later: as a fraction of the peak probability (which we have already estimated at $\sqrt{2/n\pi}$ per equation 2.12), the chance of any particular count of Heads is proportional to

$$e^{-2l^2/n} = e^{-l^2/2(n/4)} = e^{-l^2/2c} \tag{2.14}$$

where c stands for $n/4$, the variance of that count of Heads for n coins.

The following pair of figures shows this limiting behavior in two different graphics. First (Figure 2.9), the actual probabilities of encountering any total of Heads in the range of 0 to k, as k ranges from 10 to 160 coins, leads to curves on the log scale that all appear to be downward-pointing parabolas of steadily greater sharpness and lower peak height.

Second (Figure 2.10), once we correct for these two trends, the curve of log-probability converges to one invariant parabola, and so the curve of probability itself converges to the exponentiation of that same parabola. But that is just the bell curve.

On the limiting figure in the lefthand panel here the arrows indicate the "shoulders" of the bell curve, the loci at which the curve changes from

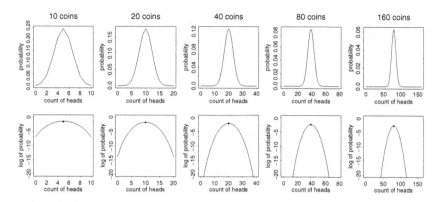

Figure 2.9 Frequencies of Heads expected from 10, 20, 40, 80, or 160 flips of a fair coin. (upper row) Raw probabilities (note changing vertical axes). (lower row) Logarithms of the curves above. These curves are approximately parabolas for which the peak falls linearly with log coin count while the vertex curvature (sharpness – second derivative of the curve there) increases as the square root of that same count. The vertical axes are now all the same scale of log p. In reading the vertical scale of the plots in the lower row, it helps to keep in mind that $e^{-10} \cong 0.0000454$ and $e^{-20} \cong 0.00000000206$. The heavy dots in this lower row actually lie on a straight line on this printed page.

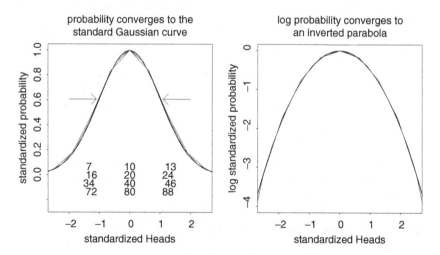

Figure 2.10 Superposition of the four rightmost curves from Figure 2.9, after scaling the vertical and horizontal separately. (left) Convergence of the probability distribution to the standard bell curve. (right) Convergence of the logarithms of those probabilities to a standard parabola. Numbers along the horizontal axis at left indicate intervals of approximately ±1.5 standard deviations from the mean in terms of counts of original Heads. The arrows indicate the inflection points of the untransformed bell at ±1 standard deviation.

convex-upward to concave-upward. These are at a distance one standard deviation from the mean in either direction. The curve has a height there that is $e^{-1/2} \cong 0.60$ of its maximum. (Drawing the shoulders at the wrong height is the most common error in students' sketches of this curve.) Notice that the log-probability plot lacks these shoulders; that form is just an ordinary parabola.

2.3.2 Milestone 2: Galton's Machine

Our **second milestone** is a physical machine that produces these curves as realizations of a random process that is physical instead of mathematical. This additional mode of generating Gaussian distributions, just as random as the coin flips of Section 2.3.1 (or the gas molecules to concern us in Section 2.3.5), corresponds closely to the notions of causation in the biology of inheritance that were just beginning to coalesce at the end of the nineteenth century.

The new line of thought began with an actual physical device invented by Francis Galton, cousin of Charles Darwin and surely the most diverse scientist that Victorian England ever produced. Galton worked, among other problems, on weather maps, fingerprints, fidgeting behavior, the efficacy of prayer, "hereditary genius," averaged photography, and eugenics. In 1877, in a letter to a Darwin cousin, Galton conveyed the design of a physical device he had built that could produce Gaussian variability while still permitting there to be "causes" of differences in the final outcome. Our attention is drawn to this clever contraption, the *quincunx* (Figure 2.11), a schematic of which I lay out in Figure 2.12. (The word "quincunx" properly refers to the X-shape of dots on the five-face of a die, or the equivalent in horticulture.) In either figure, the top is where lead shot (identical little round metal balls) enter a pattern of successive, independent left-or-right choices just like flips of a coin. Their accumulation at the bottom precisely delimits the Gaussian distribution governing such processes in the limit of many coins (many rows of a quincunx). One describes position at the bottom by the accumulated number of lefts versus rights, or Heads versus Tails, so the horizontal separation between every neighboring pair of dots in the same row corresponds to the switch of one left bounce for a right bounce, or vice versa: it is 2 units on the horizontal H-minus-T scale.

At every row past the tenth or so, these distributions are approximately Gaussian. There is no standardizing of width such as applied to show the convergence to one shared bell-shaped curve. Instead, each row has a different standard deviation (or waist, or variance). Remember that the variance of the number of Heads in flips of k coins is $k/4$, and Heads minus Tails goes

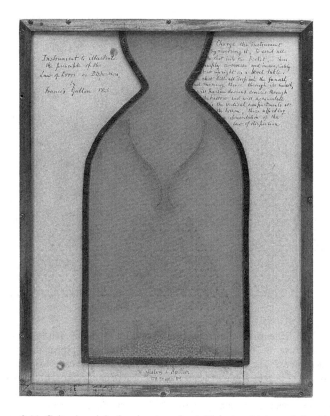

Figure 2.11 Galton's original quincunx, about 15 inches high, sealed with its lead shot still inside. The handwriting on the backing sheet conveys Galton's own instructions for its use. The rows of points visible are nails spaced almost exactly by the diameter of the shot. This is image 063 from The Galton Collection, part of the University College London Science Collections, used by permission.

as double the number of Heads, minus k. So the variance of Heads minus Tails, which is the quincunx bin variable we are looking at, is four times the variance of Heads, which happens to equal the row number of the quincunx we're looking at. Hence the distribution in row k goes as $e^{-x^2/2k}$ for $x =$ Heads − Tails. In Figure 2.12, a point is highlighted where x is $35 - 15 = 20$ for $k = 50$ (the fiftieth row). According to formula (2.14), the corresponding probability must then be reduced from the peak height of the bell curve drawn there by a factor $e^{-20^2/2 \cdot 50} = e^{-4} \cong 0.0183$, consistent with the sketch in the figure.

This description, net excess of Heads over Tails in k flips of a fair coin, can be applied at any stage of the shot's fall, not just in reference to the point

schematic of Galton's quincunx, 51 rows

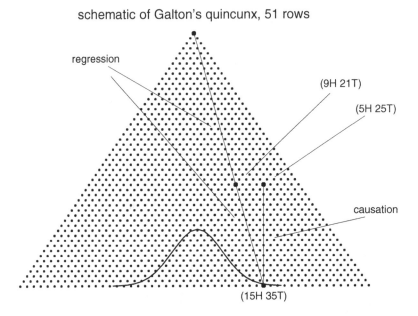

Figure 2.12 Schematic of the quincunx. Shot enter at the top and fall through each successive row of nails passing left or right with equal probability at each nail encountered. The bell curve at the bottom represents the expected Gaussian distribution of final locations of a large number of shot falling through all 50 rows. Vertical line: causation, expected (average) fall vertically downward. Oblique line: regression (what Galton called "reversion"), likeliest origin at any higher level of a lower point along the straight line connecting that lower point to the vertex of the quincunx. In this way the machine produces straight lines as part of the description of its functioning without referring to any equation from the physical sciences.

where it comes to rest. Galton's "Eureka!" moment of 1875, immortalized in a letter to his cousin (Figure 2.13), reduces to imagining the process of falling through the quincunx as the concatenation of two processes – say, falling through the first half, and then falling through the second. Imagine this as a modification of the quincunx that involves a stiff card inserted all across its width partway down, perhaps at the 30th row of the 50-row quincunx here; you then remove the card. Falling through the first half results in a normal distribution of standard deviation $\sqrt{30} \approx 5.5$. When the card is removed and each little ball in those bins is permitted to fall the remaining 20 rows, it generates its own Gaussian distribution, now of s.d. $\sqrt{20} \approx 4.5$, around its own starting position. **The composite of all of those Gaussian distributions of variance 20, weighted by the distribution of variance 30, must be identical to the actual Gaussian distribution of variance 50 (s.d. 7, waist 14) drawn**

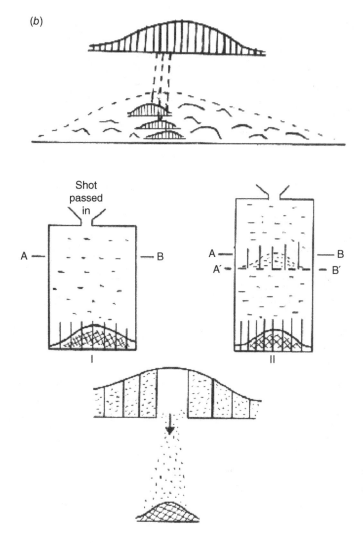

Figure 2.13 Galton's original sketches of the quincunx, from a letter to his cousin George Darwin of 1877. From Karl Pearson, *The Life, Letters and Labours of Francis Galton*, 1930, IIIB:465–466.

in the bottom row of the figure, because that is how that bottom row was actually produced in the version without any cards. (As part of this argument, Galton was exploiting the additivity of variances of independent processes that we already reviewed in Section 2.1.)

In an extension of Galton's original sketch (Figure 2.13), I present a series of simulations of this cumulative procedure (Figures 2.14–2.15). In Figure 2.14

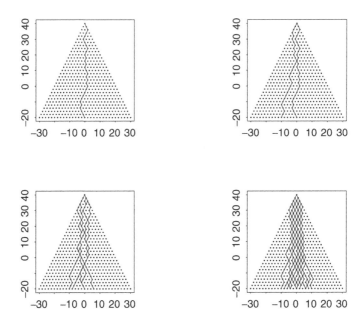

Figure 2.14 Detailed traces of progress down the quincunx for samples of 1, 2, 4, or 16 balls.

we see superimposed a set of 1, 2, 4, or 16 separate caroms of balls down the quincunx. By 16, this diagram becomes too hard to read, and it is sufficient to replace it by the distribution of the final positions of these paths as the cascade of balls arrives at the bottom of the machine. Figure 2.15 converts this display style to a histogram of the balls' final resting place at the bottom, initially with realistic levels of noise for 25, 100, 400, or 1600 balls, but finally, in the bottom panel, for a simulation involving a full one million coins (33,333 balls each running down 30 rows, with 10 left over). At this degree of precision the rendered form of the bell curve is exact to the size of the pixels used to produce this figure.

2.3.3 Milestone 3: Regression on the Quincunx

Our **third milestone** of this section is the demonstration that this machine for producing Gaussian distributions is also a machine for producing *linear dependencies* among Gaussian distributions, and hence serves as a laboratory model for the interpretation of linear dependencies as causal.

Before this insight of Galton's, Gaussian distributions had been viewed as *homogeneous*, necessarily arising from the replication of processes (flips of a coin) themselves identical over the cases of a series, and straight lines had been

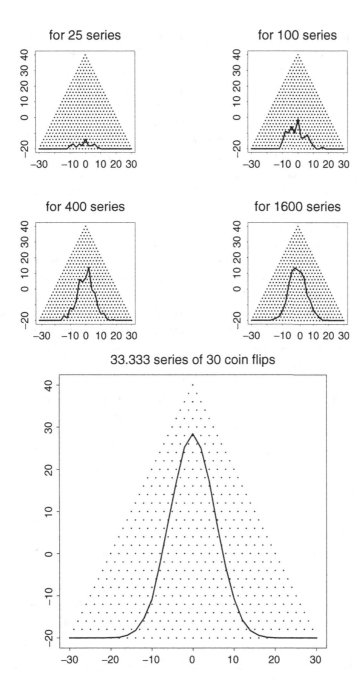

Figure 2.15 A different rendering, histogram of bins along the bottom row in which the shot ultimately come to rest. (top) For counts of 25, 100, 400, or 1600 shot. (bottom) For one million coins considered as 33,333 30-coin percolations. There is no visible deviation from the standard bell curve.

imagined to arise mainly from exactly linear theories like $s = vt$ or $F = ma$. Inherent in our third milestone is a brilliant advance in applied probability theory: a model by which a Gaussian distribution can arise from a set of initial values that are not identical but themselves variable. That is, a Gaussianly distributed pattern of outcomes – say, the weights of a batch of seeds, or the heights of British youth – can be viewed as the result of a process by which each seed or young man began at a *different* setting, the parents' seed weight or average height, and then proceeded to diffuse outward by coin flips of its or his own. (In a happy convergence of model with fact, these "coins" would later be identified – though not by Galton or Pearson – with Mendelian genes.) The overwhelming temptation, which need not be resisted, is to refer to the starting value, the location intermediate along the quincunx, as the *cause* of the value observed at the bottom. It accounts for that value *to some rigorously quantifiable extent*, by influencing the mean about which it varies by its own Gaussian noise. Hogben (1950, 1957) calls this the "the Umpire-Bonus model" and places it at the core of all valid biometrical statistics.

For an application to human heredity, which is what mainly concerned Galton, this is half of what we need – a model, free of the "hereditary particles" whose existence would not be known (outside of Gregor Mendel's monastery in Brno) for decades, for the passage from parents' scores to children's scores on any quantitative variate. The other half of the required methodology follows from a study of *reversion*, nowadays called *regression*, using this same chart.

On the quincunx, a specific score at the bottom, at the 50-coin level – say, 35 Heads, 15 Tails – could have come from, say, 25 Heads 5 Tails at level 30, or from 20 Heads 10 Tails, or from 15 Heads 15 Tails, and so on. As Galton did, take the model of causation as "falling down the quincunx": the sample of shot that enter at the top are distributed Gaussianly with variance k at the kth row downward. Let us score position in the quincunx by distance left or right from the spot directly under the entrance point: count of heads minus count of tails for the equivalent series of coin flips. After k of these binary choices, a particle is found in the yth bin of its row. Where is it likeliest to have been in the lth row, $(k - l)$ rows above?

We use Laplace's principle (Section 2.1.4) again. The shot were distributed as Gaussians in the kth row of the quincunx, and are distributed Gaussianly again in the remainder of their fall. More specifically, the probability of having been in position x in the lth row is proportional to $e^{\frac{-x^2}{2l}}$, and the probability of having fallen from position x to position y over $(k - l)$ rows is proportional to $e^{\frac{-(y-x)^2}{2(k-l)}}$. These events, the fall through the first l rows and the fall through the next $(k - l)$, are independent. Hence the likelihood of having arrived at the

yth bin of the kth row via the xth bin of the lth row is proportional (leaving out those factors of $\sqrt{\pi}$) to

$$e^{\frac{-x^2}{2l}} \times e^{\frac{-(y-x)^2}{2(k-l)}} = e^{-\left(\frac{x^2}{2l} + \frac{(y-x)^2}{2(k-l)}\right)}. \tag{2.15a}$$

To maximize this, minimize the negative of its logarithm, which is, after multiplying out by $2l(k-l)$, the formula $(k-l)x^2 + l(y-x)^2$. This is maximized where its derivative $2(k-l)x - 2l(y-x)$ with respect to the unknown x is zero. That requires $\frac{x}{y-x} = \frac{l}{k-l}$, or $\frac{x}{y} = \frac{l}{k}$, or

$$x = \frac{l}{k}y, \tag{2.15b}$$

meaning that x is just the point in its row (l) on the line between the point y of the kth row and the vertex of the quincunx. How simple this turns out to be! – the generation of a straight line not from some contingent physical law but instead as an intrinsic property of pure randomness when managed in this systematic way. The straight line is expressing the mathematics of randomness, not the physics of gravity.

With y fixed (it was the observed data, after all), the likelihood expression (2.15a), evaluated at the value of x specified by (2.15b), takes the form of just another Gaussian distribution, where the coefficient of $-x^2$ is

$$\frac{1}{2}\left(\frac{1}{l} + \frac{1}{k-l}\right) = \frac{1}{2}\frac{k}{l(k-l)}. \tag{2.15c}$$

Twice this coefficient must be the reciprocal of the variance of that x-distribution. Hence: over repeated observations (the whole set of lead shot falling down that ended in the yth bin of the kth row), the originating value x in the $(k-l)$th row is distributed around this likeliest location with variance $l(1 - \frac{l}{k})$, the variance of x reduced by the same factor $\frac{l}{k}$. (This would be an easy experiment to do using Galton's "card": after pausing the process at the $(k-l)$th row, you paint each shot there with its slot number, then remove the card.)

This would be mere intellectual play if its inferences were limited to the quincunx machine alone (Figure 2.16). But Galton found the same pattern in some actual data pertinent to human heredity. In Figure 2.17, the regression of son's height on his "midparent height" (father's height averaged with 1.08 times mother's height) appears to have been linear with an appropriate slope. In other words, the relation between the adult offspring's height and the parents' height obeys an equation of the same algebraic structure as the relation of a

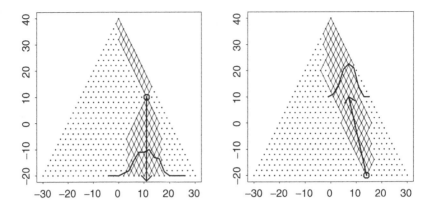

Figure 2.16 Explicit simulated Gaussians for falling halfway down the quincunx (left) and regressing halfway up (right). Gridwork on the plots covers all of the pathways taken by all of the shot involved in these distributions, but the density of coverage of each little path segment is not indicated.

ball at the bottom of the quincunx to another ball about 1/3 of the way back up toward the vertex. These processes must therefore have a great deal to do with one another. Section 2.3.6 more closely examines the ellipse superimposed over the printed tabulation here.

2.3.4 Milestone 4: A More Elegant Notation

The **fourth milestone** on our list concerns the construction of the conventional standard formula for the bell curve that is ubiquitous today in the statistical graphics of both the natural and the social sciences.

Return again to the contemplation of counts of Heads in the flip of $2m$ coins, or, rather, to their deviation l from the likeliest count, which is m. Whenever n is large enough, the distribution of l can be imagined as continuous rather than discrete – all we have to do is convert from the count $\frac{n}{2} + l$ of Heads to the fraction $\frac{1}{2} + \frac{l}{n}$ of Heads. This is the way that we get to the *standard Gaussian distribution*, the bell curve of standard deviation 1. Remember that the negative exponential factor $e^{-2l^2/n}$ in equation (2.14) was multiplying a maximum probability of $\sqrt{2/\pi n}$ corresponding to the likeliest total, which was $\frac{n}{2}$ Heads. As a fraction, this corresponds to the value 0 for $\frac{l}{n}$. But that maximum probability applies now to an interval of width only $\frac{1}{n}$, the increment of fraction-of-Heads between $\frac{1}{2} + \frac{l}{n}$ and $\frac{1}{2} + \frac{l+1}{n}$ for $l = 0$. The probability *density* at the maximum is thus actually n times that point-probability $\sqrt{2/\pi n}$; this product is $\sqrt{2n/\pi}$. For the fraction of Heads, then, the probability goes

Table 8.1. Galton's 1885 cross-tabulation of 928 adult children born of 205 midparents, by their height and their midparent's height.

Height of the mid-parent in inches	Height of the adult child														Total no. of adult children	Total no. of mid-parents	Medians
	<61.7	62.2	63.2	64.2	65.2	66.2	67.2	68.2	69.2	70.2	71.2	72.2	73.2	>73.7			
>73.0	—	—	—	—	—	—	—	—	—	—	—	1	3	—	4	5	—
72.5	—	—	—	—	—	—	—	1	2	1	2	7	2	4	19	6	72.2
71.5	—	—	—	—	1	3	4	3	5	10	4	9	2	2	43	11	69.9
70.5	1	—	1	—	1	3	12	18	14	7	4	3	3	—	68	22	69.5
69.5	—	—	1	16	4	17	27	20	33	25	20	11	4	5	183	41	68.9
68.5	1	—	7	11	16	25	31	34	48	21	18	4	3	—	219	49	68.2
67.5	—	3	5	14	15	36	38	28	38	19	11	4	—	—	211	33	67.6
66.5	—	3	3	5	2	17	17	14	13	4	—	—	—	—	78	20	67.2
65.5	1	—	9	5	7	11	11	7	7	5	2	1	—	—	66	12	66.7
64.5	1	1	4	4	1	5	5	—	2	—	—	—	—	—	23	5	65.8
<64.0	1	—	2	4	1	2	2	1	1	—	—	—	—	—	14	1	—
Totals	5	7	32	59	48	117	138	120	167	99	64	41	17	14	928	205	—
Medians	—	—	66.3	67.8	67.9	67.7	67.9	68.3	68.5	69.0	69.0	70.0	—	—	—	—	—

Source: Galton (1886a).

Note: All female heights were multiplied by 1.08 before tabulation. Galton added an explanatory footnote to the table: "In calculating the Medians, the entries have been taken as referring to the middle of the squares in which they stand. The reason why the headings run 62.2, 63.2, &c., instead of 62.5, 63.5, &c., is that the observations are unequally distributed between 62 and 63, 63 and 64, &c., there being a strong bias in favour of integral inches. After careful consideration, I concluded that the headings, as adopted, best satisfied the conditions. This inequality was not apparent in the case of the Mid-parents." Galton republished these data in 1889, where they are referred to as the R.F.F. Data (Record of Family Faculties); he then noted that the first row must be in error (four children cannot have five sets of parents), but he claimed that "the bottom line, which looks suspicious, is correct" (p. 208).

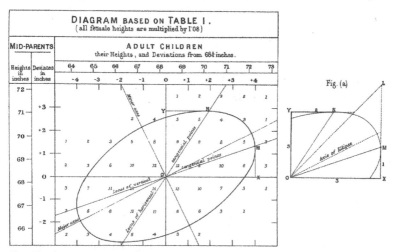

Figure 8.7. Galton's smoothed rendition of Table 8.1, with one of the "concentric and similar ellipses" drawn in. The geometric relationship of the two regression lines to the ellipse is also shown. (From Galton, 1886a.)

Figure 2.17 Galton's original published example of a correlated pair of anthropometric measurements. (above) Table of combinations of adult child height by midparent height, in bins of inches. (bottom) Interpretation as a bivariate frequency ellipse, with the regression line in both its interpretation (line of expected bin means, join of loci of vertical tangents). Source: http://galton.org/essays/1880-1889/galton-1886-jaigi-regression-stature.pdf.

as this new, properly normalized peak height times that factor of fall-off: the
product

$$\sqrt{2n/\pi}\ e^{-2l^2/n}.$$

It is customary to rewrite this formula so as to show the standard deviation
explicitly in both the premultiplying factor and the exponential term:

$$\sqrt{2n/\pi}\ e^{-2l^2/n} = \frac{1}{\sqrt{2\pi}\sigma}e^{-\frac{1}{2}\left(\frac{x-\mu}{\sigma}\right)^2}, \tag{2.16}$$

where, traditionally, the Greek letter σ, lower-case "sigma," denotes the
standard deviation – here, $\frac{1}{2\sqrt{n}}$, corresponding to the variance $\frac{1}{4n}$ in the fraction
of Heads we found in Section 2.1.2 – and $x - \mu$ renames $\frac{l}{n}$, the deviation of
the x we observe from the mean value $\mu = \frac{1}{2}$ that we "expect." The factors
in front look different but are the same. The peak of this standard curve is at
$1/\sqrt{2\pi} \cong 0.40$, and the shoulders are at horizontal coordinates ± 1 and height
$e^{-1/2}$ times that peak height, about $0.60 \cdot 0.40 \cong 0.24$.

We began all this algebra with an approximate formula for the factorial
function, but now that we are at the formal level of infinitesimals, the result is
exact:

$$\int_{-\infty}^{\infty} \frac{1}{\sqrt{2\pi}\sigma}e^{-\frac{1}{2}\left(\frac{x-\mu}{\sigma}\right)^2} = 1,$$

as it must in order to be a probability distribution, whatever the values of μ
(the mean) and σ (the standard deviation) happen to be.

It is sufficient to prove this for $\sigma = 1$. But (in a very old trick) the square of
$\int_{-\infty}^{\infty} e^{-x^2/2}dx$ is

$$\int_{-\infty}^{\infty} e^{-x^2/2}dx \int_{-\infty}^{\infty} e^{-y^2/2}dy = \int\int_{\mathbf{R}^2} e^{-(x^2+y^2)/2}dxdy = \int\int_{\mathbf{R}^2} e^{-r^2/2}r\,dr\,d\theta$$

$$= \int_0^{2\pi} d\theta \int_0^{\infty} e^{-r^2/2}r\,dr = 2\pi\left[e^{-r^2/2}\right]_0^{\infty} = 2\pi,$$

as was to be shown. This is also where the π in Stirling's Formula comes from.
The key to the mathematical cleverness here is that by writing down two copies
of the same integral we get to shift from Cartesian to polar coordinates (the
second equals sign).

Now that we have the exact formula (2.16) for the behavior of our quincunx "in
the limit of indefinitely many rows," we can compute exactly what fraction of
this probability lies above any subinterval of the range it covers that we care to
specify, by numerical integration of the formula (2.16). For instance, the total

probability between -1 and 1 is $\frac{1}{\sqrt{2\pi}} \int_{-1}^{1} e^{-x^2/2} dx \approx 0.68$; between -2 and 2, about 0.95; between -3 and 3, about 0.997.

We thereby come to a much deeper understanding of that precision of the average fraction of Heads over n coins. At the outset of this chapter, just by summing squares, we found it to improve as the square root of sample size. We have now learned that the distribution of that variation approaches one specific distribution, having a remarkably simple formula that involves the two main constants of applied mathematics (e and π), and so might have broader relevance than mere games of chance. We will see in just a moment that this same distribution arises in a wholly different context, the physics of gases. What ties them together is the notion of *randomness*, not any properties of coins.

2.3.5 Milestone 5: Other Origins of the Gaussian Distribution

This is the **fifth and final milestone** in this section's line of argument. As Galton had already sensed (see the epigraph at the head of this section), the same standard Gaussian distribution that arises from the human activity of coin flipping, which is a social process, or biparental inheritance, which is a biological process, was already woven into the logic of the universe via its relevance to the information-theoretic properties of physical disorder and the corresponding quantification, which is entropy. Of the many different origins of this same distribution (see, for instance, Rao, 1973, section 3a.1, or Hogben, 1957, chapter 7). I have selected two of particular relevance for our focus on biometrics and morphometrics. One is the argument from real statistical systems like gases or Brownian motion that produce disorder explicitly by mixing, and the other is the argument from what ultimately became information theory that the Gaussian distribution is unique in permitting no further disordering by any mechanism at all.

First: the kinematics of gases. This derivation is the older of the two here – its logic had already arrived at its present form in the hands of the British physicist James Clerk Maxwell in the 1850s.

We are going to make two assumptions, axioms really, that seem entirely verbal and hence wholly removed from any kind of mathematical argument. They apply to uniform gases (i.e., all the same molecule, separated by empty space and hence moving independently[9]) that are well mixed in containers

---

[9] Perrin (1923) notes that exactly the same equations apply to any uniform suspension in a liquid of uniform entities that can be much, much larger than molecules, and that it applies even when the particles (which he calls "inclusions") are bound to the surface of a sphere or a microscope's cover slide rather than being free to diffuse in all three spatial dimensions.

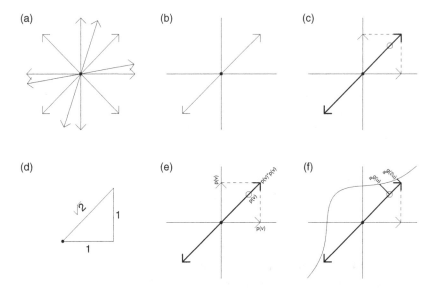

Figure 2.18 Maxwell's derivation of what is now called the Maxwell-Boltzmann distribution for speeds of gas molecules. (a) The axioms: speed distribution in all directions are the same, and speeds in perpendicular directions are independent. (b) A molecule speeding toward the northeast (or southwest). (c) Decomposition into velocity components upward and eastward. (d) The corresponding isosceles right triangle. (e) From the axioms, the probability of a speed along the diagonal must be the square of the probability of a speed along either side. (f) The Gaussian distribution is easily deduced from the equation linking the two quantities $p(v)$ and $p(v\sqrt{2})$ of panel (e). After Bookstein (2015d).

so small that the effects of gravity can be ignored. Here are the axioms (Figure 2.18, panel (a)):

- The distribution of speeds of gas molecules is the same in every direction.
- The speed of a gas molecule in any direction is independent of its speed in any perpendicular direction.

Then it follows, somewhat to our astonishment, that the distribution of the speed of all those molecules in any prespecified direction (e.g., north–south) can have only one possible form, our familiar bell curve. Such a proposition initially sounds as if it could not possibly be true – not enough has been assumed, surely, for anything at all to follow? – and, even if its truth be suspected, surely it should not be easy to prove. But it is actually quite easy to demonstrate in a remarkably elementary mathematical language that was already accessible to the lay readers of Maxwell's own time. (See the historical discussion in Strevens, *Tychomancy*, 2013. The demonstration here is a version of one conveyed in a figure within my review of that book [Bookstein, 2014a].)

Consider [panel (b)] the speed of some gas molecule that is heading in the direction that looks like "northeast" on the page. To be proceeding in the northeasterly direction, our particle must be speeding at the same rate in both of the cardinal directions, north and east [panel (c)]. Under the assumption that the distribution of speeds is the same in every direction, the rate this molecule is going in each of those two directions is related to the rate it is heading northeasterly by a factor of $1/\sqrt{2}$, as in panel (d). North–south and east–west are perpendicular, so by our second axiom these probabilities multiply. If you write v for the speed in the northerly or easterly direction, and if $p(v)$ is the probability of a particle having that speed, then $p(v\sqrt{2}) = p(v) \times p(v) = (p(v))^2$, panel (e).

Now only a little algebra stands between us and our goal. Define a new variable $u = v^2$, so that the probability $p(v)$ can be written $f(u)$. From $p(v\sqrt{2}) = p(v) \times p(v) = (p(v))^2$ we get $f(2u) = f(u)^2$. Let's write $f(u) = be^{g(u)}$ for some function g; then $g(2u) = 2g(u) - \log b$, so g has to be a linear function (we saw this same trick in Gauss's proof that if averages are maximum-likelihood the data have to have been Gaussianly distributed), and hence probability has to go as $be^{-ku} = be^{-kv^2}$, where b and k are constants (regarding which we happen to know that $b = \sqrt{k}/\sqrt{\pi}$).

But that is just the formula for a bell curve, as I have redrawn it in situ, along the northeast–southwest diagonal in panel (f). The identical curve could have been drawn along any other line through the center, but that would have cluttered up panel (a).

Second: the direct maximization of disorder. (This subsection can be skipped on a first reading.) The derivation that follows is younger than Maxwell's by about a hundred years. Although it was first guessed (in another form) in the work of Einstein during his *annus mirabilis* of 1905 (the same year that he developed the theory of the photoelectric effect whose confirmation by Milliken I mentioned a few sections earlier), it could not be formalized until the tie between entropy and information was made explicit in the papers of Claude Shannon, an American, in the 1940s. The formal proof that the Gaussian distribution is the most disorderly possible – that it maximizes the expected information content of each observation over the class of distributions with an assigned mean and variance – is terse. In fact, C. R. Rao (1973) boils it down to a proof so short that it fits in a footnote of my treatise of 2014. But an intuitive approach requires more space. Here is a development based on suggestions from the excellent posthumous course notes of the physicist E. T. Jaynes (2003).

We want to imagine any particular Gaussian distribution as a time-slice of a whole sequence of distributions that began at a single point, which we may as well set at time zero, and that thereafter evolved by an additive noise process that steadily injects uncorrelated variance at a constant rate at every point, moment by moment. The variance of the resulting distribution would have to be proportional to the time t; the question is whether it must take on the Gaussian form (or indeed any particular form).

At any given moment the situation looks like that in Figure 2.19. The evolving distribution has some form (drawn as a Gaussian, as that is what it will in fact be), and at every point we throw in some new Gaussian noise of very small variance (the tiny bell curves drawn over each point of the big one). By remembering what we just learned from the quincunx, about how Gaussian processes are generated by coin flips, we can model each of those little bell curves, in turn, as the sum of a sufficiently large number of even smaller processes that look like tiny coin flips. As in Figure 2.20, these would have the effect of "swapping" probability between any point of this distribution and one of its two nearest neighbors a distance h away. If the magnitude of one of these basic coin flips is written as h, the effect of a Head will be to increase the frequency at this central point by a quantity we can tentatively write as $f_- - f$ —

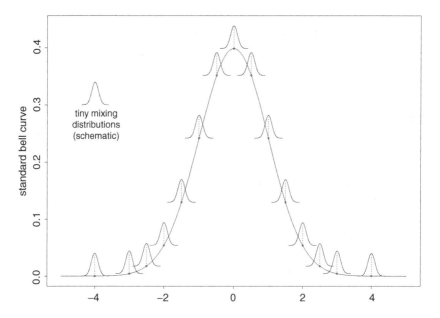

Figure 2.19 Model for instantaneous injection of noise at every moment into an existing distribution.

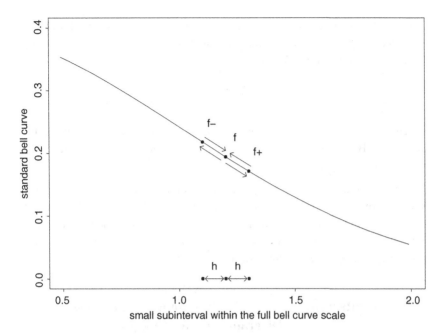

Figure 2.20 The net effect of "coin flips" at small spacings $\pm h$ along such a distribution approximates the quantity $\frac{h^2}{2}\partial^2 f/\partial x^2$, second derivative of this distribution at any particular time t. This must be equal to h^2 times the rate of change $\frac{\partial f}{\partial t}$ of the probability density at the same point as a function of time.

the difference between the gain from just left of the central point when a Head is flipped and the loss when a Tail is flipped. Likewise there is a contribution something like $f_+ - f$ from just to the right of the center point, positive if a Tail is flipped, negative for a Head. We must multiply each of these terms by $\frac{1}{2}$, however, as there is only a 50:50 chance of changing in the specified direction (a Head, if you're coming from below; a Tail, if from above). So the net expected change of the value of this distribution over this short period of time is $\frac{1}{2}((f_+ - f) + (f_- - f))$. This is a simple approximation to $\frac{h^2}{2}\partial^2 f/\partial x^2$, the second derivative of the density we are examining. But this change must lead to the value at the corresponding point in the next time interval, which is a value at a slightly larger setting of the time scale t; hence the same expected change must also equal $h^2 \frac{\partial f}{\partial t}$.

Putting this all together, we arrive at a famous equation (famous, at least, to physicists, who call it the *diffusion equation*):

$$\frac{\partial f}{\partial t} = \frac{1}{2}\frac{\partial^2 f}{\partial x^2}. \tag{2.17}$$

It is a matter of a few minutes' careful evaluation of the derivatives of products and functional transforms to confirm that this equation is satisfied by any function proportional to

$$\frac{1}{\sqrt{t}} e^{-x^2/2t},$$

which is the standard bell curve of variance t, up to the usual prefactor of $\frac{1}{\sqrt{2\pi}}$. (Both sides of the partial differential equation evaluate to $-\frac{1}{2} e^{-x^2/2t}(x^2 + t^2)t^{-5/2}$.)

In words, this means that any mixing that you inject into a Gaussian distribution increases its variance but otherwise leaves its shape alone. You cannot make it any more disorderly than it already is – it is already the most disorganized possible distribution (which is why it applies so well to gas molecules, which so thoroughly mix themselves up microsecond by microsecond).

2.3.6 "Regression to the Mean": Geometry of Regression as Diagrammed via an Ellipse

Section 2.3.5 concludes our mathematical exegesis of the formula for the bell curve, but not the geometrical formulary most pertinent to its applications. To revert to this domain, we return to Galton's ideas about the generation of *related* Gaussian scores.

Suppose x is a Gaussian variable of mean 0 and variance 1, and y is another such, independent of it. (For instance, generate twice as many samples of a standard bell curve as you need, all uncorrelated and with the same mean and variance, and then let x be the first half of the run and y the second.) Incidentally, generating samples of independent Gaussians is something we do very well because we are so good at generating uniform samples in an interval: look up the "Box-Muller method" on the Web.

We're going to be looking at patterned pairs of additive combinations of x and y, pairs like $2x + y$ and $2x - y$, because this is a good way of generating correlated Gaussian variables that have the same variance. You can think about this as a "linear model" with "predicted value" $2x$ and "error" y, but you don't have to – what is going on in regression is algebra and geometry, not science, and you don't need any of these words about models, prediction, or noise.

First, the algebra. Consider the linear composites $ax + y$ and $ax - y$ where a is some coefficient and x and y are independent and each of mean zero and variance 1. We have mean($ax \pm y$) $= 0$, var($ax \pm y$) $= a^2 + 1$ (from the Pythagorean theorem for variances), cov($ax + y, ax - y$) $= a^2 - 1$, and so the regression slope of $ax \pm y$ on $ax \mp y$ is

$$v = \frac{\text{cov}(ax \pm y, ax \mp y)}{\text{var}(ax \mp y)} = \frac{a^2 - 1}{a^2 + 1}, \qquad (2.18)$$

and (because predictor and predictand have the same variance) the correlation (to be introduced in the next section) is this same value. For $a = \sqrt{3}$, this slope is exactly $\frac{1}{2}$, a coincidence that makes the figures to follow just a little more elegant than they would otherwise be.

Draw this as a sample in the left panel of Figure 2.21. (It looks just like Pearson's actual mother-daughter data, coming in Figure 2.28.)

As the figure hints, the operation that went from the variables (x, y) to the variables $(ax + y, ax - y)$ distorted the original circle into an ellipse of axis lengths a (along the horizontal) and 1 and then rotated the ellipse from long axis horizontal to long axis at $45°$ to the horizontal. The left panel shows this scatter along with both of its regression lines, vertical on horizontal or vice versa. The symmetry is remarkable. It can be made even more obvious if one prints the entire figure twice in the same place, once as is and once after reflection in the line $x = y$ (the diagonal of the plot at right). I have also added a curve for the elliptical shape into which a circle is taken by the original transformation (original x multiplied by a, the result then rotated $45°$). With these enhancements you can see immediately that the two regression lines

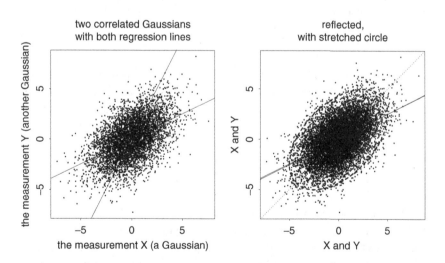

Figure 2.21 Scatterplots generated as bivariate Gaussians of the same variance look like ellipses with diagonals at $45°$. (left) A sample of points from a bivariate Gaussian distribution with means zero, variances 4, and $r = \frac{1}{2}$. Both regression lines are drawn. (right). The same figure superimposed over its reflection across the major diagonal $x = y$ (dashed line), with a concentration ellipse. After the reflection, the two regression lines appear identical.

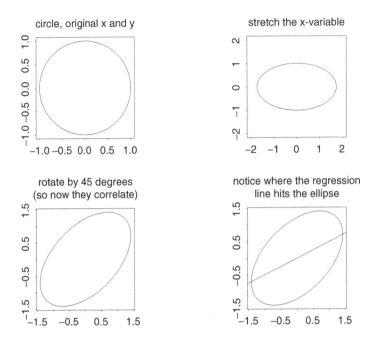

Figure 2.22 The same, without the dots. (upper left) A circle, indicating a bivariate sample of uncorrelated Gaussians of the same unit variance. (upper right) The horizontal variance a^2 is stretched by a factor of 3. (lower left) Rotation by $45°$. (lower right) The regression line, of slope $\frac{a^2-1}{a^2+1} = \frac{1}{2}$, intercepts this ellipse where the tangent is vertical.

are now absolutely indistinguishable – they print atop the same pixels along nearly their entire length. We don't really need the simulated data any more to drive this plot; we can proceed using only its algebra, using any one of those concentric elliptical curves. The construction goes as in Figure 2.22.

And now one might notice something remarkable (which is one of the ways that one generates the conjectures that become theorems: see Pólya, 1954): the regression line cuts the ellipse just where the tangent to the ellipse seems to be vertical.

This was a special value of the regression slope, $\frac{1}{2}$. Perhaps it was that particular value that engendered some special symmetry like the one we just noted. Let's try some other values of a, then (Figure 2.23). The place where the regression line hits the ellipse has vertical tangent in *all* these examples, even the bare circle (the example with $a = 1$, upper left). The figures also show the other regression, x on y, in each frame; these lines all hit the ellipse in the mirror-image loci with tangent lines horizontal (the mirror would be along the diagonal in all frames).

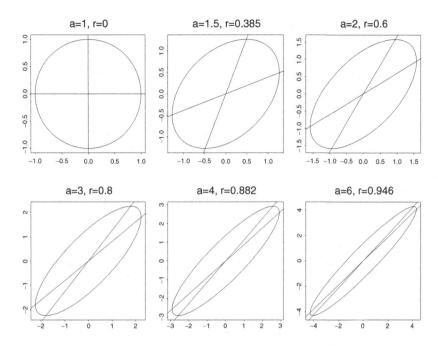

Figure 2.23 The same for six more values of a (and thus six more correlations).
In all panels, the regression lines intersect the ellipse at the loci of vertical or
horizontal tangents.

So it *always* seems to be the case that a regression line for any Gaussian
bivariate distribution cuts an ellipse of constant probability density for that
same distribution at the location where the ellipse's tangents are vertical (and
the regression in the other direction, where they are horizontal). Notice, too,
that the direction of the regression line seems to be the same as the direction
of the tangent to the ellipse at the points directly above and below its center.
This is one geometric expression of the *conjugacy* of these two directions,
that of the regression line and that of the vertical on the page: when either is
drawn through the center of the ellipse, the tangents at the points of intersection
between line and curve are parallel to the *other* direction. We will encounter
another example of this conjugacy when we discuss relative eigenanalysis in
Section 4.3.

Galton noticed this around 1875, and got a colleague to prove it in 1877. (It
only takes a mathematician a few minutes, but Galton was no mathematician.)
Figure 2.24 is a demonstration that I find particularly accessible. The locus of
tangent vertical *after* the 45° rotation of the stretched ellipse is the locus of a

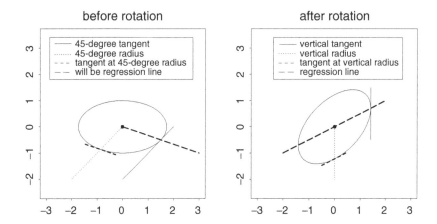

Figure 2.24 Proof of the property demonstrated in Figure 2.23, by explicit computation of the slope $-1/a^2$ of the corresponding line before the 45° rotation, and also for the claim of conjugacy (see text).

tangent line at 45° to the horizontal *before* we rotated that stretched ellipse. Now back to high-school analytic geometry: the equation of this stretched ellipse is $x^2/a^2 + y^2 = c$, where the value of c doesn't matter. So the tangent direction dy/dx must satisfy the equation $2x\,dx/a^2 + 2y\,dy = 0$. Rearranging, we have $dy/dx = -x/ya^2$. If this is the direction $(1,1)$, we have to have $\frac{y}{x} = -\frac{1}{a^2}$. Rotating by the 45° we actually used rotates this direction from $(a^2, -1)$ to $(a^2 - 1, a^2 + 1)$ – but this **is** the computed regression slope. So we have just confirmed what Galton noticed: the regression line goes through the point where the tangent to the ellipse of constant concentration is vertical. As for the claim of conjugacy, the same equation $2x\,dx/a^2 + 2y\,dy = 0$ can be read in the opposite direction: if we require $x/y = 1$, the 45° line before rotation, we must have $dy/dx = -1/a^2$. This *tangent* at the intercept with the 45° line must be parallel to the *diameter* through the point with tangent line at 45° to the horizontal. But after rotation, the first of these is the tangent at the intercept with the vertical axis, and the second is the regression line; so they must be in the same direction, too.

It follows, then, that you can approximate regression lines for Gaussian scatters by hand, just by connecting the pair of points either side of the centroid where the isolines of the distribution appear to run vertically. This can apply as well to cross-tabulated approximations, as we already saw in Galton's earliest example: the regression still runs through the two locations where your approximating curve, adequately smoothed, appears to be running vertically.

This locus, the vertical tangent, is always below the diagonal of the ellipse: hence "regression to [meaning: toward] the mean." But it is also "below" that diagonal when we reflect the whole picture, *including that regression line*, in the main diagonal: so whether we regress x on y or y on x, there is a "regression towards the mean."

In other words, *whenever* a regression is linear in this way, predicted values are less extreme than their predictors. Back in Figure 2.17, the figure where Galton first intuited the relevance of the ellipse we have been speaking of, one can convert this same phenomenon into words as follows. From the table, we see that the parents of the taller children are typically not as tall as their children, but also the children of the taller parents are not as tall as their parents. In an example published some years later, Pearson's analysis of families from which the data of Figure 2.28 were adapted, tall mothers have daughters averaging shorter than their mothers, and at the same time, tall daughters have mothers averaging shorter than their daughters. Either way, this comes from the geometry of ellipses, and has nothing whatever to do with causation. Rather, it is a necessary consequence of the arithmetic by which we have implemented the computation of a prediction in this context of bivariate Gaussian noise – which is, as we have seen, not a causal concept at all. On average, predicted values in linear systems like these are closer to the mean than the predictors regardless of whether prediction goes in the direction of causation or in the opposite direction. Galton actually discovered this in the course of an even older study, the inheritance of "eminence" (Galton, 1869). For a sample of "eminent" Victorian gentlemen, the fractions of eminent fathers and eminent sons were about the same (roughly 50%), the fractions of eminent grandfathers, grandsons, and uncles about the same at 25%, and so on. This phenomenon affects the findings of predictive analyses whenever a group has been assembled based on its extremeness on some indicator. For a famous example in the context of American social research, see Donald Campbell's discussion of the "Connecticut crackdown on speeding," Campbell and Ross (1968) or Campbell and Stanley (1963), or consult the discussion of this example in Section L4.6 of Bookstein (2014).

Summary of Section 2.3

- Milestone 1. As the count of coins being flipped increases, the probability distribution of the count of heads as a deviation from its maximum, appropriately scaled, tends to one common pattern. This is the familiar Gaussian distribution or bell curve, the logarithm of which is just a downward-pointing parabola.

- Milestone 2. Bell curves can be produced physically by Francis Galton's clever device, the quincunx, which simulates the flips of arbitrarily many coins arbitrarily many times.
- Milestone 3. "Regression" on the quincunx – the tracing of any particular outcome state at the bottom of the instrument upward to its likeliest location at any intermediate level – is linear. Thus the quincunx provides us with an unusually simple example of the emergence of a linear equation in the absence of any formal physical law, just as a result of random chance when constrained by a very clever experimental setting.
- Milestone 4. Leaving behind this context of coin flips and counting, we can convert the equation of the bell curve with mean μ and variance σ^2 into the celebrated formula $\frac{1}{\sqrt{2\pi}\sigma}e^{-\frac{(x-\mu)^2}{2\sigma^2}}$ that was already introduced in Section 2.1.
- Milestone 5. There are several other randomizing physical systems that produce bell curves, of which two of the most important are the Maxwell-Boltzmann distribution of the velocities of gas molecules and Einstein's law of diffusion.
- When a bivariate scatter is represented by any ellipse of constant probability, the regression line cuts the ellipse at the two loci with tangent line vertical. When variances are the same, the two regression lines are mirror-images with respect to the diagonal of the ellipse. That the standardized regression prediction is thus always less than the standardized value doing the predicting is the phenomenon usually called *regression to the mean*.

2.4 Correlation

2.4.1 Galton's Other Insight

The quincunx that concerned us in Section 2.3.2 was getting wider and wider (counts of Heads minus Tails more and more variable) with every row. This hardly ever matches real phenomena in the world of natural science. To circumvent this inconvenience, divide each bin index, x or y, by the standard deviation of the distribution of Heads-minus-Tails in its row, $\sqrt{l}$ or $\sqrt{k}$, respectively, and call these *standard scores*. The "standard score" z_y of y, in the kth row, is $y/\sqrt{k}$, and the "standard score" of x, in the lth row, is $x/\sqrt{l}$, and now every row has the same variance of 1 as well as an unvarying mean of 0. See Figure 2.25, which also copies in the two lines from Figure 2.12, one for regression and one for causation. The phenomenon of "regression to the mean" (Section 2.3.6) is even clearer in this geometry inasmuch as now both

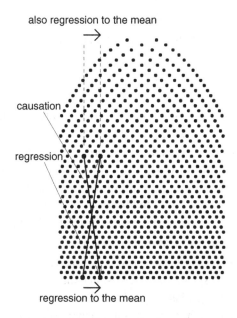

also regression to the mean

causation

regression

regression to the mean

horizontal is now normalized to constant variance

Figure 2.25 Revised version of Galton's quincunx standardizing for the variance of the rows. Lines labeled "causation" and "regression" are as in Figure 2.12. In this new coordinate system they are mirror-images of one another in a vertical axis. Each one falls by the same ratio (here, about 30%) of its original distance from the axis of symmetry, a ratio that is one minus the square root of the ratio of row values involved. That squared ratio is r, the correlation (here, 0.5) of the values in the two indicated rows.

prediction lines, that for the fall down the quincunx and that for the inverse inference upward, are tipped equally toward the midline of the diagram.

Now the equivalence of the two regression lines is geometrically obvious: they have the same slope with respect to the x-axis for the two different orientations (upward or downward) of the y-axis. The linear least-squares prediction of x from y was $x \sim \frac{l}{k}y$, so the prediction of z_x is

$$z_x = x/\sqrt{l} \sim \frac{\frac{l}{k}y}{\sqrt{l}} = \frac{\frac{l}{k}(z_y\sqrt{k})}{\sqrt{l}} = \sqrt{\frac{l}{k}}\, z_y.$$

And the prediction of y from x was $y \sim x$, so the prediction of z_y is

$$z_y = y/\sqrt{k} \sim \frac{x}{\sqrt{k}} = \frac{z_x\sqrt{l}}{\sqrt{k}} = \sqrt{\frac{l}{k}}\, z_x,$$

which is exactly the same formula but with x and y interchanged. In terms of the crossproduct formula (2.8) the computed slope is now

$$\Sigma z_x z_y / \Sigma z_x^2 = \Sigma z_x z_y = \Sigma (x/\sqrt{\Sigma x^2})(y/\sqrt{\Sigma y^2}) = \frac{\Sigma xy}{\sqrt{\Sigma x^2 \Sigma y^2}} \equiv r_{xy}, \quad (2.19)$$

where now the symmetry between x and y is obvious. (The symbol $\equiv$ means either "is a definition of" or "is defined as.")

For the remainder of this section, I will drop the z-sub- notation. What had been z_x is now written just x, and similarly y. With this change, we have *standardized* for the (increasing) variance of the position of the lead shot as we go down the quincunx. Now the prediction of cause by effect (x by y) and the prediction of effect by cause (y by x) have the same slope: $x \sim ry$ or $y \sim rx$, with $r = \sqrt{\frac{l}{k}}$, the **correlation** between position in the kth row of the quincunx and position in the lth row above it. In other words, a correlation is just a regression between standardized scores, in either direction. *That* is why correlation tells you nothing whatsoever about cause. In Figure 2.28 the slopes for the two regressions, mother's height on daughter's and daughter's height on mother's, are nearly the same because their variances are nearly the same. So each of those slopes was very nearly a correlation already, and we have already verified that indeed, by virtue of this symmetry, the relationship tells us nothing at all about causes.

The probability of either standardized observation is distributed about this predicted value with variance $1 - \frac{l}{k}$, the famous "$1 - r^2$" of *unexplained variance*. The complementary fraction r^2 of variance is what is "explained," namely the variance of the standardized prediction $y \sim rx$ or $x \sim ry$. Because the predicted part and the residual part are uncorrelated, their variances must add to 1, the variance of either standardized variable, and so the variance of the residual must be $1 - r^2$, the difference of the variances of y and rx after the standardization. Why are they uncorrelated? This is an algebraic check: if x and y are both centered of variance 1, then the covariance of y, say, with $x - ry$ for $r = \Sigma xy / N$ is $\text{cov}(x, y) - r \text{var}(y) = r - r = 0$. Before we standardized, one regression coefficient was $\frac{l}{k}$ and the other simply 1. The product of these two coefficients is $\frac{l}{k}$, and $r^2 = \beta_{y.x}\beta_{x.y}$ – the correlation coefficient r is the square root of the product of the regression coefficients in the two directions – whether variables were standardized or not.

We sum all this up in another cross-reference-able equation:

$$1 - r^2 = \text{var}(y - \beta_{y.x}x)/\text{var}(y) = \text{var}(x - \beta_{x.y}y)/\text{var}(x), \quad r^2 = \beta_{y.x}\beta_{x.y}. \quad (2.20)$$

Yet the words "explained" and "unexplained" here are remarkably misleading, because the variable x finds itself "explained" to exactly the same extent as y, regardless of any actual scientific understanding achieved. Evidently explanation here is not in the sense of scientific explanation, but instead in some weaker sense beholden more to the numbers than to the phenomena. It is the *relation* between x and y that is explained in the context of this particularly powerful stochastic model, the quincunx. There are some settings, notably the agricultural experiments in which this terminology originated, within which the two uses of the word "explanation" are reasonably consistent; but the formulation for correlations and "explained" variance apply regardless of whether that phrase makes any scientific sense. We will delve much more deeply into the connection between line-fitting and explanation when we discuss *multiple regression,* regression on more than one predictor, in Section 3.1.

This second version of the quincunx, the one with the rows normalized, shows "the paradox of regression to the mean" quite clearly. Extreme causes produce, on the average, less extreme effects; but also, extreme effects are produced, on the average, by less extreme causes. As the figure makes clear, the slopes are in fact the same: the two lines drawn are symmetric with respect to a vertical line (not drawn) that runs between them through their point of intersection. It was this same paradox that first started Galton puzzling over the tie between causation and bell curves, when he noticed that the parents of tall children, though tall on average, were nevertheless not as tall on average as those tall children; and yet the children of tall parents, while tall on average, were likewise on average not as tall as those tall parents. The "paradox" arises because the standardized regression coefficients r are identical, not reciprocal, for prediction in the two temporal directions. For standardized variables, or indeed any pair of variables having the same variance, this shared regression slope must lie between -1 and 1.

2.4.2 Example 2.3: Pearson's Study of Limb Lengths: Every Family Member, Every Limb

Examples 1 and 2 in Section 2.2.3 dealt with quite highly correlated pairs of variables. A historically important example dating from the earliest years of biometrics instead dealt with data for which the prediction error was a large fraction of the actual numerical signal, and so helps us reconstruct the bioscientific context in which these methods were first disseminated for practical use. The following material is adapted from Pearson and Lee, 1903, a paper that, because of the prominence of the journal in which it appeared, is available from the web via the scholarly journal archive JSTOR in spite of being from the turn of the previous century.

In this paper, Karl Pearson, the follower of Francis Galton and the single greatest innovator in the history of biometrics, set to generalizing the phenomena that Galton had noticed in fragmentary data sets from the 1870s like the one in Figure 2.17. (Following Galton's lead in the study *Hereditary Genius* of 1869, this methodology would also be extended to the domain of "psychic characteristics" – see the nearly contemporanous publication [Pearson, 1903] purporting to analyze some personality data by the same methods.) Pearson set about to systematically gather a sample of *families* – mother, father, and at least two offspring – and carry out the same fundamental anthropometric measurements on both generations, to see if indeed the apparent agreement between parent–child statistics and sibling–sibling statistics could be more rigorously demonstrated than Galton had done a quarter-century earlier. From the "data card" reproduced in my Figure 2.26 we can see the full structure of the data set: three length measurements, each to the nearest quarter-inch, for mother, father, and up to four adult offspring. Pearson reports *all* of the bivariate analyses that are possible given this sampling design.

The scatterplot not yet having been invented, Pearson published his raw tabulations as just that – tables. Figure 2.27 reproduces a typical one of these, Pearson's table 31 of mother's height by daughter's height in one-inch bins. The fractions are for measures reported in whole-number inches, which had to be split between two or four bins. Note that daughter's height runs vertically downward instead of upward as in the current convention.

Following a suggestion of Sanford Weisberg, who calls this data set to the reader's attention in his regression textbook of 2005, we "jitter" the data for visibility and then present the regression lines and the class means in the same plot. For my own pedagogic purposes, Figure 2.28 extends that diagram to show the regression in both directions, not just the direction of biological inheritance.

I present the class means here because Pearson had already done so in 1903. To interpret this remarkable arithmetical pattern, Pearson had to intuit what is perhaps the single most salient contingency in the entire domain of regression analysis as we see it today: the requirement that the class means computed using subsets of the data conform, up to sampling variation, with the regression line computed using all the data. The implication is obvious in one direction – if the Gaussian regression prediction applies to the data set as a whole, it must also apply subset by subset – but in fact the reverse implication is true as well. This is a theorem that Pearson guessed but that was not formally proven for about fifty years more (the earliest proof I can find in the literature is Fix, 1949). We see Pearson's care for this concern in a lengthy range of plots pair by pair of measures similar to the two in Figure 2.29 for diverse choices of measure and parent-child or sibling-sibling pairs.

Sample of filled in Data Card of Family Measurements.

One Family only		Height*		Span of Arms		Left Forearm	
		Feet	Inches	Feet	Inches	Feet	Inches
Father... ... ... (Not step-father)		5	9¼	6	1½	1	7¼
Mother ... ... (Not step-mother)		5	0¾	5	2	1	4¼
	Age						
Son ...	26	5	7¼	5	11	1	6½
Son ...	—	—	—	—	...	...	—
Daughter	30	5	4¼	5	5	1	4½
Daughter	24	5	5¼	5	6¼	1	5

Name and Address of Recorder (not to be published in any way, but for convenience of reference).

Miss A. L. Robinson,

Blounts Court Mansions, Kensington, S.W.

....

Both father and mother are absolutely necessary and should not be over 65 years of age.

All the measures are to be recorded to the nearest quarter of an inch. Before measuring read the notice circulated with this card, and kindly return the card as soon as possible to

[Name of individual collector was here inserted]

or to Professor Karl Pearson, University College, London, W.C.

* Put B against numbers if measure is taken in boots. If any person measured has ever broken a leg, arm or collar-bone, put L, A, C against all his or her measurements.

Figure 2.26 Data card format for the Pearson-Lee (1903) study of anthropometrics of family members.

TABLE XXXI.

Mother's Stature and Daughter's Stature.

Mother's Stature.

Daughter's Stature.	52–53	53–54	54–55	55–56	56–57	57–58	58–59	59–60	60–61	61–62	62–63	63–64	64–65	65–66	66–67	67–68	68–69	69–70	70–71	Totals
52–53	—	—	—	—	—	—	—	·5	—	—	—	—	—	—	—	—	—	—	—	·5
53–54	—	—	—	—	—	—	—	·5	—	—	—	—	—	—	—	—	—	—	—	·5
54–55	—	—	—	—	—	—	1	—	—	—	—	—	—	—	—	—	—	—	—	1
55–56	—	—	—	—	—	1	—	—	—	—	—	—	—	—	—	—	—	—	—	1
56–57	—	—	—	—	—	1	·25	1·5	1·25	·25	·25	—	—	—	—	—	—	—	—	4·5
57–58	—	—	—	—	1·5	1·25	1·5	1·25	1·5	3·25	1·25	1·25	·75	1	—	—	—	—	—	14·5
58–59	—	—	—	—	·5	2·25	1·5	2·25	4·75	2·5	·25	·5	·25	·75	—	—	—	—	—	15·5
59–60	—	—	—	—	—	3·5	5·75	12	11·25	9·25	3	1·5	·75	·25	1·25	—	—	—	—	48·5
60–61	·25	·25	—	—	2·75	4·75	9·25	15	19·5	15·75	17	7·75	3·25	1·75	1·5	·25	1	—	—	100
61–62	·25	·25	·25	·25	·75	2	8	18·5	18·25	34	27·25	15	8·75	6	3·25	·25	—	—	—	143
62–63	·5	—	·25	·25	·25	4	11·5	19·75	33·25	34·75	34·75	24	12·75	10·25	2·75	1	·5	—	—	190·5
63–64	·5	—	—	—	·75	3·75	6·25	17·5	29	41·5	46·5	33·5	18·25	10·25	3·75	·5	·5	—	—	212·5
64–65	—	—	—	—	—	2·5	4	6·25	23·75	32	38·5	40	27·75	18·75	3·5	1·5	·5	—	—	199
65–66	—	—	—	—	—	—	·25	1	5·75	10·5	18	27·5	35	26	16·5	12·25	3·25	·5	—	156·5
66–67	—	—	—	—	—	·25	1·25	3·25	10·25	14·75	23	29·25	21·75	16·25	15·75	2·75	2	·5	·5	141·5
67–68	—	—	—	—	—	—	—	1·5	5·5	7·75	7·75	15	14·25	11·25	8·25	5	1·25	·5	1	79
68–69	—	—	—	—	—	—	—	—	—	—	·5	1·5	6·5	5·75	5·75	4·75	3·25	1	1	35
69–70	—	—	—	—	—	—	—	—	—	—	—	1	2·5	5·25	3·25	3·25	1·5	·75	1	18·5
70–71	—	—	—	—	—	—	—	—	—	—	—	·5	1	1	1·25	1·25	2	1	1·5	9·5
71–72	—	—	—	—	—	—	—	—	—	—	—	—	—	·5	·75	·75	·5	·5	1	4
72–73	—	—	—	—	—	—	—	—	—	—	—	—	—	—	—	—	—	—	—	—
73–74	—	—	—	—	—	—	—	—	—	—	1	—	—	—	—	—	—	—	—	1
Totals	1·5	·5	·5	2·5	8	24	51·5	108·5	168·5	212	235	213·5	145·5	101·5	61·5	22·5	9	5	4	1375

Figure 2.27 Data on stature for 1375 mother-daughter pairs, from Pearson and Lee (1903). The apparent margin of the nonzero table entries here and in Figure 2.17 appears to be adequately summarized as an ellipse.

This degree of discipline, implicit in the prophylaxis of "regression diagnostics" that we teach our students of statistics and biostatistics today, would be admirable in *any* research project here in the twenty-first century. All the more remarkable, then, that these examples are more than 110 years old.

From the resulting large collection of analyses, all mutually consistent, Pearson compiled a useful summary table that I reproduce in Figure 2.30. (The standard errors reported here do not appear to be consistent with his formula from 1898 that I will derive in Section 4.1; the assistant seems to have counted all family members, not family units.)

And indeed his computations provide an excellent example, probably the first one ever published, for the systematic inspection of a multivariate data set of morphometric lengths. (The example of Sewall Wright's in the next section, for instance, is 20 years younger.) Pearson checked that all these regressions are adequately linear, so that all the pairwise distributions can be seen as Gaussian, just the finding that his mentor Francis Galton had guessed. (In fact, to get a little ahead of our story, all it takes is for the principal components to be independent (linearity there is precisely horizontal) – this is what Lukacs's [1956] theorem actually shows.) But Pearson completely missed the deeper meaning of Galton's displays – the Gaussianity is unrelated to causation, much less indicative of the probable success of "breeding," which is to say, intervention.

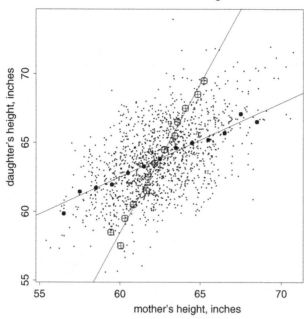

Figure 2.28 A resampling from the table in the preceding figure, with uniform noise of range 1 inch added for visual clarity. Both regression lines are shown and also both sets of class means, in bins at integer spacing, except for the extreme tails of the two directional distributions. Note, as Pearson did, how closely the class means of the more frequently encountered classes approximate the straight-line regressions they are intended to model.

Pearson's own summary. Pearson was fearless in his preaching of scientific method as he construed it. His textbook on this subject, *The Grammar of Science,* went through three editions during his lifetime (1892, 1900, 1911) and is still in print. Just a few years after the publication of the paper I am reviewing here, in a eulogy (Pearson, 1906) on the premature death of his great collaborator W. F. R. Weldon, he wrote:

> Science, no less than theology or philosophy, is the field for personal influence, for the creation of enthusiasm, and for the establishment of ideals of self-discipline and self-development. No man becomes great in science from the mere force of intellect, unguided and unaccompanied by what really amounts to moral force. Behind the intellectual capacity there is the devotion to truth, the deep sympathy with nature, and the determination to sacrifice all minor matters to one great end.

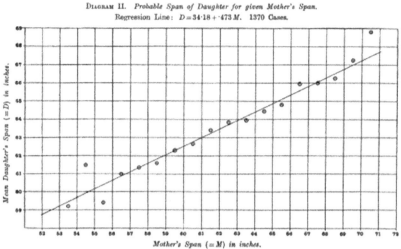

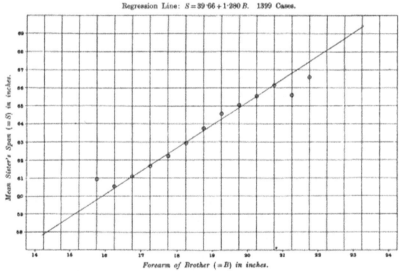

Figure 2.29 Two of Pearson's charts of class means, from Pearson and Lee
(1903), indicating their centrality to his logic of biometrical inference.

What Pearson was referring to here was mainly his own recent work on the
inheritance of both physical characteristics and "civic worth" in Victorian
England. He believed, incorrectly, that the progress he had made in biometrics
of limb lengths bore enormously important implications for the survival of

TABLE IV.

Coefficients of Heredity. Parents and Offspring.

Character	Father and		Mother and	
	Son	Daughter	Son	Daughter
Stature	·514 ± ·015	·510 ± ·013	·494 ± ·016	·507 ± ·014
Span	·454 ± ·016	·454 ± ·014	·457 ± ·016	·452 ± ·015
Forearm	·421 ± ·017	·422 ± ·015	·406 ± ·017	·421 ± ·015

Figure 2.30 Pearson's tabular summary of the central tendency of his computed correlations, which are restricted to a range of only about ±0.05 around 0.46.

British civilization. These misunderstandings of his own work on human heredity are brought into sharp focus in the course of those research papers themselves.

In the case of the document we have just been examining, his paper with Lee (whoever that was) of 1903, Pearson crisply reviews his empirical findings (pages 395–396) but then turns to a peroration, a call to action, that is wholly unjustified by any findings that preceded. Regarding those findings, it is impossible to read Pearson's own words today without profound dismay. Yes, bell curves suffice to describe the distribution of the chief physical characters in man; the regression between pairs of blood relations is linear; the coefficient of parental heredity has a mean value of about .46; fraternal correlation for the physical characters is also close to .5. This is all fair enough; we would say the same of his data today. But then Pearson launches off into an inference that is purely ideological and, in light of the history of Europe through mid-twentieth-century, a hideously embarrassing fragment of testimony by the founder of my field:

> The values of the parental correlations determined for man show that two or three generations of selection would suffice to raise the mean of the offspring to the selected standard. Further with quite reasonable values of the grandparental correlations no regression would take place, and the stock breed true. The result is of extreme importance, for two reasons: (a) It illustrates the absurdity of the prevalent biological conceptions of regression as a constant factor, ... (b) It emphasizes the all-important law that with judicious mating human stock is capable of rapid progress. A few generations suffice to modify a race of men, and the nations which breed freely only from their poorer stocks will not be dominant factors in civilization by the end of the century.

There seems to be no escaping the ferocious historical irony that the great innovator of correlations, the chisquare, maximum-likelihood estimation, and principal components, among other tools – my intellectual grandfather, as it were – was also an uncompromising eugenicist preaching the same explicit racism that would come to be indelibly associated with Nazism during his own lifetime. The dangers of seduction of theory by numerical inference were never more clearly exposed than in this very paper of Pearson's that introduced all of today's best methods for the confirmation of a linear theory in the biometric context. For more discussion of this episode in the history of statistical science, see Bookstein (2014).

2.4.3 Example 2.4: Wright's Chickens: All 15 Pairwise Relationships

Although there are hints in the right direction as early as Karl Pearson (1900), the modern setting of our topic as an important application of applied pattern analysis began a couple of decades later with a famous data analysis of Sewall Wright's dealing with six measurements on 276 leghorn chickens. The measurements are Skull length, Skull breadth, and the lengths of four limb bones (femur, tibia, humerus, and ulna, four of the same six that you have). As Figure 2.31 shows, the six measures all correlate positively among themselves. We already studied one of these fifteen scatterplots in Section 2.2.3.1. There we deleted one specimen because of an outlying value for the length of the humerus; here another outlying case is deleted also, owing to badly typed data for the length of the tibia.

Here are the correlations:

$$\begin{pmatrix} 1.000 & 0.583 & 0.567 & 0.602 & 0.623 & 0.603 \\ 0.583 & 1.000 & 0.515 & 0.550 & 0.590 & 0.525 \\ 0.567 & 0.515 & 1.000 & 0.930 & 0.883 & 0.879 \\ 0.602 & 0.550 & 0.930 & 1.000 & 0.887 & 0.903 \\ 0.623 & 0.590 & 0.883 & 0.887 & 1.000 & 0.945 \\ 0.603 & 0.525 & 0.879 & 0.903 & 0.945 & 1.000 \end{pmatrix} \quad (2.21)$$

The following can be noted:

- All of the pairwise scatterplots look a lot like the prototype in our Pearson study except that most of the ellipses are narrower (i.e., the correlations are higher). It is reasonable to presume that they are all close enough to Gaussians for arguments from regression to apply cogently.

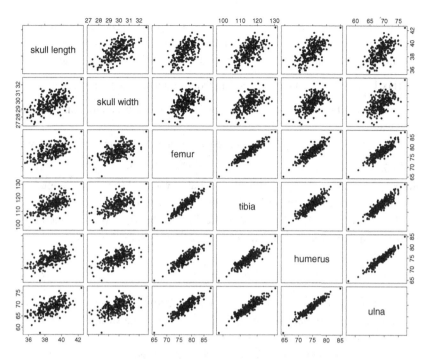

Figure 2.31 A graphical matrix of correlations among all pairs of skeletal measurements for all but two of Sewall Wright's sample of 276 leghorn chickens. Specimen 101 has been disregarded as in Figure 2.7, and also specimen 5, which has a typo for length of tibia.

- Limb measurements correlate more with other measures of the same limb than anything else in this little data set, and they correlate much more with measures of the *other* limb than they do with either measure of the skull. This suggests a nested system of biometrical control: forelimb or hindlimb *within* the general system of the limbs *within* the scaling program of the organism as a whole.

A good deal more can be said about this simple example, which was crucial at the birth of biometrical factor analysis. See the more extended discussion in Wright 1932 or in Chapter 4.

2.4.4 Working Backward from One Single Correlation

We have seen that one single covariance $\sigma_{st} = \Sigma (s - \bar{s})(t - \bar{t})/N$ does not have any obvious scientific meaning. Nevertheless, the normalization $r = \sigma_{st}/\sigma_s \sigma_t$

is often meaningful. So scientific interpretability must inhere somehow in the set of three quantities $\sigma_s, \sigma_t, \sigma_{st}$ taken all at once. In Chapter 4 we will see how this meaning can be expressed in a new formalism, the 2×2 **matrix** $\begin{pmatrix} \sigma_s^2 & \sigma_{st} \\ \sigma_{st} & \sigma_t^2 \end{pmatrix}$, that can be generalized for data sets numbering more than two variables. For now, let us try instead to "run the previous construction backward."

For x and y both independent Gaussians of mean zero and variance 1 we had $\sigma_{ax\pm y}^2 = a^2 + 1$ and $r_{ax\pm y, ax\mp y} = \frac{a^2-1}{a^2+1}$. So **given** data s, t with $\sigma_s, \sigma_t, \sigma_{st}$ all preassigned, how do we get back to suitable x and y? In another language, how do we *standardize* the ordered pairs (s, t) with which we began?

If in the data we were handed it is already true that $\sigma_s = \sigma_t = \sigma$, then it is enough simply to find the a for which $r = \frac{a^2-1}{a^2+1}$. This is for $a^2 r + r = a^2 - 1$ or

$$a^2 = \frac{1+r}{1-r}. \tag{2.22}$$

If $s = ax + y$ and $t = ax - y$, then $y = (s - t)/2$ and $x = (s + t)/2a$. We can check that indeed, under the assumption $\sigma_s = \sigma_t = \sigma$, the variances of x and y are equal and their covariance is 0.

In the preceding text we had characterized the transformation of x and y to s and t as a stretch of x followed by a sum-and-difference operation, but we could just as well think of the sum-and-difference part as a *rotation*. We went from variables y and ax to new variables

$$s = \sqrt{2}(y \cos 45° + (ax) \sin 45°), \quad t = \sqrt{2}(-y \sin 45° + (ax) \cos 45°). \tag{2.23a}$$

Now break the symmetry of that assumption $\sigma_s = \sigma_t$. We proceed by freeing the *angle* in the preceding formulas. Given σ_s, σ_t, and r, we want to compute an angle θ, at present unknown, such that if we compute x and y by "unrotating" – by rotating the two derived measures s and t "backward" by the same (unknown) angle θ – the new variables

$$y = (s \cos(-\theta) + t \sin(-\theta)), \quad ax = (-s \sin(-\theta) + t \cos(-\theta)) \tag{2.23b}$$

now have covariance zero (but, in general, different variances: hence the unknown ratio a of standard deviations in the formula).[10]

But from the requirement of zero covariance we can compute θ explicitly by simple trigonometry. Remember, from high-school math, that $\sin 2\theta = 2 \sin \theta \cos \theta$ and $\cos 2\theta = \cos^2 \theta - \sin^2 \theta$. From equations (2.23), the

---

[10] In Chapter 4 we will see that this amounts to the *orthogonality* property of the principal components.

covariance of y and ax is $\sigma_s^2(\cos\theta\sin\theta) + \sigma_t^2(-\cos\theta\sin\theta) + \sigma_{st}(\cos^2\theta - \sin^2\theta)$. Two times this is $(\sigma_s^2 - \sigma_t^2)\sin 2\theta + 2\sigma_{st}\cos 2\theta$. For this to be zero, we must have

$$\tan 2\theta = \frac{\sin 2\theta}{\cos 2\theta} = -2\frac{\sigma_{st}}{\sigma_s^2 - \sigma_t^2}. \qquad (2.24)$$

For the moment this is as far as we can get without matrix notation (see Section 4.3), but we can already check a pair of special cases. If $\sigma_s = \sigma_t$, the sum-and-difference case where we started, we have $\tan 2\theta$ infinite, $2\theta = 90°$, $\theta = 45°$. This is the angle we were using before. In the "opposite" situation, with one of s or t having variance much larger than the other – say, $\text{var}(s) >> \text{var}(t)$ – we can drop the smaller variance from equation (2.24). We then see

$$\theta = \frac{1}{2}(2\theta) \approx \frac{1}{2}\tan 2\theta \approx -\frac{\sigma_{st}}{\sigma_s^2} \qquad (2.25)$$

and so the direction we seek takes the line we already computed in Figure 2.32, the regression line of t on s, and just rotates it back down to the horizontal. See Figure 2.32.

We will use this property in Section 4.3.5 when we interpret the results of the principal-component computation in Procrustes form space. Usually allometries take this form there, with the role of X being played by the variable we will be introducing under the name of Centroid Size.

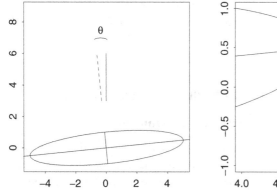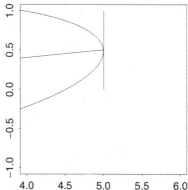

Figure 2.32 In the limit of one variable having variance a great deal larger than a second, the standardization of their scatterplot (here iconified into one of its ellipses) by rotation to uncorrelated variables sends to the new x-axis the direction of slope nearly the same as the regression slope we have been considering all along.

Summary of Section 2.4

- When we change the shape of Galton's quincunx so that every row has the same variance, the slope of the "causation" line downward from row l to row k and the slope of the "regression" line upward from row k to row l have the same value, $\sqrt{l/k}$, a number less than 1.
- For a general pair of variables X and Y, we arrive at the same number, the *correlation* r of X and Y, by taking the square root of the product of the two regression coefficients, that for X on Y and that for Y on X. The equivalent formula is $r = \text{cov}(X, Y)/\sqrt{\text{var}(X)\text{var}(Y)}$.
- The phenomenon of "regression to the mean" arises as an artifact of the correlation's being always less than 1 in absolute value.
- A remarkable paper by Karl Pearson guessed at the theorem that true class means lie on both regression lines (X on Y and also Y on X) only if the (X, Y) distribution is bivariate normal, the result of rotating, scaling, and stretching the scatterplot of some pair of independent Gaussian variables. He illustrated this using some of his own data about family resemblances in Victorian England.
- As shown in an almost equally old example from the geneticist Sewall Wright, patterns of larger or smaller correlations among measured lengths can sometimes correspond to explanations in terms of *morphological integration*, the accounting for correlations by factors common to subsets of one's measurements or to all of them.
- If one variable X has much greater variance than another variable Y, then the regression line for Y on X lies very nearly along the direction of the linear combination of X and Y that has the greatest variance for unit sum of squares of coefficients.

2.5 Further Useful Formulas for This Setting

2.5.1 Acrobatics on the Quincunx

Using this same isomorphism between quincuncial patterns and linear regressions, we can go on to compute the regression relating *consequences of the same cause*. (This was actually the question with which Galton originally began: a regression relating the heights of pairs of brothers, modeled as if they were generated by falling down a quincunx from a point corresponding to midparent height at some upper row.) On the quincunx, these are pairs of shot on lower rows (not necessarily the same lower row) that arise from the same starting position some rows above. In effect, a pair of shot fall from the top of the quincunx while tied together down to some position x in the kth row. At that moment the tie is broken and they thereafter fall separately, one l_1 rows further and one l_2 rows further. Denote the counts of Heads minus Tails for these two lower falls as $\varepsilon_1, \varepsilon_2$, and let x denote the position at the kth row. Then the regression relating the position of the two shot at the lower rows has numerator $\sum (x + \varepsilon_1)(x + \varepsilon_2)$, and since the expected product of either ε multiplying anything, including the other one, is zero, this is just the variance of x, the same as the row number k we've been using all along. The denominator is still the variance of the $(k + l_2)^{th}$ row, the predictor variance in the regression; this is the same as its row number. Hence the regression coefficient for the l_1-row descendant on the l_2-row descendant is thus

$$k/(k + l_2) \qquad (2.26)$$

independent of the value of l_1. The earlier result for the pure inverse inference, predicting the cause from the effect, is the case of this formula for $l_1 = 0$.

Figure 2.33 demonstrates this equation for the case of two evaluates in the 30th row of the quincunx having a common cause halfway up, at the 15th row.

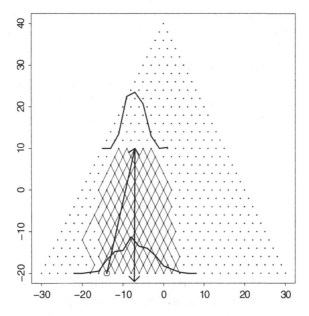

Figure 2.33 Paths traversing the quincunx in mixed directions. A value of -15 in the last row (open circle) regresses to a Gaussian distribution around a mean of -7.5 (upward arrow and Gaussian) and then falls (on average) straight downward, resulting in the wider Gaussian back at the bottom row again. As the mean there is the same -7.5, the regression coefficient must be $\frac{1}{2}$.

For any observed row-30 outcome (e.g., the point drawn in the open circle), the predicted distribution of another "effect" of the same cause at row 15 is the Gaussian curve shown, the one that is centered, back down in the 30th row, just halfway back from the selected value toward the (vertical) axis of symmetry. Hence the regression coefficient of either sibling on the other is 0.5, just as formula (2.26) would have it ($\frac{k}{k+l_2}$ for $k = l_2 = 15$).

As another example, often helpful as a practical analogy, consider a different situation in which $l_1 = l_2 = k$ — three independent, identically distributed (i.i.d.) Gaussian processes x_i, $i = 1, 2, 3$. Then the regression coefficient of $x_1 + x_2$ on $x_1 + x_3$ is $\frac{1}{2}$.

For the case of the common cause, after standardization, the regression coefficients $\frac{k}{k+l_1}$ and $\frac{k}{k+l_2}$ relating l_2-row and l_1-row descendants of a common ancestor in the kth row become the correlation coefficient

$$\frac{k}{\sqrt{(k + l_1)(k + l_2)}}. \tag{2.27}$$

But this is the same as the product $\sqrt{\frac{k}{k+l_1}} \sqrt{\frac{k}{k+l_2}}$ of the correlations linking the cause (the row-k value) to the two effects separately: one factor for the regression "up" and a second one for the passage back "down." Just as the correlation pays no attention to the direction of causation, so this product pays no attention to the fact that one prediction is along the direction of causation while the other is in the opposite temporal direction. In practice, we are asking the following question, which corresponds to a good many practical questions in today's applied natural and social sciences: How can one reasonably predict the consequence of an imperfectly observed cause? If all errors are Gaussians like these, the answer, according to this maximum-likelihood style of argument, is the simple formula I've just given you. The regression of one effect on another is by the product of their two separate correlations on their common cause, once these effects are variance-standardized themselves. If we use a different topology of causation, row k to row l to row m in steady downward order, then the product of the separate correlations involving row l is

$$\sqrt{\frac{k}{l}} \sqrt{\frac{l}{m}} = \sqrt{\frac{k}{m}}, \tag{2.28}$$

which is just the regular formula applied to the full interval from row k to row m. Causal chains on a quincunx behave the way they ought to.

A related question. Suppose one has observed a suite of positively correlated variables $x_1, x_2, \ldots, x_m$, and that it is reasonable on scientific grounds to imagine all of them as caused by the same underlying hidden variable Y.

(For instance, the x's might be a collection of size measurements, all of which are caused by a variable Y that stands either for the passage of time, if this is a growth study, or else for net weight or some other summary measure.) We might wish to model the collection of x's as points on m different levels of the quincunx all descending from an unobserved variable Y at some level higher than all of them. Let this hypothetical Y be at level k of the quincunx and the x's lie below it at intervals $l_i, i = 1, \ldots, m$.

In this setup, the correlation of each x_i with Y would be $\sqrt{\frac{k}{k+l_i}}$, and the correlation of x_i with x_j, more concisely written r_{ij}, would be $\frac{k}{\sqrt{(k+l_i)(k+l_j)}}$ $= \sqrt{\frac{k}{k+l_i}}\sqrt{\frac{k}{k+l_j}}$, product of one factor in i only and another in j only. If there are only three variables, we have enough information to compute all the ratios involved: $\frac{k}{k+l_1} = r_{12}r_{13}/r_{23}$ and the others like it. There is, however, no guarantee that this product of correlations is positive or that it is less than 1 in value: some 3×3 correlation matrices cannot be modeled on the quincunx. For more than three x's, the model fits just when $r_{ij}r_{kl} = r_{ik}r_{jl}$ for all i, j, k, l without duplicates – the so-called *tetrad criterion*. We return to this subject in Chapter 4 when we talk about factor analysis.

2.5.2 Tukey's Approximation

Our basic formula for a regression coefficient, equation (2.7), requires that we compute a sum of crossproducts. We might not have the patience for this extent of multiplications (especially if we are working with pencil on paper far from a computer). Is there some way to arrive at a good approximation to a regression coefficient only by adding and subtracting? Yes, if one is willing to (1) sort the set of all the predictor (x) values, from low to high, and (2) accept a loss of efficiency of about 8%. Though I cannot locate the relevant citation, I believe the following trick was suggested by John Tukey.

Assume a true linear model $y \sim a + bx$ defined for a predictor x that, by virtue of some experimental design, is spaced uniformly over some range, say, -1 to 1 every 0.01. Assume a sample size N sufficiently large that we needn't worry about small fractions. Take prediction error as uniformly distributed with mean zero and constant variance σ^2.

Assume, finally, that we are so lazy in our approach to univariate regression that we don't actually want to compute any of the formulas in Section 2.1, not even Edgeworth's formula that gives us the coefficient as a weighted average of slopes. We ask instead if there is one *single slope* that could do most of the job for us. One good guess for that single slope would be the slope between the centroids of the data for the two subsamples shown in Figure 2.34. Here k is

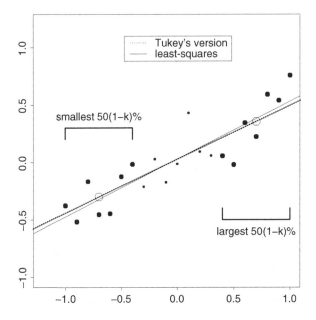

Figure 2.34 Diagram of John Tukey's method of outer thirds for estimating a regression coefficient without computing a crossproduct. The estimate is the slope of the line connecting the two centroids shown by the open circles. What value should k take?

some fraction between 0 and 1, which we use to define the "k-tails" of the predictor distribution. We average the observations y for x between k and 1 — call this $\bar{y}^{+k}$ — and again for x between $-k$ and -1 — call this average $\bar{y}^{-k}$ — and agree that we will estimate the true regression coefficient by the simple ratio

$$\frac{\bar{y}^{+k} - \bar{y}^{-k}}{1 + k}, \tag{2.29}$$

which is the slope of the line connecting the two points plotted with open circles in the figure. (The difference between the horizontal coordinates of the centroids of the two subsamples, on this assumption of a uniform distribution of the x's, is just $1 + k$ — that's where the denominator comes from.) What fraction should we use for k? The combination of these two samples covers the whole range of x's except for the region right around their average of zero – and ignoring that central interval for purposes of the slope estimation is indeed a sensible strategy according to the argument we have already noted in Section 2.1.

Because the numerator of (2.29) is the average of a collection of $N(1 - k)$ values of y all with the same standard error σ and coefficients of ± 1, its variance is just $\frac{\sigma^2}{N(1-k)}$. To get the variance of the slope, we divide this by $(1 + k)^2$, the square of the denominator of equation (2.29). Since N and σ are constants, by assumption, our problem reduces to a straightforward task, minimizing the ratio $\frac{1/(1-k)}{(1+k)^2}$, or, equivalently, maximizing $(1 - k)(1 + k)^2 = 1 + k - k^2 - k^3$ as a function of k between 0 and 1. The extrema are where the derivative $1 - 2k - 3k^2$ of this expression is zero. This is for $k = \frac{1}{3}$ or -1. Only the first of these values is meaningful. So the short-cut we are looking for divides the segment $(-1, 1)$ exactly into thirds. We average the y's from the upper third of the x-range, subtract the average of the y's from the lower third of the range, divide by $2 \times \frac{2}{3}$ (i.e., multiply by $\frac{3}{4}$), and that is Tukey's slope estimate (the dashed line in the figure, which happens to be for the optimal value of k as long as x stays scaled to range 2 in this way). Notice that this arithmetic completely ignores the data from values of x in the middle third $(-\frac{1}{3}, \frac{1}{3})$ of the x-range.

This estimate is a valuable tool for anyone who ever has to guess at regression slopes by hand. From the formula $\text{var}(\hat{\beta}) = \sigma^2/(N\text{var}(x))$ (equation 2.10), together with the facts that the variance of $\pm\frac{2}{3}$ is just $\frac{4}{9} = \frac{12}{27}$, whereas that of the uniform on $\pm(\frac{1}{3}, 1)$ is $(\int_{1/3}^{1} x^2 dx)/\frac{2}{3} = \frac{13}{27}$, we deduce that the efficiency of the Tukey procedure is $\frac{12}{13}$, about 92%, of the efficiency of the covariance-divided-by-variance method for the same data subset.[11] In other words, the slope estimate you get by Tukey's method has a sampling (error) variance about $\frac{13}{12}$ times that for the optimal method, and it does not require computing any crossproducts at all, just averages. So you can actually "compute" it by running your pencil over a scatterplot, as long as the points don't cluster too obviously.

2.5.3 The Hat Matrix

We would like to be able to classify individual observations as inconsistent with our expectations. (For instance, they might be telling us that something

---

[11] The comparison to the least-squares estimates comes under the authority of the *Cramér-Rao inequality*, which states, roughly, that under reasonable assumptions, such as that the linear model is true and that appropriate error terms are Gaussian, the machinery this chapter is exploiting for linear models is maximum-likelihood and so must have the smallest variance (or, equivalently, will require the smallest sample size for a given precision of estimate) for any unbiased estimator (meaning, any formula that is expected to give you the correct average value over an indefinitely long series of repeated samples from the same population distribution). So the fraction $\frac{12}{13}$ here really *is* the extent to which we have approached the best possible procedure. By way of comparison, the efficiency of the ordinary median (middle value) as the estimate of the mean of a Gaussian distribution is only $2/\pi \cong 0.637$.

has gone wrong with our measuring equipment, or they might be informing us about unusual circumstances that have induced a breakdown of the principal theory under consideration.) Here is one elementary approach to accomplishing just that.

Rephrase everything in terms of errors in the equations (remembering this is how the computations actually proceed), not those cascading errors in measurement. So now we are *starting* with an equation like $y_i = a + bx_i + \varepsilon_i$ with $\text{var}(\varepsilon) = \sigma^2$, all i, by assumption. Here a and b are unknown "true parameters," and the ε are the true (but unknowable) error terms in the model. After we get through all the rigmarole of fitting the least-squares line, with estimated intercept $\hat{a}$ and estimated slope $\hat{b}$, we have apparent residuals $e_i = y_i - \hat{y}_i = y_i - (\hat{a} + \hat{b}x_i)$, and the variance of *these* residuals is no longer σ^2 but instead σ^2 times $\frac{N-2}{N}$, where N was our original "degrees of freedom" and the 2 subtracted are the two "degrees of freedom" that we "used up" when we fit a two-parameter model to our data. This can make a whole lot of difference – if we are fitting a line to four points, for instance, the variance of the apparent error is half of the true value. What is going on here, and why does the number 2 not depend on anything else about the problem setup?

The following demonstration is one relatively straightforward way to get to this result. And if you can follow it for this simple case of a line fit, you are well prepared for the general case, which we will take up in the next chapter.

So, let us write out the line-fitting procedure that we just reviewed a little while ago, in the matrix notation that you may have seen before. If X stands for the $N \times 2$ matrix $\begin{pmatrix} 1 & x_1 \\ 1 & x_2 \\ \cdot & \cdot \\ \cdot & \cdot \\ 1 & x_N \end{pmatrix}$, then the fitted model is $\hat{Y} = X\beta$ with $\beta = (X'X)^{-1}X'Y$, where $X'X$ is the 2×2 matrix of sums and crossproducts $\begin{pmatrix} \Sigma 1 & \Sigma_i x_i \\ \Sigma_i x_i & \Sigma_i x_i^2 \end{pmatrix} = N \begin{pmatrix} 1 & \bar{x} \\ \bar{x} & \bar{x^2} \end{pmatrix}$ and $X'Y$ is the column vector $\begin{pmatrix} \Sigma y_i \\ \Sigma x_i y_i \end{pmatrix}$ of length 2. We got this just by setting the derivative of $Y - X\beta$ to zero for every element of β (in this case, there were only two of them).

It is surprisingly helpful to write this as $\hat{Y} = X\beta = HY$ where H, the **hat matrix**, equals $X(X'X)^{-1}X'$. We verify, trivially, that $HX = X$ and that $H^2 = H$. (Matrices satisfying $H^2 = H$ are called *idempotent*; they most often arise as projection matrices in contexts like these. Here H projects Y onto the column space of X. Least-squares analysis, remember, is just geometry.) Then, using the definition above of the ith "apparent" residual, we have $e_i = y_i - \hat{y}_i$ for every i and so the whole vector e of all the e_i's satisfies $e = Y - \hat{Y} =$

$(I - H)Y = (I - H)\varepsilon$, since $HX = X$. The expected sum of squares of e – the variance of the apparent residuals – is then, because the elements of ε are independent by assumption, just the sums of the variances of the e_i separately. The ith of these is equal to the ith diagonal element of $I - H$ times the variance σ^2 of each original ε.

But we can compute those diagonal entries explicitly. If $H = X(X'X)^{-1}X'$, then the ith element of its diagonal is

$$\begin{pmatrix} 1 & x_i \end{pmatrix} \begin{pmatrix} \Sigma 1 & \Sigma_i x_i \\ \Sigma_i x_i & \Sigma_i x_i^2 \end{pmatrix}^{-1} \begin{pmatrix} 1 \\ x_i \end{pmatrix} = N^{-1} \begin{pmatrix} 1 & x_i \end{pmatrix} \begin{pmatrix} 1 & \bar{x} \\ \bar{x} & \overline{x^2} \end{pmatrix}^{-1} \begin{pmatrix} 1 \\ x_i \end{pmatrix}.$$

We use the simple identity $\begin{pmatrix} A & B \\ B & C \end{pmatrix}^{-1} = \begin{pmatrix} C & -B \\ -B & A \end{pmatrix} / (AC - B^2)$, and for

the preceding matrix we note that $AC - B^2 = \overline{x^2} - (\bar{x})^2 = \mathrm{var}(x)$. Then

$$H_{ii} = (N\mathrm{var}(x))^{-1} \begin{pmatrix} 1 & x_i \end{pmatrix} \begin{pmatrix} \overline{x^2} & -\bar{x} \\ -\bar{x} & 1 \end{pmatrix} \begin{pmatrix} 1 \\ x_i \end{pmatrix}$$

$$= (N\mathrm{var}(x))^{-1} (\overline{x^2} - 2x_i\bar{x} + x_i^2)$$

$$= (N\mathrm{var}(x))^{-1} (\mathrm{var}(x) + (\bar{x})^2 - 2x_i\bar{x} + x_i^2)$$

$$= (N\mathrm{var}(x))^{-1} (\mathrm{var}(x) + (x_i - \bar{x})^2)$$

$$= \frac{1}{N} + \frac{(x_i - \bar{x})^2}{N\mathrm{var}(x)}. \tag{2.30a}$$

Then, finally,

$$E(e'e) = E(\varepsilon'(I - H)\varepsilon) = \sigma^2 \Sigma_i \left(1 - \left(\frac{1}{N} + \frac{(x_i - \bar{x})^2}{N\mathrm{var}(x)} \right) \right)$$

$$= \sigma^2 \left(N - \frac{N}{N} - \frac{N\mathrm{var}(x)}{N\mathrm{var}(x)} \right) = \sigma^2(N - 2), \tag{2.30b}$$

which was the point of this derivation. (The quadratic form collapsed from an $N \times N$ matrix to just the diagonal because, by assumption, the ε's are independent, so $E(\varepsilon_i \varepsilon_j) = E(\varepsilon_i H_{ij} \varepsilon_j) = 0$ for $i \neq j$.)

More interestingly, we learn the variance of each apparent residual e_i separately: it is

$$\sigma^2 \left(1 - \left(\frac{1}{N} + \frac{(x_i - \bar{x})^2}{N\mathrm{var}(x)} \right) \right) \tag{2.31}$$

and hence is largest for residuals of cases with x_i at the grand mean and smallest for cases whose x-value is farthest from the grand mean. Once a regression is actually fitted, the ratio of each residual e_i to that case-specific standard deviation (square root of the formula for H_{ii} above) is called its *studentized residual* (after "Student," the pseudonym W. S. Gosset used when publishing the original papers about the t-distribution), and cases of particularly large ratio are of interest for their improbability on the declared model.

I could have shortened the last part of the previous derivation by using the theorem that if matrix products AB and BA both work then $\mathrm{tr}(AB) = \mathrm{tr}(BA)$, where "tr" is the *trace operator* that sums the diagonal entries of a square matrix. (Chapter 4 has more to say about traces.) Apply this to H with $A = X(X'X)^{-1}$, $B = X'$ and one gets $\mathrm{tr}(H) = \mathrm{tr}(AB) = \mathrm{tr}(BA) = \mathrm{tr}(X'X(X'X)^{-1})$ $= \mathrm{tr}\begin{pmatrix} 1 & 0 \\ 0 & 1 \end{pmatrix} = 2$, which is where the 2 in equation (2.30b) comes from. It is a count of the columns of X, not a geometric quantity at all. Chapter 3 will deal with regressions on two predictor variables instead of one; there, the variance of the apparent residuals e will divide the variance of the true residuals ε by $\frac{N-3}{N}$, and so on.

Figure 2.35 is a simulated example of a regression on 21 cases that are far from Gaussianly distributed. The regression line for this sample is drawn in the

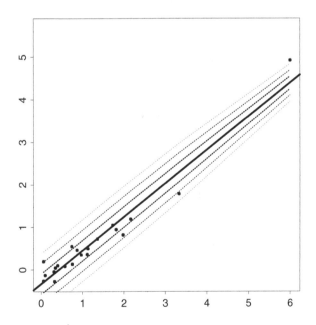

Figure 2.35 Diagram of loci of standardized residuals 1, 2, or 3 standard deviations from the regression line for a simulated data set of 21 points including a very long tail. The bowing of these curves is quite obvious over this wide range.

heavy solid line; the lunes of ± 1, ± 2, and ± 3 times the imputed standard error of the fitted points are drawn in the series of steadily lighter dashed lines. The rightmost point is seen to fall outside the limit of $+3$ standard deviations, and is thus suspect on any reasonable inferential logic. A point of equal and opposite deviation, the second from the right, is not to be viewed quite so skeptically – it falls below the line by just a little over twice its standard error because it is so much closer to the mean of the predictor, and according to the formula in the text, the curves of equal expected e produced by the hat matrix method bow outward toward the center $\bar{x}$ of their domain and inward toward the extremes.

Most of the machinery of significance testing in linear models follows pretty much the way this decomposition of variance in the hat matrix proceeds. In essence, it can be traced to an elegant and fundamental theorem due to William Cochran in the 1930s. If $Y = (y_1, y_2, \ldots y_k)$ are i.i.d. Gaussian variables of mean 0, and if $YY' = \Sigma y_i^2 = \Sigma_j YH_jY'$ for some list of idempotent matrices H_j, then the YH_jY' are independent, and each YH_jY' is $\chi_m^2 \sigma^2$ where m is the rank of H_j, and the total of the m is the net degrees of freedom, k, of the sum of squares YY' that, up to a factor of σ^2, defines the χ^2 distribution in the first place. The proof is a deep consequence of the information-theoretic properties and symmetries of the Gaussian distribution. Since the YH_jY' are independent, then by definition their ratios are all F-ratios, and that is where all the F-tests of the linear model actually come from. (Here χ_m^2, read "chisquare on m degrees of freedom," is the distribution of the sum of m squared standardized Gaussians. Chapter 4 will have more to say about chisquares.)

Example 2.5: Tetrahymena, one experimental condition. We exemplify this useful computation using an example from an organism without hard parts: a protist (single-celled animal) that is found in freshwater ponds and in biomedical research labs. We will use it to exemplify analysis of covariance, one of the special cases of multiple regression that will be introduced in Chapter 3. Here in Chapter 2, half of the data set, considered on its own, is a useful introduction to one aspect of biometrical regression, the possibility of meaningful transformations of dimension. My attention was called to this example by Andersen and Skovgaard (2010). These data are included in this book's online resource.

Consulting Hellung-Larsen et al. (1989), we learn that these data arose from an experiment, not any sort of random sample of *Tetrahymena* colonies found floating in a pond somewhere. The experiment controlled glucose, temperature, initial concentration, and other measures, and measured final concentration and final diameter (an approximation of the cube root of volume).

Have a look at the left panel of Figure 2.36. These are the actually measured data for one of the conditions (high glucose). This is certainly not a promising

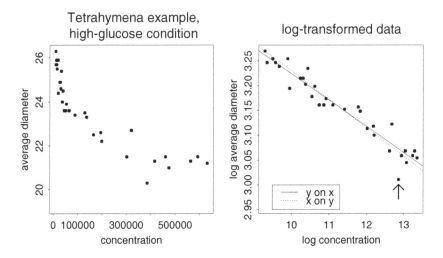

Figure 2.36 Joint analysis of concentration and diameter for one of the two experimental conditions of the *Tetrahymena* experiment. (left) Original data, very difficult to interpret in this form. (right) After log transforms of both axes. The linearity is obvious, and the coefficient can actually be reduced to a convenient integer in the course of a narrative report. The arrow indicates a possible outlying datum (see text).

beginning for a quantitative study. The data appear enormously heterogeneous from left to right end of the plot. At the left, concentration appears to hardly change as diameter falls from 26 to below 24. Then there is a sudden change of behavior whereby the roles of concentration and diameter appear, if anything, to reverse. The formulas we imagined to apply to the motorcar example in Section 2.1 obviously gain us nothing useful here.

When data look like these, the log-log transformation often linearizes them, because processes in biology often follow power laws $y = ax^b$ that appear linear on the log scale. (This is a property of the data, not of the method. The usual argument for the log-transform is that it normalizes "prediction error" in cases where the variance of that error is proportional to the predicted value; but that is not the reason for invoking it here.) The transformation worked wonderfully, as you see over at the right. At the upper left, now we can make some visual sense of the trend instead of just seeing points falling down a ladder. In fact, the regression looks linear throughout the range of the experimental results, and the correlation ($-.963$) is close enough to -1.0 that the two regression lines, log concentration on log diameter and log diameter on log concentration, are practically indistinguishable. (The figure shows them both. The one for log concentration on log diameter is the dotted line.)

We noted that correlation need not be interpreted causally, and indeed this is a good example of such noncausal language. What the experimenter was managing was instead probably a system under *homeostasis,* meaning some kind of search for equilibrium. The different experimental runs here (made under different starting conditions) result in different colonies that appear to be obeying an equation that, from the regressions, takes the form log diameter $\sim$ -0.054 log concentration, or log diameter $+ 0.054$ log concentration $\sim$ constant, or, since the volume of a sphere goes roughly as the cube of the diameter,

$$6 \log \text{volume} + \log \text{concentration} \sim \text{constant.} \qquad (2.32)$$

In our field it is always good to reduce coefficients to integers when you can. In keeping with that rule, one might report the present situation as follows: the volume of the typical protist seems to scale as concentration to the minus one-sixth power.

There is one more symbol on this plot that is worth attending to: the arrow at lower right, pointing to the unusually large negative residual at the indicated point, seventh from largest on the concentration scale. To judge this point it is convenient to consider the regression through all the *other points,* and then refer the residual at this point to the normalization by position along with the variance of the *other* residuals, the computation we previously called "studentizing" (it is the variant called *external studentizing*). The residual for this seventh point in terms of the distribution of residuals from the other points works out to -3.812 times its estimated standard error. It is fair to ask how often we would observe any residual this large from data that are truly generated by adding Gaussian noise to a truly linear regression. Samples from a bell curve with the standard error actually observed here produce a value this extreme, the tables tell us (or routines with names like pnorm in the standard statistical packages), about 69 times in a million. But that standard error itself was observed with error (after all, it was based on only 31 other cases). The standard error of a standard error, we will see in Chapter 4, is approximately a fraction $\frac{1}{\sqrt{2N}}$, about 13%, times that standard error itself. Here N is about 30, and $1/\sqrt{2 \cdot 30}$ is about 0.13, so that extreme residual could easily have been "only" as extreme as $-3.812 \times 0.87 = -3.32$ times the standard deviation of the others, a deviation that a bell curve will generate about 45 times in a hundred thousand.[12] Because we selected it as the extreme among all 32 in

---

[12] The argument here is an informal substitute for the more common derivation of a probability using the *t-statistic,* which takes the full distribution of the standard error into account, not just the conservative adjustment I mentioned. That more precise $p(t_{30})$ is 0.00032, but given that we have no assurance that residuals are actually Gaussian, this value is only a rough guide about the "unlikelihood" of the extreme.

this high-glucose group, it is appropriate to carry out a *Bonferroni correction*, multiplying its probability by 32; there results a recalculated p of just under 0.015. Hence what we are seeing at the point indicated by the arrow is, in fact, a relatively unlikely deviation from the regression line if all the data were equally likely to have arisen from this loglinear model with measurement errors that all came from the same Gaussian distribution. Figure 3.13 will suggest that the likeliest explanation is a miscoding of the glucose level: the problematic point actually lies close to the line for the study's *other* experimental group, which I haven't mentioned yet.

Summary of Section 2.5

- The correlation between two variables that are each predictable as regressions on a third one, plus independent error, is the product of the corresponding separate correlations, regardless of whether that third variable is their common cause or instead an intermediate in their causal chain.
- The slope of a regression on evenly spaced predictors can be estimated nearly as well by connecting the centroids of the top third and bottom third of predictor values and observed outcomes as by the extended least-squares formula. This is *John Tukey's approximation by thirds.*
- Prediction errors that all had the same variance before a regression computation now have different variances, which are smaller for predictor values that are farther from their average.
- A transform to logarithms often linearizes the relationship between a pair of variables that are associated with some biophysical process or constraint.

2.6 Other Data Structures

All the preceding advice is sound as long as your data set arose as a representative random sample of some population. But data sets appropriate for exploring most of the really interesting questions in biology do not arise from designs like that. We are trying to study the processes and forces that hold organisms together over space or over time. To get at aspects of their integration, the logic of the associated comparisons must be built into the data collection protocols just as deeply as the methodology.

The assumptions governing the overwhelmingly most common sampling framework, random sampling of putatively independent specimens, badly fail to accommodate the designs of the best studies in quantitative biology. Organisms that are followed over time yield measures that are no longer independent, and measurements made on different parts of the same organisms or the same ecosystem cannot be expected to be independent – if they are, it is an occasion for great disappointment. The same criteria that lead to success in the physical sciences – the mastery of independence of successive measurements of stars, rocks, or coin flips – and likewise in the social sciences (independence of successive cases of a random sample) – has the paradoxical effect of working to block progress in quantitative biology, where nearly all of our interest deals with the persistence, indeed the perseveration, of signals across the millennia, across the ecosystem, and across the embryo. We are interested in the quantification of the patterns that encode these persistences, not merely their existence, which goes without saying. (This point has been made before in much greater generality by Walter Elsasser [1998] when he noted that whereas the physical sciences concentrate on three principal aspects of the world – space, time, and energy – biology needs to add a fourth, **memory,** as well. Memories, whether declarative or structural, cannot be modeled as independent in any useful way.)

Successive coin flips are independent. So can be research samples from a museum's collection of fossils, Pearson's London of Victorian two-parent families, or a hospital's records of people with a rare and sporadic disease. But the same independence that makes much of statistical theory so algebraically tractable – sums of squares, exponentials of these sums, straight lines as theories – severely impoverishes our biometrical arguments. Independence of samples demolishes the sort of factors that we actually rely on for our most powerful explanations: factors like growth and development, selection and speciation, or ecophenotypy. The power of *all* our biometric statistics, both the elementary and the advanced, is scaled upward enormously when the independence assumption is replaced by incorporating these real biological factors at the root of a sample design.

Chapter 2 closes, then, with introductions to three of these alternative data structures: growth series, random walks, and the phylogenetic branching that we know characterizes evolution above the species level at all the relevant time scales. It is the presence of these higher levels of data organization, which inevitably entail measurement redundancy for both functional and structural reasons, that requires this book to extend over three more big chapters.

2.6.1 Growth Series

Growth series represent one of the enduring concerns of biometrics, specifically the aim that bursts out of the museum to involve serial measurements of actual living material at a time scale larger than cycles (gait, respiration, seasonality) but smaller than the full life span. Appropriate statistical methods must accept the persistence of individual differences, with the corresponding "tracking" seen in growth plots like ours, right alongside the hoped-for independence of sampling of the organisms that are actually going to be repeatedly measured in this intentionally correlated way. Superimposed over the longitudinal measurement pattern there might be another crossed factor for multiplicity of actual measures. For the Berkeley data set, our first example to follow, these are the four formally unrelated measurement channels of height, weight, leg girth, and strength. For the example after that, Melvin Moss's "Vilmann data set," the material was less refractory (having not originated in human children). These data are a much more strenuously controlled suite of 16 Cartesian coordinates representing the locations of eight anatomically homologous landmark points (Section 5.1), most of them interosseous, as jointly digitized in radiographs at eight ages of 18 growing male rodent skulls. Good analyses of growth data always exploit the additional longitudinal structure of the data and, whenever possible, the measure-to-measure redundancy as well. The corresponding graphics concentrate on enhancements of the standard scatterplots that serve to emphasize the visual connections among alternate measures of the same organisms across times, measurement protocols, or both.

These two examples thus span the extremes of this domain of data formats. The Berkeley Guidance Study affords the possibility of longitudinal analysis but hardly anything else. In Chapter 3 it will be exploited as one example of the technique of added-variable plots for the detection of additional information beyond single fits of explanatory lines. The Vilmann rodent data, in contrast, will prototype the highest and best applications of the morphometric tools to be introduced in Chapter 5. The tools that it will help us demonstrate can exploit relationships among multiple measurements, not just their correlations but also their geometry, just as deftly as relationships across multiple times of observation.

Example 2.6: The Berkeley Guidance Study. This example can serve as an introduction to the concerns of "the classic anthropometry of growth." The principal reference is Tuddenham and Snyder (1954), the extended monograph about these data by the original investigators. It includes an appendix that lists all the original measurements subject by subject.

The Berkeley Guidance Study (BGS) was one of a series of grand schemes of *longitudinal data analysis* begun at various times in the twentieth century all across America. The Bolton–Brush study and the University of Michigan University School Study both centered around data from carefully positioned x-rays of the growing human head. There was also the Terman Study of the

Gifted Child, which, like the Berkeley study, followed some California children born between the world wars. Later there came the Seattle Longitudinal Study (founded by the Pennsylvania psychologist K. Warner Schaie in 1956 as part of his doctoral dissertation, and still in progress [the study, not the thesis] at the University of Washington), and, from 1974 through 2008, the Seattle Longitudinal Study of Pregnancy and Offspring Development (an entirely independent investigation, in spite of the similarity of names and in spite of actually sharing a building with the Schaie study for a while). Studies like these overlap a good deal concerning issues such as initial recruiting, loss to follow-up, subjects who miss their appointments, advances in measurement strategies or statistical tactics, the secular trend of steadily larger people of nearly every age in the United States over time, responses to changes in the social and medical contexts of the life courses under study, and, for Terman and Schaie, natural deaths of the subjects, none of which I have the space to talk about in this book.

The main BGS study produced physical measurements of up to 7 quantities on 66 boys and 70 girls at each of 34 ages between 3 months and 18 years. I will be working from a subset that Sanford Weisberg extracted and has publicly posted as a resource associated with his textbook of 2005: the measurements of weight and height at three ages (2, 9, and 18 years) and two more measures, leg (calf) girth and "strength," at ages 9 and 18 years only. There is also a summary age-18 rating, "somatotype," that is worth a Google look in its own right.[13] These data also appear as part of this book's online resource. (Another subselection of data, height [only] at 31 ages, forms the contents of another publicly available data archive, part of the online R resource library "fda" associated with the book *Functional Data Analysis* by James Ramsay and Bernard Silverman.)

The structure of this data set is thus realistically rich. We have two sexes, three ages (out of 34, as I noted), and variously two, four, or five variables. We can therefore talk about how the measures relate to each other at a single time, how they predict their own values across time, how they predict *other* values across time, or how any or all of the quantitative scores predict this mysterious categorical twelfth variable, the "somatotype" observed at the time of "skeletal maturity."

A typical simple biometrical investigation is carried by the four panels of Figure 2.37. Shown here are the data for height and weight at three select

---

[13] This "measure," arising from an essentially crackpot theory of W. H. Sheldon that begins with examination of nude photos, made the news a couple of decades ago when it turned out to have been used in another study, Wellesley College freshmen in the 1960s, one of whose subjects, then named Hillary Rodham, ended up as the wife of America's 42nd president, a Secretary of State under Barack Obama, and the runner-up in the 2016 election.

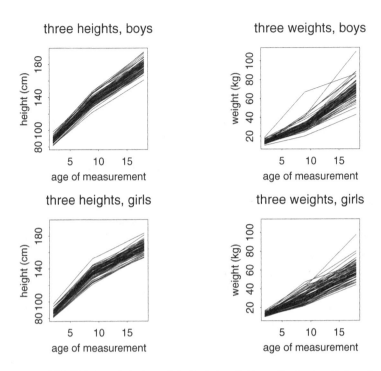

Figure 2.37 Height–weight data of the Berkeley Guidance Study, ages 2, 9, and 18 years, first version. Segmented lines connect consecutive observations for each of the 66 boys or 70 girls.

ages, graphed as growth curves separately by sex. In these graphs, however, the horizontal direction is mostly wasted – that direction was not measured, but serves only to label the ages (whose numerical values we already know). In other words, the information along the horizontal axis does not increase with sample size the way the information along the vertical axis does.

The considerably more useful plot in Figure 2.38 combines the fundamental measurements as vertical and horizontal of a single scatterplot, with the ages again linked by lines. At the same time, to circumvent the evident systematic divergence of these curves as the children become larger, I converted both measurements to the logarithm. In these panels, the heavy marginal dashes along the horizontal and vertical axes indicate the means of log height or log weight, plus and minus one standard deviation, separately for each age for each sex, and the light dashes intercalated between these are the same for the two changes of log height or log weight, respectively. (The standard deviation of the natural logarithm of a positive quantity is approximated by a possibly more familiar numerical summary, the *coefficient of variation*, which is defined as the ratio of the standard deviation to the mean.)

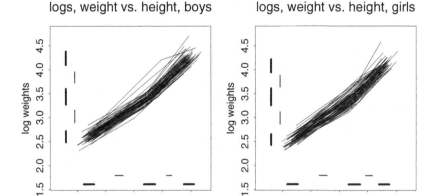

Figure 2.38 Berkeley Guidance Study, second version: log height and log weight are now plotted on orthogonal axes. Heavy dashes in the margins are means plus or minus one standard deviation for the separate ages; light dashes, mean changes plus or minus one standard deviation of the change.

There is more information available than just these means and standard deviations, of course; there is also the matter of the intercorrelations among these variables. Here are all of them.

For the 66 boys :

	HT2	HT9	HT18	WT2	WT9	WT18
HT2	1.000	0.704	0.574	0.618	0.522	0.380
HT9	0.704	1.000	0.878	0.525	0.707	0.501
HT18	0.574	0.878	1.000	0.458	0.523	0.461
WT2	0.618	0.525	0.458	1.000	0.605	0.360
WT9	0.522	0.707	0.523	0.605	1.000	0.722
WT18	0.380	0.501	0.461	0.360	0.722	1.000

For the 70 girls :

	HT2	HT9	HT18	WT2	WT9	WT18
HT2	1.000	0.743	0.669	0.653	0.549	0.409
HT9	0.743	1.000	0.813	0.611	0.750	0.652
HT18	0.669	0.813	1.000	0.462	0.452	0.547
WT2	0.653	0.611	0.462	1.000	0.706	0.439
WT9	0.549	0.750	0.452	0.706	1.000	0.731
WT18	0.409	0.652	0.547	0.439	0.731	1.000

Correlations within the log height block or log weight block are higher for the girls than for the boys with the exception of the prediction of HT18 from HT9. This change, although greater in its typical ratio, actually shows noticeably less variability among the boys than the girls. (In the language of

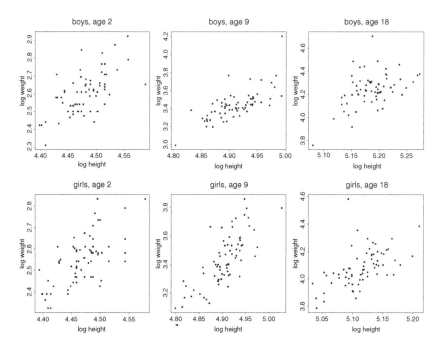

Figure 2.39 Log height–log weight scatters at each age, corresponding to some of the correlations in the tables in the text. Note the one very small boy at ages 9 and 18.

Tanner and Davies [1985], the boys show a greater average spurt in height, but the girls are more variable.) Girls have the higher height–weight correlation at all ages, corresponding to the scatterplots in Figure 2.39.

The preceding series of three diagram styles typifies the biometric approach to data that come as growth series in individuals from different groups. In the context of this book's main theme, the articulation of arithmetic with understanding, the most promising of these composite plots is probably the second set (Figure 2.38), which indicates a very strong shared linear trend about which there is a small bend that shows slight differences between the sexes. Dimorphisms like these tend to be interpreted as owing to differences in sex-specific hormonal environments or some other implication of having a Y chromosome versus a second X chromosome. The scatterplots of change are simply too disorderly to align with theory (although they are certainly relevant to the practical problems of predicting future body size; see, again, Tanner and Davies, 1985), and the initial plots use the display area too inefficiently to count as cogent for the purpose of scientific comparisons.

Comment on an index. There is a conventional approach to standardizing the data in Figure 2.38: the *Body Mass Index* (BMI), traditionally taken as the formula Weight/Height^2 where weight is traditionally measured in kilograms and height in meters. The quotient for an individual is referred to standards that involve thresholds for categories such as "underweight, normal, overweight, obese," where "normal" is typically in the range of 25 or so. Many publications report correlations between these scores and various indicators of health, morbidity, and mortality.

The units of BMI as stated are evidently kg/m^2, which is a unit of pressure. This does not make any scientific sense as a measure of body habitus. Instead, it follows as a formula for a transformed residual in a conventionalized regression of log weight on log height, a regression for which the estimated coefficient is near 2.0 for a range of reported samples.

Consider the panels in Figure 2.40 (top row, analyses for the Berkeley Guidance Study boys; bottom row, for the girls). In the left column are the conventional BMI scores at ages 2, 9, and 18. There is a good deal of scatter at the latter two ages in both sexes, atop a central band of probability density that appears to stay approximately horizontal for the first two ages and then rise to the third.

The design of this pair of figures is not as helpful as that for the pair in the middle column. There the relatively wasted age axis has been reassigned as the height axis and the vertical to weight. For this combination of ages, the scatters can be plotted together on one common set of axes without any overlap. Scribed atop this scatter are level lines for values b of the formula Weight = $b \cdot$Height^2 that correspond to equal values of the BMI. These are a family of nested parabolas that would all intersect at the point $(0, 0)$ if either figure extended that far to the lower left (i.e., to include zygotes, as I will mention in Chapter 3 in connection with some prenatal ultrasound data). You can see how the central tendency of the set of scatters jumps up about two of these level lines (an increase by about one-third of the earlier value) from age 9 to age 18. However, there is an obvious tail of these points toward high values that interferes with the perception of pattern.

Better than either of these displays is the version in the rightmost column, which replaces the raw height and weight measures by their logarithms. Notice how the highest tails of the distribution in the middle column have been brought much more effectively under control by this maneuver. When the data are logged, the lines of equal BMI become ordinary straight lines of slope 2. As straight lines, these loci can be usefully compared to straight lines of another sort, the linear regressions between log weight and log height age by age. For each sex there are three of these lines, one for each age, plotted in three

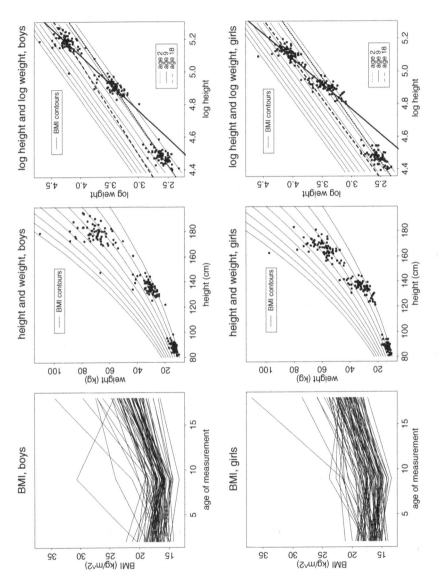

Figure 2.40 Graphical analysis of the Body Mass Index (BMI). This ratio goes better as a coordinate system (center and right columns) than as a quantity (left column). In that capacity the associated regressions are far more informative after the data are transformed to the logarithm (right column).

120

different line weights (dotted for the age-2 data, solid for the age-9 data, and dashed for the age-18 data).

Three facts about these lines render them of particular interest for the understanding of the Berkeley children's growth. First, two of the lines, that for age 2 and that for age 18, have slopes indistinguishable from the value of 2 encoded in our isolines of BMI: that is, the formula exactly suits the data for these two ages. Second, the slope of the fitted relationship at age 9 is distinctly different, having a value of 3.0 for boys and 3.24 for girls. Third, for each sex separately, these regressions at age 9 cut across the level lines for BMI in a geometry that *precisely* matches the change of mean level actually observed in the data between ages 9 and 18.

The result is that each of the lower two regression lines turns out to be predictive after all. The line fitted to age-2 data predicts the mean of the age-9 data, and the line fitted to the age-9 data predicts the mean of the age-18 data. This data set does not extend past age 18 as published, but one suspects that the same trend might continue: the age-18 regressions, which are parallel to the BMI isolines, appear to be suggesting a BMI trend that is likewise horizontal, at least over the next few years of age. This simple equivalencing of within-group to between-group regressions does not obtain for the data to the original scales, without the logging (figures not shown). The interpretation of these coincidences might be straightforward: perhaps some of the age-9 children had already begun their growth spurts, and the coordination in *their* height-weight changes anticipates the changes we will see later in most of the others.

Example 2.7: Vilmann's rat skull data. Around 1982, a group of Columbia University faculty, including Richard Skalak and Melvin Moss, learned of a very interesting data set of images from the laboratory of Henning Vilmann of the Royal Dental College, Copenhagen: sagittal x-rays of the skulls of 21 homogeneous laboratory rodents images eight times each, at ages 7, 14, 21, 30, 40 60, 90, and 150 days. A sagittal x-ray is an x-ray of the head that is, as precisely as feasible, straight on from the side. Bilateral structures are blurred thereby, but outlines in the head's plane of symmetry right up the middle, the *midsagittal plane,* are usually very clear. Taking advantage of this clarity, Moss digitized the eight landmarks shown in Figure 2.41 on all 168 of these radiographs. The resulting data have been the domain of many different investigations into the methodology of morphometrics: first, the tensor methods of Bookstein (1984); then, the thin-plate splines to be reviewed here in Chapter 5; then the mathematical-statistical theory of shape propounded by Ian Dryden and Kanti Mardia in 1998; then the investigations of spatial gradients in Bookstein (2004); quite recently the demonstration of developmental patterns

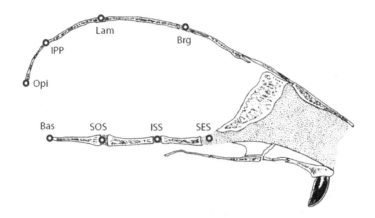

Figure 2.41 Schematic of the midsagittal neural skull of a laboratory rat as seen in H. Vilmann's lateral cephalograms. Landmarks: *Bas,* Basion; *Opi,* Opisthion; *IPP,* Interparietal Suture; *Lam,* Lambda; *Brg,* Bregma; *SES,* Spheno-ethmoid Synchondrosis; *ISS,* Intersphenoidal Suture; *SOS,* Spheno-occipital Synchondrosis. For operational definitions of these points, see Bookstein, 1991, table 3.4.1.

in covariance structures (Mitteroecker and Gunz 2009) that will concern us in Section 5.4; and just a few months ago the introduction of a method of factor analysis for landmark coordinate data (Bookstein 2017b and Figure 5.100 of this book). The data themselves – the actual coordinate values Moss marked on his tracings of the x-rays – were published as an appendix to Bookstein (1991). A listing is also included in this book's online resource.

Of the $8 \times 8 \times 21$ potentially visible landmark points of this exercise, Moss failed to locate a total of four on 3 of the 21 animals. To "complete" these forms is well within the competence of current approaches to such so-called "missing-data problems" (see, e.g., Gunz et al., 2009), but this topic would distract us from our purpose here. Instead, I simply deleted all the data from these three animals, leaving a data set of 1152 points on 144 images in a perfectly crossed design, 8 ages by 18 animals by 8 anatomical loci.

It is not a bad idea to begin an analysis of a region with important contents by extracting the ordinary area of the octagon of landmarks in the figure. Area is computed easily from the coordinate data (x_i, y_i) of p points numbered in counterclockwise order by way of the formula

$$A = \frac{1}{2}((x_1y_2 - y_1x_2) + (x_2y_3 - y_2x_3)$$
$$+ \cdots + (x_{p-1}y_p - y_{p-1}x_p) + (x_py_1 - y_px_1)). \qquad (2.33)$$

Figure 2.42 plots these 144 values in four different ways: by age class of the animal (upper left panel), by the log of that age (upper right panel), or

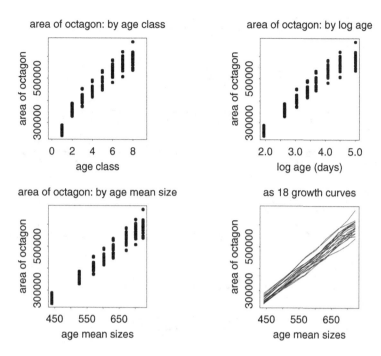

Figure 2.42 Four graphical representations of the growth history of the area of the octagons of landmarks, 18 rats, 8 ages. (upper left) By age class number. (upper right) By log of age. (lower left) By average Centroid Size per age class (root mean square of all the pairwise interlandmark distances). (lower right) As segmented lines linking successive observations.

by the average size of the animals in the relevant age class plotted either as a point scatter (lower left) or as growth curves (lower right). The third version, which exploits the variable *Centroid Size* to be introduced in Section 5.3, evidently gives an almost perfectly linear representation (which is in fact what it is designed to do). At lower right, the same data are plotted as growth curves animal by animal. These lines interweave a bit but mostly remain in approximate rank order. Correlations of areas at one age against areas at another age range from 0.927 downward to 0.633 only.

A display of this design is still not an effective prod to biological understanding. Figure 2.43 shows that, although every possible length that can be measured between a pair of vertices of this octagon grows as a function of the same shared summary Centroid Size, nevertheless some of these graphs curve upward, and others downward, while only a few fortunate candidates are linear with respect to the summary predictor. Information about variances of shape is roughly conveyed by the thickness of these curve packets. Some are of constant variance over age, while others show increases or decreases over this sample

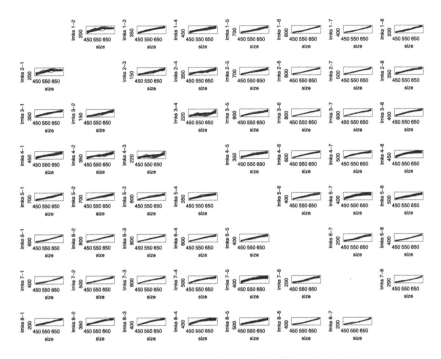

Figure 2.43 Displays of the trajectory of each of the 28 interlandmark segments
separately. Their diversity is impossible to comprehend in this format.

of 18 animals. If these traces had all been linear on the average, we would be
observing the happy circumstance called *isometric growth*, but that situation
does not in fact obtain. The plot in Figure 2.44, which shows all the average
interlandmark distance growth ratios over the full 143 days of the study, age 7
to age 150 days, is likewise too complex to parse in this format. At least we
can state that they are not all the same: the rates of increase of length range
nearly fivefold, from 23.4% to 121.2%.

More powerful tools are required if we are to make developmental sense
of this composite pattern. For the details of the better methods and their
justification, you will have to wait until Section 5.2.

2.6.2 Random Walks

Take any single trajectory of one of those little lead balls as it falls down
Galton's quincunx. Let it leave a track of lead dust behind it, such as appears in
the left panel of Figure 2.45. Now turn this whole image sideways, panel (b).
The same track now appears as a history of jumps of a line up or down, one
unit at a time, over a chronicle of 30 such steps. This is another specific data
scheme, known for over a century under the name of *random walk*.

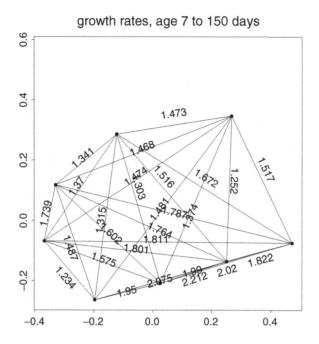

Figure 2.44 First attempt at a spatial representation: growth ratios of all 28 interlandmark segments, averaged, from age 7 to age 150 days. Plots like these correspond to the approach called *Euclidean distance matrix analysis* (EDMA), to be discussed in Section 5.2.

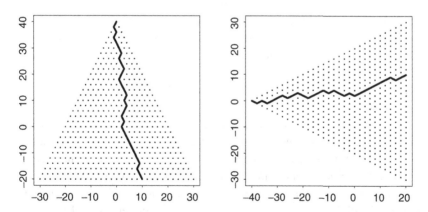

Figure 2.45 From the quincunx to random walk. (left) One trajectory down the quincunx. (right) The equivalent random walk, ending 10 above its starting level.

As the count of elements is substantially scaled up, we tend to misperceive nearly every example of random walk in a manner that is curiously impervious to the ordinary scientific intuition. Figure 2.46 presents twelve instances

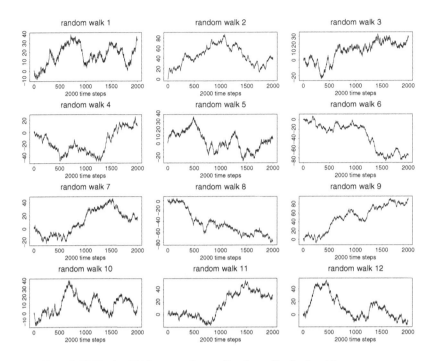

Figure 2.46 Twelve 2000-step random walks of step distribution ±1 at every step. These traces are quite a challenge to the intuition, which struggles to find them *without* meaning in most contexts. Note that every vertical scale is different.

of such walks of length 2000. They show jumps, trends, gaps between "zero-crossings" (successive values of zero), reversals, and extrema that all strongly suggest the possibility of meaningful scientific interpretation. Yet all these examples are completely random, that is to say, uninformative about any conceivable real process under physiological or other experimental or mechanistic control.

The elements of these series certainly cannot be thought of as independent, since the best predictions of any single observation are the observations to its left and right. Every successive observation must be within ±1 of its predecessor, as it must in fact have one of those two specific values. But there is *no other information* available to sharpen this prediction – no available explanations like "runs," "trends," or "preferences": all these are just superstitions. As the advertisements say, "Past performance does not predict future prospects" – that nonpredictability is the main reason for the mathematical and practical usefulness of random walk in the first place.

If the individual elements of the series are available, the analyst would choose simply to subtract each observation from its predecessor, so as to re-express the data as the *increments* that, on the model of random walk, should have been independent and identically distributed. An explanation like that is tested as a potential two-factor model after the fashion of the faceted models in Section 2.6.1: data that are labeled by animal and by time, where we look for effects of both, separately or together, on the mean value of the increment or its variance. But if the data were not so closely observed, this analytic pathway is blocked. For example, if the data are collections of fossils, we cannot get back to individual genealogies – the count of generations separating any two "consecutive" observations might be in the millions.

The mathematicians have had more than a century to develop methods appropriate for dealing with data schemes like these, and they have done so. The earliest statistical treatment, the doctoral dissertation of Louis Bachelier (1900), dealt with financial data (to be specific, stock prices), as exquisitely reviewed in the autobiography of Benoit Mandelbrot (2013). Since then there have been developments both scientific and mathematical, such as my two expositions (Bookstein, 1987, 2013b) for paleobiologists.

As one example, if your data arose from a serial measurement on a complex organized system, and if the positive or negative extremum of their value is located near one end or the other of the series, and if the trend over the range is not obviously linear or obviously sinusoidal, it is always reasonable to suspect the possibility that the data may have been integrated by a serial summation of zero-mean increments in this way. (In effect, this becomes a plausible alternative theory to any biological process the scientist who requested the regression computation might be claiming.) One easy test is to ascertain the timing of that extremum and match it to the theoretical distribution for random walks that was derived only in 1939, which is startlingly recent for mathematics so elementary and fundamental. It is usually expressed in the form of the *Arc-Sine Law* graphed in Figure 2.47. The cumulative probability distribution of the timing of any such extremum goes as $\arcsin(\sqrt{x})$ where x is the fraction of the entire series length at which the extremum was encountered. Expressed in the form of a probability distribution, the formula for $p(x)$, the probability density for the occurrence of an extremum at the fractional position x of the full time range of the walk, is

$$p(x) = \frac{2}{\pi} \frac{1}{\sqrt{x(1-x)}}, \tag{2.34}$$

from which the arcsine formulation follows as the indefinite integral of $1/\sqrt{x(1-x)}$. Equation (2.34) looks symmetric in x and $1-x$, the initial and final segments of the walk. The function $\arcsin(\sqrt{x})$ must have a comparable symmetry, as shown in Figure 2.47.

Of course, all bets are off if you decided to start or finish your examination of the data at a location that looked extremely low or extremely high. This is another version of the "regression to the mean" discussed earlier in this chapter.

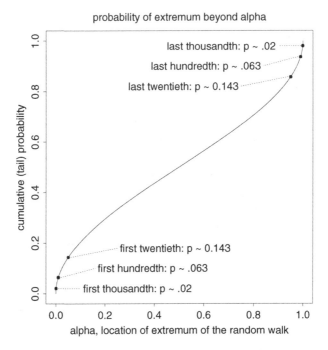

Figure 2.47 The Arc-Sine Law, distribution of the locus of the extremum of a random walk as a fraction of the length of the walk. The mathematics of this curve is startlingly recent.

It is odd but true that exactly the same arcsine distribution applies to the quantity that is the fraction of time that the cumulative sum remains above the zero line. See Feller, 1957, chapter 3.

Example 2.8: Jean Perrin's verification of Einstein's theory of Brownian motion. The first appearances of random walk in the natural sciences preceded Bachelier's by many decades: the two-dimensional random walks first reported by the botanist Robert Brown in 1827. This is the phenomenon we call *Brownian motion*. Brown could comment only on the motion's total irregularity, a circumstance that was easily verified in a series of nineteenth-century studies. The first quantification in the natural sciences came nearly 80 years later at the hands of two of the twentieth century's great physicists: first, Albert Einstein, who announced what proved to be the exact theory of this phenomenon, including the component of particle rotation, in 1905; shortly afterward, the experimentalist Jean Perrin, who confirmed every aspect of

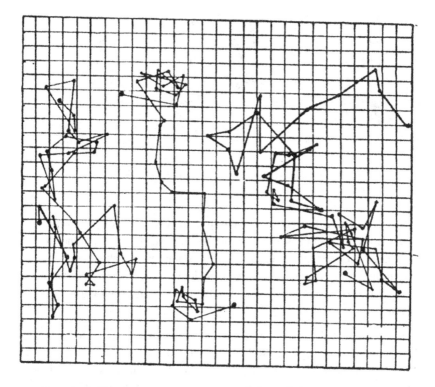

Figure 2.48 One of the earliest published examples of a biological random walk: three histories of Brownian motion from transcription of a microscope image. From Perrin, 1923:115.

Einstein's hypothesis in work first published in 1908 that, like Millikan's a decade later, won him a Nobel Prize in the 1920s.

Figure 2.48 reproduces one of Perrin's figures showing three random walks, each of which arose by following one single particle in a microscope and recording its position by eye and hand every few seconds using a graticule (a coordinate grid superimposed a microscope image). Perrin invented all the elementary ways of demonstrating the underlying Gaussian explanation that we still rely on. Here are three, all beginning with the perception of the "total irregularity of the walk" in any measureable aspect of theincrements:

1. Projections on any direction are Gaussian.
2. Squared length of a step in two dimensions is distributed as the sum of squares of *two* Gaussians (the distribution that we have already named "a χ^2 [chisquare] on two degrees of freedom").

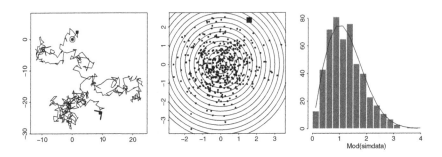

Figure 2.49 Perrin's first experimental confirmation of Einstein's law of diffusion:
a schematic of the argument. See text.

3. The cumulative distribution of the step lengths in any direction (point 1
   above) is linear in the square root of time. Equivalently, the variance of
   squared net step lengths regardless of direction (point 2 above) (i.e., the
   expected value, averaged over many random walks, of squared distance
   from the first point of a random walk to the last point) is proportional to
   time.

Perrin presented versions of all three of these confirmations for data like
the random walk in Figure 2.48. I will attend to the second and third of these.
Regarding item (2), the distribution of step length, Perrin offered a version of
this confirmation in tabular form, but it goes better as the graphic at right in Figure 2.49. The left panel here is a simulation that I selected out of several candidates for its unusual legibility: the cumulative trace of 500 increments each
distributed as Gaussian of mean 0 and variance 1 independently in the x- and
y-directions. The starting position is given by the dot inside a circle at upper
center, and the position after the first time step is at the large square plotting
symbol to its northeast. The walk appears to be following a striking (but
entirely meaningless) pattern involving, first, a trend to the left, then twice as
far to the right, then back toward the left, all the time it is drifting slowly downward. The final position is shown by the heavy arrow at lower center (after a
final step that is relatively short – it began at the dot in the crotch of the arrow).

The middle panel is the representation that bears the weight of interpretation: the scatter of all 500 increments of the process, equivalently, a
sample of 500 from a circular Gaussian distribution of variance 1 in every
direction. That first step printed as a black square in the left panel, for
instance, is copied here as the black square at upper right. (It turns out to
have had an unusually large amplitude, which is what made this particular
simulation suitable for pedagogic use here.) A variety of tests can be applied
to this display – a test of circularity (the same variance in every direction),
for example (see Section 4.3.1), or a simple regression test for directional

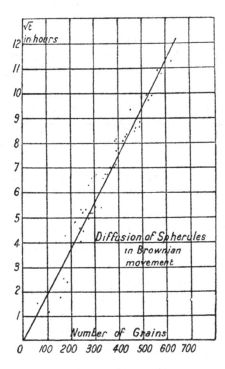

Figure 2.50 Perrin's experimental confirmation of Einstein's law of diffusion by linearization against the square root of time. From Perrin, 1923:131.

drift – but let us simply replicate what Perrin himself checked in 1908, the appropriate distribution of the actual distance moved per unit time interval.

The right-hand panel displays a histogram of this distance, binned by equal radial steps per the circles in the central panel (rings spaced every 0.25 of step length; the first thirteen of these proved nonempty). Superimposed over this histogram is the corresponding theoretical distribution, a χ (chi) variate – square root of a chisquare – on two degrees of freedom. The fit is good enough, and the graphical representation conveys this fact more effectively than the columnar tabulation offered by Perrin so long ago.

Figure 2.50 reproduces Perrin's own version of the confirmation of claim (3), the scaling of diffusion by the 0.5 power of time. Interestingly, he chose to convey this scaling "like a physicist" – by a diagram involving a straight-line fit of net diffusion to an axis that, as you see from its label, is evidently in units of $\sqrt{\text{hours}}$, an unusual unit of measurement indeed. Notice too that the fitting is by hand, not by formula.

For a more extended discussion of the relation of these innovations to the contemporary philosophy of quantitative science, see the discussion in Bookstein (2014, Sec. E4.3), or Perrin's own book (English translation, 1923), which is still in print. One specific application of these ideas is to the theory of repeated evolutionary shocks. Jonathan Weiner's review of the work of the Grants on Darwin's finches (Weiner, 1995) discusses this possibility explicitly, and William Calvin's exploration of the role of climate variability in human evolution (Calvin, 2002) considers but rejects the same hypothesis in favor of a "climate ratchet," a pattern of shocks leading only to increases in brain size, not to decreases. For one explicit methodological experiment in the application of all these quantitative models to hominid evolution, see the formal statistical theory in Bookstein (2013b).

A separate model, the *Ornstein–Uhlenbeck walk,* combines a random walk for one or several traits with another classic notion, that of *stabilizing selection.* In this scenario, a random walk is tempered by a very weak but continual trend back toward the peak of a very broad fitness surface shaped like a paraboloid (for just a single measurement, a parabola) opening downward. Figure 2.51 shows two different variants of this model. In the left panel, the two measurements change independently over time. In the right panel, their changes are dependent, and a startling cyclic structure emerges that goes beyond the verbal formulation of stabilization for which the model was supposedly appropriate. The emergence of spiraling in the right-hand panel is a genuinely counterintuitive surprise analogous to the emergence of periodicity in the *Lotka–Volterra* equations of ecology. Ornstein–Uhlenbeck models (mainly of the first kind, independent changes) have been the subject of intensive biomathematical investigation ever since their first promulgation by Lande (1979), but the profession has not yet agreed on any method for checking their implications by elementary numerical formulas.

2.6.3 Data on Phylogenies

Another data structure of great importance to the organismal biologist, a scenario more sophisticated and more demanding of auxiliary information than the time series in Section 2.6.2, organizes the empirical measurements around a *true phylogeny.* This is a branching diagram in which the tips of the branches are the living species that sustained the measurements, while the lines connecting them represent patterns of descent from common ancestors (usually, extinct species). These diagrams come in different flavors depending on the additional information they convey beyond the simple fact of speciations. The version on display in this subsection will presume that each bifurcation of a phylogenetic tree is accompanied by a geological date.

Let's begin with an obviously artificial example: two measurements X and Y that turn out to be identical over a little data set of ten species. Suppose the

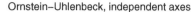

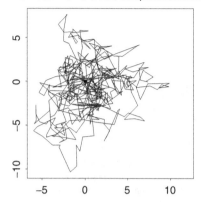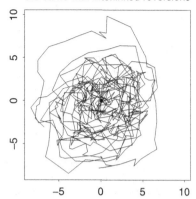

Figure 2.51 Ornstein–Uhlenbeck walks: simulations of an alternative to Brownian motion. (left) Two measurements carrying out independent O–U walks along an evolutionary trajectory. (right) The same when the dimensions are not independent, but rather changes in either have regressions on both. Compare either of these figures to the true Brownian motions in Figures 2.48 and 2.49.

measurements turn out to be $X = (0, 0, 0, 0, 0, 0, 0, 0, 0, 1)$ and Y exactly the same. Then the correlation between X and Y is 1.0, which seems pretty big. But still we can ask the reasonable question of how often we would see this correlation "by chance." The best way of answering that question, at least for small populations like the one in this parable, is the method of *permutation testing*. Imagine that we had lost track of which species was which between the measurement of the X-character and the measurement of Y. Then how often, out of all the 3,628,800 possible pairings between the two sets of 10 measurements, do we get this same correlation of 1.0 (the maximum)? The answer is 362,880 times, exactly one-tenth of all those permutations. The "p-value," if you can't help talking that way, is 0.10.

Let me now make the example somewhat more realistic by replacing those scores of 0 with a random set of nine numbers averaging zero in a way that is uncorrelated between X and Y. Also, to make the arithmetic specific, I will set the standard deviation of these variations equal to 10% of the mean difference between the subset of nine species and the tenth. This might correspond to an actual phylogeny drawn for either variable, X or Y, as panel (a) of Figure 2.52. There results the data scatter in panel (b) of the figure, where the value B should be taken equal to 10 (our purported sample size) and there are nine points scattered around the center of the little circle shown with means of zero and variances of 1 in every direction.

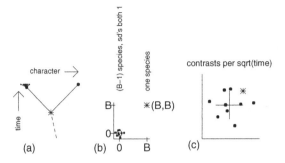

Figure 2.52 Why we need a phylogenetic correction when we study evolution across species (deep time). (a) A "true phylogeny" for one morphometric character measured on ten extant species. Horizontal, measured character; vertical, geological time (the present is along the top). Arbitrarily assume that the ratio of the duration of the adaptive radiation at upper left to the temporal divergence of the left genus from the right genus is 100. (b) Schematic of an analogous analysis for two characters. Regression and correlation analyses along the lines of this chapter are potentially sensible only when modeled in light of the true phylogeny, panel (a). (c) When character differences are scaled by the square root of net evolutionary time, the roles of regression and correlation are far less implausible.

Then formulas from the early sections of this chapter produce variances and covariances as follows. The variance of either variable, X or Y, equals its mean-square minus the square of its mean. The sum of squares on either axis has been set to $9 + B^2 = 109$, for a mean-square of 10.9, and either mean is just 1, so the variance of either axis is 9.9. The covariance is the mean crossproduct of X and Y, which works out to $B^2/10 = 10$, minus the product 1.0 of those same means, so the covariance is 9. Then the correlation in this population is expected to be 9/9.9, or 10/11.

The "statistical significance" of this association remains close to the value of 10% we computed in the $(0, \ldots, 0, 1)$ case. But the approach via the formulas of the next chapter would give us a spectacularly misleading answer for the same question. Formula (3.19) there, which would surely be valid had this same correlation arisen from a random (i.e., independently selected) sample of data distributed according to a pair of bell curves, gives us a Fisher's z-statistic of $\frac{1}{2} \log \frac{1 + \frac{10}{11}}{1 - \frac{10}{11}} = 1.522$, which is to be "tested" as a Gaussian with zero mean and a variance of $1/\sqrt{7}$. The result is a "significance level" of 0.00003, which is quite a long way from the actual probability of $\frac{1}{10}$ that we confirmed by explicitly testing the claim of a meaningful association. To know a true phylogeny is, in this context, to know a causal model of the the empirical data that is completely unrelated to the assumption of "independent sampling from a common distribution" on which the first five sections of this chapter, along with all those formulas for standard errors, tacitly relied.

Another way of thinking through this knot, which we will rely on in the course of our mammalian evolution example driving Figure 5.61, is to recall that one version of a regression slope is as a weighted average of component slopes such as the nine in Figure 2.52(b) that link each of the points around zero to the point at (10, 10). In the exposition of Section 2.2.2, these slopes, written $\frac{y_i - y_j}{x_i - x_j}$, were characterized by an error variance inversely proportional to the square of the *predictor* interval $x_i - x_j$. For present purposes, we would assert instead, based on the models of Section 2.6.2, that the errors of *both* numerator and denominator would each be *directly* proportional to the *time interval* over which the fragment of evolutionary history in question had accumulated. Assuming that the branch at the bottom of panel (a) is 100 times as far from the descendants at upper left as is their immediate common ancestor, as shown, we estimate the real evolutionary regression of one character on the other correctly only if we scale the contrast between the value B and all the others by the square root of its elapsed evolutionary time, which is to say, if we shrink its values of *both* measures by a factor of $\sqrt{100} = 10$. There results the scatter shown in panel (c) of the figure, for which a computed correlation or regression would be indistinguishable from zero. For an extended example involving this correction, along with the niceties of geometric morphometrics sketched in Section 5.4.6, see the discussion of Figure 5.60 in Chapter 5.

In short, this chapter's standard versions of regression analysis and correlation analysis seem just as inappropriate for data that arose from an evolutionary phylogeny (Figure 2.52a) as they were for data arising from a random walk (e.g., Figure 2.46): which is to say, they are inappropriate for just about any investigation of evolutionary patterns in deep time. The resolution of this impasse (here I summarize the far more detailed rationale in Felsenstein, 2004) is to model not the values of characters species by species, but instead their *contrasts*, meaning their differences along the various evolutionary paths conveyed by the phylogeny. One suitable model, for example, is the *Brownian diffusion*, which imputes to every comparison along a phylogeny an expected value of zero (that is, no selective gradient, on the average) with a variance proportional to the net geological time over which these putatively independent changes have accumulated. (In Figure 2.52, if B has a value of 10 as averaged over a very large number of quantitative characters, we would expect the ratio of divergence times between the two branching events shown (the bush at upper left, versus the higher-level bifurcation at the asterisk, lower center) there to be about 100. (On this argument, see also Bookstein, 2013b.) On the

Brownian model of the preceding subsection, differences between sibling species can be as "statistically significant," conventionally speaking, as you like, and still be completely without evolutionary meaning. (Of course, they might still entail functional consequences.) In studies of evolutionary process per se, the appropriate level of interrogation of the data is not about group mean differences but about contrasts as a function of evolutionary time, environmental variability, selection gradients, or other supraorganismal aspects of the process.

Summary of Section 2.6

- When your data come as the same measurement carried out at a fixed series of ages, often it is useful to inspect their relationships in sets of consecutive triples. When there is also more than one measurement, scatterplots can be more enlightening than line plots for this purpose, or else each measurement can be graphed or regressed against a summary score of the complete set.

- The exponent of height in the denominator of the familiar *body mass index,* weight divided by height squared, is close to the actual regression slope of log weight on log height in the human children of the Berkeley Guidance Study both in early childhood and in late adolescence, but not around the age of 9.

- The physical model of *random walk,* which applies equivalently to individual paths of shot down Galton's quincunx and to real Brownian motion, generates statistical series that can look like regression lines but have entirely different typical behaviors often described by the Arc-Sine Law instead of the Gaussian distribution.

- When the list of cases of a regression analysis has been generated by a process of branching with memory (for instance, a biological phylogeny), the corresponding prediction errors should not be taken as independent (as in Section 2.2). Instead, according to Joe Felsenstein's method of *contrasts,* one should analyze the innovations of each entity or branch with respect to the entities on the entities or branches nearby, using a weighting factor equal to the reciprocal square root of the net elapsed evolutionary interval from the last common ancestor of the branches in question.

3

Multiple Regression, in General and in Special Settings

Chapter 2 showed how to use the simple geometry of ellipses and the elegant algebra of line-fitting mainly to predict one single measurement by another in the presence of measurement variation. When this variation is just measurement noise of small amplitude, the interpretation of the situation can profitably focus on the *slope* of the straight line the data nearly fit. But when the variation is substantial, as is usually the case when it comes from real biological variability, the interpretation more likely deals with the pattern of the prediction *errors,* and how they do or do not look like a Gaussian distribution centered on the line and of constant error variance, rather than with the prediction slope per se. For example, the standard arithmetic of equation (2.7) always gives you a straight line as the prediction whether or not the class means actually lie along it (Figure 2.29) – but it is those class means, together with the variation around them, that actually bring you the information about organisms you were after.

A related setting had been familiar to natural scientists for a hundred years before Pearson and Galton. The methods of *geodesy,* the least-squares "relaxation" of networks of interpoint distance and elevation measurements, had been used since the French revolution to improve the accuracy of mapped point-locations on Earth's surface. Geodetic analyses are targeted to the estimation of rigorous physical constants (e.g., the exact location of the top of Mount Everest; see Keay, 2000) up to the inevitable measurement errors that, equally inevitably, diminish as instruments improve over the decades. In this context, what we need to know about measurement error is mainly how to compute its variance (so as to be realistic about its implications, such as the locations of legal boundaries). Unlike the situation in biology, geodetic measurement error is not telling us about any true variability pertinent to the underlying phenomenon of interest; it only tells about the accuracy of that year's measuring machines.

In effect, then, we have been talking about two different types of scientific explanation that happen to have the same algebra. One of them, beloved of physicists, involves more and more exact estimates of the coefficients of an exact law in a situation of steadily less instrument noise decade after decade. The other, exemplified in the Pearson example (Figure 2.28), instead is concerned with least-squares prediction in the presence of large variation that, in the course of most of the examples here, arises instead as real biological variability. In this second context the main factors of increased precision are increasing sample size – there is an N in the denominator of formula (2.10) – and approximate linearity of the formula chosen, and what is particularly important to the credibility of the arithmetic is the match of the resulting coefficients from measure to measure, experiment to experiment.

We can imagine two different ways of generalizing this arithmetic. In one thrust, there is no single focus of prediction, but rather it is the pattern of *all* of the bivariate relationships that is of interest. That setting requires the methods for examining whole patterns of covariances that are the subject of Chapter 4. In the other thrust, one particular outcome measurement is of the greatest concern, but we know in advance about more than one possibly important predictor. In this setting, we need to combine the predictors into a more accurate (or informative, or suggestive) overall formula. It is this task that is the concern of the present chapter.

For this second, more limited type of investigation, a corresponding arithmetic coalesced in the method of *multiple linear regression* first propounded by another British statistician, G. Udny Yule, just before the turn of the twentieth century. The data sets he studied tended to come from the social sciences, agriculture, or medicine. But the new technique quickly caught the attention of applied statisticians across a wide range of fields. By 1918 it had moved deeper into biometrics in the hands of Sewall Wright, an American whose work along these lines is reviewed later here. Next the focus of this toolkit shifted back into a social science, econometrics, in the work of the Cowles Commission in the 1920s and 1930s. A final metamorphosis led to the standard statistical notation in today's textbooks of linear modeling, through the pedagogics of C. R. Rao and others beginning in the 1950s.

By now this toolkit is so established a part of the conventional curriculum that considerations of the type raised in this chapter, investigations of the foundation of epistemology and inference at the root of the method, are hardly ever raised any more. Even now, in 2018, more than a century after all the fundamental innovations, it is appropriate to broach these basic issues anew for today's quantitative scientists. The distractions of high-dimensional pattern detection and "data mining" should not exempt us from the obligation to examine the language by which we use data patterns to explain things, and linear explanations ("the more X, or the more Y, the more Z"), when not misleading, remain by far the simplest to report and act on. Even complex situations *sometimes* accord with this simple linear statistical language.

This chapter is concerned with assessing the quality of simplifications like those and with properly communicating the valid inferences about organisms that follow from them. A rhetoric of "the more the ..., the more the ..." is not enough; indeed *it should not be enough* to persuade a principled skeptic however constructive. The slopes of the implied regressions must be robust and stable across multiple predictors measured across multiple studies, and they must be in at least rough agreement with the arithmetic of the same processes when observed using data measured at other levels, e.g., cell division rates as one underlying mechanism for physical growth. This chapter deals mainly with the simultaneous consideration of multiple "the more X, the more Z" statements for a common Z. The following chapter will broaden its purview to the setting of different Z's as well.

To begin, Sections 3.1 and 3.2 present the most general scheme, least-squares prediction of one continuous measurement by multiple others. Section 3.1 introduces the three quite different languages that you can use to report the same arithmetic, depending on your application and your scientific epistemology. The example worked here is a generic one involving three measurements of 35 sparrows that are part of a data set collected in 1898 for a quite different purpose. This general approach extends to a good special-purpose graphic, the *added-variable plot*, for deciding when any predictor "adds information" to the analysis based on some preexisting shorter list. As Section 3.2 explains, the added-variable method can alternatively be construed as a way of forcing the noncorrelation of predictors at the level of explicit scores instead of regression slopes, which had been the concern of Section 3.1. The pair of techniques is then exemplified in two settings. Example 3.1 is a matter of human public health (the effects of passive smoking on two common diseases); Example 3.2, a practical obstetrical concern, the forecasting of birthweight by prenatal image measurements.

The remainder of the chapter surveys five special cases, each with an example or two. The first of these, analysis of covariance, is illustrated by Example 3.3 in Section 3.3. Here we extend Example 2.5 on the protist *Tetrahymena* and continue with an overview (Example 3.4) of a long-standing dispute in vertebrate evolution, the development and systematics of the brain weight – body weight ratio. The examples are accompanied by the dissection of a classic fallacy, the *ecological fallacy*, that often greatly interferes with valid reports of this type of computation. A second special case, growth curve analysis, is the topic of Section 3.4 as illustrated in Example 3.5 by the data from the Berkeley Growth Study that we encountered once before when we didn't have the added-variable plot device yet, and also by Example 3.6, the Vilmann rodent skull data, likewise expanded from Chapter 2. The third and fourth special cases are both versions of what is usually called *discriminant analysis*, the assignment of specimens to groups. Section 3.5 is about *linear discriminant analysis*, a tool introduced in the 1930s by R. A. Fisher. It is the main tool used in Example 3.7, which concerns a much older published data set on the mortality of sparrows caught in a snowstorm (the original scientific context of the data used for Section 3.1). Another algebra of discrimination, *quadratic discriminant analysis*, is demonstrated using two data sets of my own, Examples 3.8 and 3.9, about the effect of high prenatal alcohol exposure on one particular part of the human brain.

3.1 The General Logic of Multiple Regression

The mechanism of Galton's quincunx is simple indeed. There is only one physical process at work, "falling down the quincunx." Conceptual difficulties enter as soon as we imagine there to be more than one separate process at work – it is quite difficult to imagine, for example, two separate "directions" of gravity. An experimentalist would surely design a study carefully enough that it highlighted just one mechanism at a time. Nevertheless, today's statistically minded researcher typically tries to work instead with the less optimal data resources that, in place of the discipline and invasiveness of the true experiment, compensate by considering multiple explanations at the same time. In these contexts, success consists in winnowing that list of possible explanations so that at most one or two from the set of alternate explanations plausibly apply.

In keeping with David Freedman's pessimism about the prevalence of good multiple regressions (see Section 3.1.4), it is surprisingly difficult to find sound examples of the fundamental geometrical setup here. For teaching purposes I have extracted a subset of three variables from a data set that will be introduced in Section 3.5 in its original scientific context, which was a test of Darwin's "hypothesis" in the course of a natural experiment involving a Rhode Island snowstorm. That data set, listed in this book's online resource, will involve 59 adult male sparrows altogether, each measured in nine different morphometric ways. To demonstrate one actual multiple linear regression, I limit the data to just the 35 birds that survived the snowstorm (since the nonsurvivors had different averages) and to total length, wingspread, and femur length only. One might focus down on a restricted measurement list like this in order to explore a question like the following: Given a pleiotropic measurement like "total length," presumably the summary of a great many different genetic and epigenetic influences and factors, is it more reflective of other pleiotropic measures, such as wingspread, or instead of measurements like femur length that are of lesser scope but greater immediate functional relevance? (But remember that this was not Bumpus's actual reason for collecting these data.)

In addition to this actual Bumpus 1898 data subset – call it **Version 1** – we will be considering a fictional **Version 2** where total length and wingspread will be taken as uncorrelated: being high on either will not alter the average value of the other. In both versions, there will be a **true model** by which wingspread and femur length jointly predict total length according to the following equation:

$$\text{total length} = \text{constant} + 0.2237 \times \text{wingspread} + 2.5188 \times \text{femur length} + \varepsilon,$$
(3.1)

where "constant" is some centering scalar whose value is of no particular interest at this time (but which is crucial to the study of the snowstorm effect per se; see Section 3.5), and ε is, as usual, a *residual* (regression error) uncorrelated with both of the predictor scores and averaging zero. Such a design is tacitly accommodated by the layout of Figure 3.1, which treats wingspread and femur length symmetrically (as Cartesian axes, which are a proper substrate for linear combinations) but displays total length as a number instead of a coordinate, suggesting that it will have a different logical role. All measurements are in millimeters. The correlation of total length with wingspread is 0.610; of total length with femur length, 0.694; of wingspread with femur length, 0.591.

Figure 3.2 draws out the geometry of equation (3.1) as it would apply to Version 1. The oblique lines in the figure are contours of equal predicted total length according to the model in equation (3.1). These lines are precisely straight and evenly spaced millimeter by millimeter. You interpret them just as a hiker would interpret the analogous lines of constant height on a contour map of a mountain – these are the paths that involve no change in level. Perpendicular to them is the direction of steepest descent or ascent, the *gradient* of the height field. This gradient direction is (0.0885, 0.9961), the unit vector along the vector (0.2237, 2.5188) of the actual regression coefficients to come. (Perpendicularity is in the geometry of this figure, which implicitly normalized the ranges of the two dimensions plotted.)

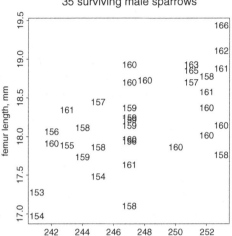

total length (mm) by wingspread and femur length
35 surviving male sparrows

Figure 3.1 Three measured lengths for 35 living adult male sparrows revived after a snowstorm in Providence, Rhode Island, in February 1898. Wingspread and femur length are plotted along the axes; total length is the printed number inside the scatterplot itself. Total length and wingspread were originally measured to the nearest millimeter. Femur length was originally reported in thousandths of inches; I have converted those data to millimeters for this analysis.

Figure 3.3 shows the same geometry for Version 2, the fictional data instead of the data actually measured. The contour lines are the same, but now they fit the fictional data of total length exactly.

In real applications, the geometry of the contours in Figure 3.2 or 3.3 is not incidental to the method but an absolute mandate. Perhaps it is more clearly viewed as the three-dimensional construction in Figure 3.4, a tilted plane in projected view instead of a contour map. If the following algebraic computations are to have any scientific meaning, the surface (or hypersurface, if there are more than two predictors) representing averaged values of the outcome over clusters of jointly specified predictor values must at least approximately manifest the symmetries indicated in the diagram. Specifically: for the coefficients of a multiple regression equation to correspond to what one would reasonably expect from an actual *intervention* on the system under study, whether experimental or hypothetical (e.g., historical), the observed effect of any incremental change in any single predictor value must be independent of the values of *all* the predictors. As Lieberson (1985) notes, it

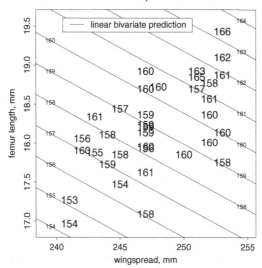

Figure 3.2 Contour map for the linear regression model of equation (3.1) superimposed over the scatter in Figure 3.1 (Version 1). Integers in large print, measured total lengths; other integers, levels of equal predicted value according to equation (3.1).

must also be the case that intervening by *raising* the value of a predictor must have precisely the opposite effect of intervening by *lowering* the predictor to the same extent, or, putting the same point another way, if you intervene to set the value of a predictor to 4, it cannot matter whether you brought it up from 3 or down from 5. Moreover, the *error* around this prediction must be independent of the values of *all* the predictors. Geometrically, any cut of the surface by a vertical plane parallel to one of the predictor axes must result in a curve of *conditional expectation* that takes the form of a straight line never varying in slope regardless of how the sectioning plane is translated. For more than two predictors, these statements about intervention and independence apply to all of the possible combinations.

These assumptions are demanding. Usually, too, they are hidden from the reader's scrutiny by concealment under a meaningless phrase such as the Latin *ceteris paribus*, "other things being equal." For more on the underlying epistemology, see, for instance, Freedman (2009) or Mosteller and Tukey (1977). Much of our praxis in the examples of this chapter concerns their conscientious verification caveat by caveat.

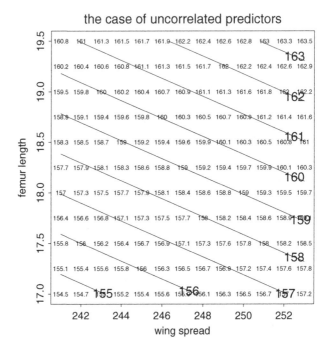

Figure 3.3 Fictional data set for Version 2 of the sparrow lengths example: 143 artificial "specimens" constrained to a correlation of precisely zero between wingspread and femur length, together with a total length that is exactly as predicted by equation (3.1), without any prediction error. Light solid segments are isolines of total length according to equation (3.1). Now the large numbers index these segments, while the small numbers are individual values of total length assigned in this fictional setting. These values fit the equation without error before they were rounded to print to one significant digit.

3.1.1 Interpretation 1: The Counterfactual of Uncorrelated Predictors

The approach to multiple regression that makes the most sense begins with the relationships between these two predictors and their joint outcome *separately*. For Version 2 these are plotted, each with its corresponding regression line, in the left panels of Figures 3.5 (for the wingspread predictor) and 3.6 (for the femur length predictor).

In these left panels one sees the linear structure of the prediction modeled in equation (3.1) along with the balanced nature of this version of the data set: the distribution of residuals around the regression line is the same at every separate value of the predictor. The slopes of the regression lines shown are

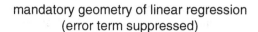

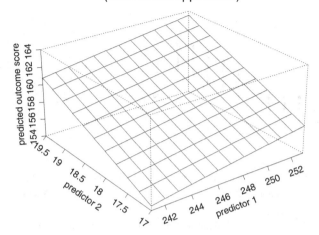

Figure 3.4 Exact geometry of multiple regression in this two-predictor case. The actual regression equation treated as an error-free account: a flat conditional mean surface over the plane of the predictors. See text.

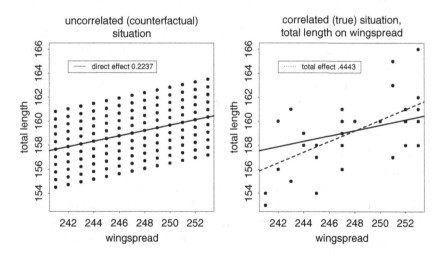

Figure 3.5 Two regressions for total length on wingspread. (left) Version 2, fictional predictors uncorrelated and without prediction error, as explained in the text. (right) Version 1, actual data (correlated predictors and actual prediction error). Heavy solid line, both panels: the true direct path. Dashed line at right: the "total effect," which requires a correction for predictor correlation.

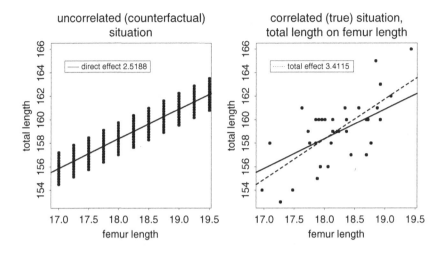

Figure 3.6 The same for predicting total length by femur length.

exactly those of equation (3.1): 0.2237 for wingspread (Figure 3.5), 2.5188 for femur length (Figure 3.6). The coefficient for femur length is much larger in part because that average length itself is much smaller (as per the axis ranges in Figure 3.1).

Version 2, you recall, involves a fictional data set where, as promised, there is no correlation between the two predictors of total length. Instead, each one covers its full range with perfect evenness regardless of the value of the other. This is called the case of **orthogonal** or **uncorrelated** predictors, hence the title of Figure 3.3. In Figures 3.5 and 3.6 we see that the corresponding univariate regressions yield precisely the correct slopes – for wingspread, 0.2237; for femur length, 2.5188. Here "correct slopes" are slopes that equal the coefficients in equation (3.1) that generated the data being modeled.

But when we change from the unrealistically symmetrical scheme of Version 2, Figure 3.3, back to the real situation in Version 1, Figure 3.2, we alter the regressions for the plots of the *actual* total length against the *actual* predictors. As Figures 3.5 and 3.6 show, these regressions shift from the solid lines to the dotted lines, which evidently have different, thus *incorrect*, slopes even though they still pass through the centroid of the data scatter.

The main purpose of **multiple regression analysis** in such applications is to make possible the recovery of the correct coefficients when the competing predictors are no longer uncorrelated. In practice, one uses a computer for this. In the environment of your favorite statistical package (I am using one called

"Splus," but today it is more common to use a close analogue called "R") you type a command like

```
summary(lm(bumpus.male.using[,"TotalLength"]~
bumpus.male.using[,c("Wingspread","FemurLength")]))
```

where "lm" is an acronym for "linear model." Seemingly instantaneously you receive a response[1] that will include the following information:

```
           Value Std. Error t value Pr(>|t|)
(Intercept) 57.7798 21.6852 2.6645 0.0120
Wingspread   0.2237  0.1078 2.0757 0.0460
FemurLength  2.5188  0.7276 3.4619 0.0015
Residual standard error: 1.955 on 32 degrees of
   freedom
Multiple R-Squared: 0.5435
F-statistic: 19.05 on 2 and 32 degrees of freedom,
   the p-value is 3.552e-06
```

For a regression like this one with both predictors so far from zero, the line labeled "(Intercept)" does not concern us. In the third and fourth lines, the first number printed is the estimated direct effect (see below) and the second is its standard error under sampling variation (equation 2.10). The third column is the ratio of the first column to the second. The values here, 2.08 versus 3.46, suggest that the dependence of predicted total length on femur length is calibrated nearly twice as precisely as its dependence on wingspread. The fourth column sets out the "tail-probability" of either of these effects against a "null hypothesis," an approach I will deprecate throughout this book as of absolutely no scientific importance in any well-designed morphometric study. (The column headed "$Pr(> |t|)$" is generated by computations that assume some linear model is true and that regression error is distributed as a Gaussian: see footnote 12 in Chapter 2.) The same is true of the content of the bottom line, the "F-statistic." This is the ratio of explained variance to what is expected on a hypothesis of complete noncorrelation between total length and either wingspread or femur length. But that hypothesis is entirely irrelevant to any rational investigation of this data, as shown by its p-value of 0.00000355 according to this same line.

---

[1] This is one example of the only actual computer printed output format included in this book. For all other computations I will be demonstrating, there is no consensus about the format or contents of printouts like these. Any program I might supply would surely be superseded early in the lifetime of a published volume like this one. The formulas, on the other hand, will endure permanently.

The analysis thereby becomes of some scientific use. The correlation between predicted and observed total length (which is also called the "multiple correlation of total length on wingspread and femur length" – it is usually written with a capital R) is the square root of 0.5435, or .737, which is larger than the correlation of total length with either wingspread (0.61) or femur length (0.69) separately. The estimated standard deviation for the prediction error of total length is 1.955, which compares favorably to its observed standard deviation of 2.807. In the conventional language of "explained variance" (although in this book the goal is always to explain biological processes, not variance) we have reduced the variance to a fraction $1 - r^2 = 0.4565$ of its original value. The lowest predicted length, about 154, is 1.8 standard deviations below the mean (159) of the variable being predicted, and the highest predicted value, about 163, is more than 1.4 standard deviations above that mean. So we have learned something important about total length in terms of its scaling with other meaningful measurements of these flying systems.

Now return to Figures 3.5 and 3.6 to see exactly how the multiple regression corrected for the failure of noncorrelation of the predictors. First, recall what failure of the simple scatters it is that requires correcting. At right in Figure 3.5 is the partial analysis for the prediction of total length by wingspread alone. The dots correspond to the real data in Figure 3.1, with the horizontal axis the same as the wingspread plotted there and the vertical the value of total length that was printed on the earlier plot. This right-hand panel presents two lines. One copies the true regression of total length on wingspread, as already sketched on the left (which was in turn copied from the regression fit to be justified in a moment). The other represents the apparent regression slope computed from just this subset of the data, ignoring the data of femur length and its correlation of 0.59 with wingspread.

It is clear that the slopes of the partial predictions in the rightmost pair of plots have changed from those in the uncorrelated case *even though the model, equation (3.1), is the same*. Because wingspread and femur length are positively correlated, the points at the left of the wingspread range have a lower average femur length and thus a lower average total length than would be predicted from their wingspread alone. The opposite bias applies for the points at the right of the wingspread range, where large wingspread goes with long femur length and thus results in a higher average total length than is accountable to the high wingspread alone. By virtue of the combination of these two shifts, the dashed regression line here has been tipped upward with respect to the true model. Its slope is now 0.4443, versus the value of 0.2237 that is the biologically meaningful value according to equation (3.1).

Similarly, as the right-hand panel of Figure 3.6 demonstrates, the *same* correlation between wingspread and femur length accounts for a similar upward bias in the partial prediction of total length by femur length. As the points of lowest femur length are associated with narrower wingspreads, they average lower total lengths than would be appropriate for their femur length per se. Similarly, the subjects of highest femur length average a larger wingspread than the others, and thus have an average total length that is elevated beyond what is appropriately attributed to that high femur length alone. The regression slope that ought to have been 2.4155 is incorrectly computed as 3.5188 instead.

Hence whenever predictors of positive slope are themselves positively correlated, both slopes are overestimated by regressions like those at the right in Figures 3.5 and 3.6 – but these are just the predictions by the actual predictors taken one at a time. (An exactly analogous argument would apply if both predictors had negative slopes, whereas if their slopes were of opposite sign, then the logical problem here serves to drive them toward one another. All these tendencies reverse should the correlation between the predictors be negative.)

To understand our data correctly, we are obliged to compensate for the double-counting of the correlated effects of femur length and wingspread – to reduce the estimate of each back from the right-hand panels to the corresponding left-hand panels, which, as we have already noted, are correct. In other words, our job is to recover the **true values** 0.2237 and 2.4155 of equation (3.1) from the data of Figure 3.1 with its realistically correlated predictors.

We need a notation for the quantities we're trying to compute. It is customary to call them the **direct effects** d_{Wing}, d_{Femur} of the predictor variables. While this language sounds magisterially wise, it merely means that these are the coefficients that will appear in equations like (3.1) intended to quantify the separate mechanisms of ultimate scientific interest. Though there may indeed have been two processes that together underlie the data actually encountered, apparently they have been commingled – superimposed by the organism itself – before anything was measured. The quantities we extracted from the correlated-predictors figure are the (numerically different) **total effects** t_{Wing}, t_{Femur} expressing only the separate regression slopes of the outcome measure upon the predictors, not any deeper understanding of the quantitative situation.

The total effect t_{Wing} of wingspread exceeds the direct effect d_{Wing} we're interested in by the amount that is **indirect via femur length.** A rise of 1 unit in wingspread, according to this logic, is "associated" (we are making no claim as to how, and may actually remain clueless as long as we wish) with a rise of some number of units $b_{Femur.Wing}$ of femur length. (The dot in the subscript notation is read as the word "given," so the subscript is "femur length given wingspread"). That rise, in turn, produces the "extra" effect $t_{Wing} - d_{Wing}$ that we are trying to subtract out of t to arrive at d. We get this value of b (and also its counterpart, the reverse regression coefficient $b_{Wing.Femur}$ that we will need presently) from the analysis of Chapter 2 as applied to the pair of predictors by themselves, as in Figure 3.7.

The slope $b_{Femur.Wing}$ that we need is just the ordinary regression slope for the prediction of femur length by wingspread. This slope turns out to be 0.0876: on the average, increase of wingspread by one millimeter is associated with an increase in femur length of about 0.09 of that amount. To repeat, there is no associated claim of causality here. This quantity 0.0876 is the net effect on femur length of the variation induced in wingspread by *all* the causes of

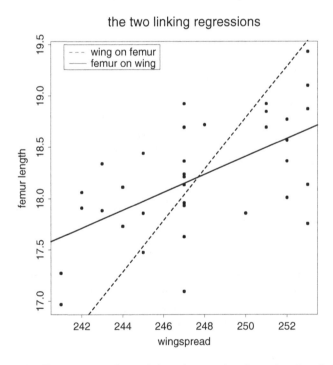

Figure 3.7 The two regressions relating wingspread to femur length and vice versa, one for each of the normal equations. We saw this construction before in Figure 2.28. The intersection of the two lines is at the centroid of this scatterplot, $\overline{wingspread} = 247.7$, $\overline{femurlength} = 18.2$. These data might indeed be plausibly taken as elliptical with linear class means, in keeping with the assumptions of the Wright path interpretation.

wingspread that also have effects on femur length – it is those unknown "joint causes" that are abstractly held responsible for the correlation we see.

So we get **one equation** relating the two d's:

$$d_{Wing} + 0.0876 \times d_{Femur} = 0.4443. \tag{3.2}$$

This is called the first **normal equation,** a name you have seen before.

Similarly, to correct the total effect 3.5188 of femur length on total length, Figure 3.6 (right), for the indirect path through wingspread (even though we still have no theory as to why they covary), we first extract an adjustment factor for the rise in wingspread associated (whether explicably or inexplicably) with a rise in femur length. We get this adjustment from the *other* regression in Figure 3.7, the dashed line, which is the regression of wingspread on femur length. This slope is 3.9902, resulting in the second normal equation:

$$3.9902 \times d_{Wing} + d_{Femur} = 3.4115. \tag{3.3}$$

Copy the first one again:

$$d_{Wing} + 0.0876 \times d_{Femur} = 0.4443.$$

Just as in Section 2.1, these equations are solved by determinants:

$$d_{Wing} = (0.4443 \times 1 - 0.0876 \times 3.4115)/(1 \times 1 - 0.0876 \times 3.9902)$$
$$= 0.2237,$$
$$d_{Femur} = (3.4115 \times 1 - 0.443 \times 3.9902)/(1 \times 1 - 0.0876 \times 3.9902)$$
$$= 2.5188.$$

The computation checks, of course: we recover the coefficients of the dashed lines in Figures 3.2–3.3 as $0.4443 = 0.2237 + 2.5188 \times .0876$, $3.4115 = 2.5188 + 3.9902 \times 0.2237$ (all arithmetic carried out to seven digits, not the four printed).

In this way **we have recovered the coefficients of the uncorrelated-predictors figure from the data of the correlated-predictors figure.** Geometrically, we have recovered the slope of the coordinate plane *sections* in Figure 3.4 from slopes of its coordinate plane *projections*. All those logical assumptions pertaining to the method were necessary for the subterfuge to succeed. These coefficients are called **multiple regression coefficients**, or sometimes **beta weights** (because many textbooks write them using the Greek letter β, beta).

Pause now to try and decide what it means to "get back to the uncorrelated-predictors figure" from data that started out looking like the correlated-predictors figure. The coefficients 0.2237 and 2.5188 are usually phrased as "the effect of wingspread holding everything else [in this case, femur length] constant" and, symmetrically, "the effect of femur length holding wingspread constant." What that means is, precisely, a conversion of the explanation to the scenario of the uncorrelated-predictors figure, in which the predictors have been forcibly **un**correlated by some abstract cancellation, such as an experimental intervention, of *all* of the common causes they actually share. Nothing is in fact "held constant" in any real sense. It is all an "as if": the fiction of uncorrelated predictors, exploited in order to guess at the effect of an intervention that was not actually carried out.

Therefore, although the coefficients 0.2237 and 2.5188 enter into a least-squares prediction of the value of total length from the values of wingspread and femur length (as we shall see in a moment), this is an accident of algebra. What these numbers really represent is **a kind of explanation,** one that philosophers of science call a *counterfactual.* **If** wingspread were found to be uncorrelated with femur length, in some alternate world (or alternate data set, perhaps as the result of some genetic knockout), **then** their separate predictions of total length would be the numbers we just computed. In that world you could change wingspread without changing femur length, or vice versa, and the effect of the wingspread change would then be 0.2237 mm of additional total length per millimeter change in wingspread, or 2.5188 mm of additional total length per additional millimeter of femur length. It is because we cannot guarantee the invariance of femur length over that change of wingspread, and vice versa, that these expectations are counterfactual, which is to say, biologically unreal.

Two more diagrams help us tidy up our understanding of this complex situation. In Figure 3.8, actual total length is plotted against its multivariate prediction from equation (3.1). The regression line is necessarily $Y = X$, diagonal of the square, and there are no gross deviations from ellipticity such as will be seen in Figure 3.13. The relation of that diagonal to the implicit ellipse bounding this scatter distribution echoes the geometric theorem about its tangency at piercing points that was introduced and proved in Figure 2.24.

It is also worth checking whether additional geometric terms beyond the linear would improve our prediction in this setting. Figure 3.9 shows the result of a fit that incorporates additional terms in wingspread squared, femur length squared, and wingspread times femur length. While the rotation of the corresponding contour lines from lower left to upper right is suggestive, the net effect of the additional three terms is to actually *lower* the strength of the evidence. (Likelihood in the multiple regression model is roughly proportional to sample size times the log of the root mean square residual. But that estimated root mean square prediction error actually *increases* a bit when we augment the linear predictors by those three quadratic terms – the unexplained variance

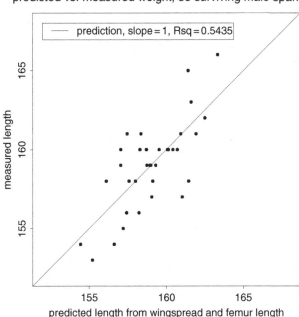

predicted vs. measured weight, 35 surviving male sparrows

predicted length from wingspread and femur length

Figure 3.8 Predicted versus observed total length. The regression of observed on predicted must be the diagonal line drawn.

drops more slowly than the divisor $(n-k)$ in the formula analogous to equation (2.30b) – meaning that there is no evidence here against the decision to pursue understanding via the two coefficients of the multiple linear regression alone.)[2]

3.1.2 Interpretation 2: The Path Analysis

The preceding was analysis by regressions, but one can rework the same argument using correlations instead. (In other words, assume that all variables have mean 0 and variance 1, so I can write all slopes using the same letter r

---

[2] The claim is *not* that the rotation from lower left to upper right in the contours of Figure 3.9 is not biologically real. Rather, what we are inferring from the stability (nonshrinkage) of this residual sum of squares is that the present sample is much too small for adequate quantification of any such trend, together with any insights that might follow from knowing its magnitude. An appropriate analysis would require a substantially different experimental design, perhaps one with twelve times as many birds. (In a sample twelve times the size of this one, an effect of the magnitude shown in the figure would be more than three times its own standard error.) There is an excellent discussion of this point, the wisdom of *not* speculating on effects of small magnitude in studies that were not intended to estimate them, in D. R. Anderson (2008).

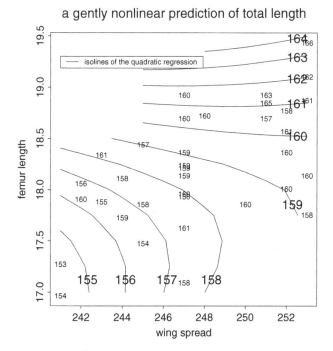

Figure 3.9 The same contour representation for a convenient nonlinear surface fit (a quadratic regression). Integers in small font represent data; those in large font, contour levels. The slope of the lines in Figure 3.2 is not obviously invalid as a key to the "expected" total length.

instead of the letter t, total effect, I have been using up to this point.) Let the predictors be X and Y and the dependent variable be Z, and write r_{XY}, r_{XZ}, r_{YZ} for the three correlations among these three variables. Then, as Figure 3.10 diagrams, we want to estimate coefficients $d_{Z.X}, d_{Z.Y}$, the *direct effects* of X or Y on Z, where, in words,

the total effect r_{XZ} on Z of a unit change in X is the sum of its direct effect $d_{Z.X}$ and its *indirect effect via Y*, which is r_{XY}, the expected rise in Y given that same unit change in X, times the direct effect $d_{Z.Y}$ of Y on Z;

or, in an equation,

$$r_{XZ} = d_{Z.X} + r_{XY}d_{Z.Y}. \tag{3.4a}$$

Similarly, in words (not shown) and then in a second equation,

$$r_{YZ} = d_{Z.Y} + r_{XY}d_{Z.X} = r_{XY}d_{Z.X} + d_{Z.Y}. \tag{3.4b}$$

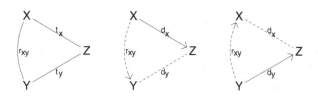

Figure 3.10 The logic of multiple regression as a path analysis is expressed well in the form of a diagram indicating the observable quantities (left panel) and the two compound paths (center and right panels) that are intended to account for them.

It is convenient to be able to talk in terms of these competing processes, but no such rhetorical advantage comes for free: one must be able to argue persuasively that the distinction between the two is at least potentially real. There must be arguments, for instance, that it is at least conceivable to mount an intervention on one path but not the other, or that they correspond to nonoverlapping mechanisms at some lower level of explanation. The didactic example just concluded, on how wingspread and femur length jointly predict total length, comports with that requirement in two ways. First, the effect of wingspread is pertinent to one functional domain, flying, whereas the effect of femur length is pertinent to the quite different domain of hopping or grabbing hold of branches. One can imagine selection gradients customized for one or the other. Second, the embryological compartments entailed in these two length measurements are quite distinct, both as regards average extent (mean lengths differing by a factor of more than ten) and as regards proportions down the proximal–distal axis. It would be as reasonable to search for a gene affecting one of these but not the other as, say, it was reasonable in Hallgrimsson's study of murine facial form (Hallgrimsson, 2015) to search for a gene affecting brain forward projection without direct effects on other neurocranial dimensions.

Ultimately, the claim that a multiple regression is a valid part of the study of any complex organized system rests on demonstrations of causality in experiments specific to the entangled processes one by one. Any nonlinearity of the relation among one or more pairs of putative "causes" would violate the ostensibly reasonable accounting for indirect paths that was shown in Figure 3.10. That and other failures of our linear assumptions would render the claims of multiple pathways quite insecure even had the data been collected in an appropriately randomized experiment. One should also be skeptical of the biases that might have been induced by sample selection criteria (here, the requirement that the birds in question did not freeze to death during the snowstorm, and that Prof. Bumpus saw them lying on the ground on his walk to work that day). Indeed, few published multiple regressions can withstand the scrutiny that we are here devoting to this specific example. But that is no reason to ignore those requisites. Rather, we are obligated by today's professional ethics to keep them in mind in order that our reports can be intellectually honest and modest. In particular, every multiple regression rests on an explicit defense of the reality of the direct and indirect paths it implicitly presumes.

In this respect the example at hand, though entirely pedagogical in its purpose, will closely parallel the reanalyses of two published claims to follow. The topic in Example 3.1 is the multiplicity of pathways by which an environmental condition (passive smoking) might alter the rate of heart attacks, and the corresponding multipath logic rests on the retrieval of an experimentally confirmable mechanism (platelet aggregation) corresponding to a numerically similar estimate of the same direct effect, in a design that itself ignored "everything else," all those correlations of smoking with other criteria of heart health or heart risk (diet, exercise, etc.). These correlations can remain unexplained (why, indeed, do smokers eat fewer carrots?) and yet the path analyses (e.g., Figure 3.11) are reliable calibrations of the main effect

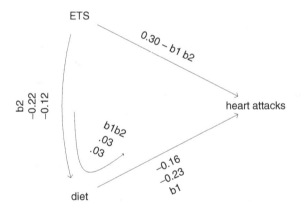

Figure 3.11 Path model for the analysis of the joint effects of environmental tobacco smoke (ETS) and diet on the risk of heart attacks in the nonsmoking wives of smokers. A raw effect size of 0.30 (excess risk 30%) is reduced by the net magnitude of an indirect effect combining the effect of smoking on fruits and vegetables in the diet, which is negative (the more smoking, the less fruit), and the effect of net fruits and vegetables in the diet on heart attacks, which is also negative (the less fruit, the more heart attacks). The indirect path evaluates to about +0.03 in two different ways (upper numbers, according to the fruit data; lower numbers, the vegetable data). b_1, predicted change of diet for 1 s.d. of change in ETS; b_2, predicted change in heart attack risk for one s.d. of change in diet; $b_1 b_2$, indirect path, of magnitude about 3%, for correcting the predicted change of 30% in heart attack risk for their joint association with diet.

of concern, and the original authors' interpretation ("the rate of heart attacks [among spouses of smokers] is a serious environmental hazard, and one that is easily avoided") is a sound pointer to a potentially important intervention.

Such a reanalysis with its one dominant path is more robust than the reanalysis in Example 3.2, the prediction of a baby's birthweight. In this second example the duality of the two predictive paths is considerably clearer – the paths are separate just *because* the physical mensurand (body weight) sums over the contributions of multiple separate components – and yet the take-home message for practitioners turns out not to have overlapped much with the findings of the multiple regressions.

3.1.3 Interpretation 3: Least Squares

Now start all over, temporarily ceasing all talk about scientific reality but just sticking to the arithmetic. For whatever reason, imagine we are trying to fit a plane "$Z \sim d_{Z.X} X + d_{Z.Y} Y$" to some data about X, Y, and Z by least squares. If you want you can think of this as a model $Z = d_{Z.X} X + d_{Z.Y} Y + \varepsilon$ for a least-squares estimated ε, a calculation that will be maximum-likelihood if the model is true and the real ε is normally distributed, etc. For convenience, let N stand for the number of cases and assume X, Y, and Z have all been set to mean 0 and variance 1 before we started calculating, so that $\Sigma X^2 = \Sigma Y^2 = N$ and $\Sigma XY = Nr_{XY}$, $\Sigma XZ = Nr_{XZ}$, $\Sigma YZ = Nr_{YZ}$. Our task is to minimize

$$Q = \Sigma(Z - d_{Z.X} X - d_{Z.Y} Y)^2 \tag{3.5}$$

as a function of its two unknown parameters $d_{Z.X}$ and $d_{Z.Y}$.

To minimize Q, set to zero its partial derivatives with respect to those two d's:

$$\frac{\partial Q}{\partial d_{Z.X}} = -2\Sigma X(Z - d_{Z.X} X - d_{Z.Y} Y) = 0, \tag{3.6i}$$

and likewise

$$\frac{\partial Q}{\partial d_{Z.Y}} = -2\Sigma Y(Z - d_{Z.X} X - d_{Z.Y} Y) = 0. \tag{3.6ii}$$

These are called the **normal equations** for the bivariate regression. If we had not assumed $\bar{X} = \bar{Y} = \bar{Z} = 0$, there would be a third normal equation $\Sigma 1(Z - d_{Z.X} X - d_{Z.Y} Y) = 0$, meaning that the prediction plane has to pass through the point $(\bar{X}, \bar{Y}, \bar{Z})$, the centroid of our data scatter.

The two normal equations are equivalent to the rearranged equations

$$d_{Z.X} \Sigma X^2 + d_{Z.Y} \Sigma XY = \Sigma XZ,$$
$$d_{Z.X} \Sigma XY + d_{Z.Y} \Sigma Y^2 = \Sigma YZ.$$

Cancelling the N in every term of both equations, in view of our assumptions about variances, we get

$$r_{XZ} = d_{Z.X} + r_{XY}d_{Z.Y},$$
$$r_{YZ} = r_{XY}d_{Z.X} + d_{Z.Y}. \tag{3.7}$$

But those are the same as the two equations (3.4a, 3.4b) at which we arrived at the end of the path analysis. So the path analysis, which is explicitly causal, gets us to the same coefficients as the ordinary least-squares fitting of the linear model, which, as usually set down, does not sound like it entails causality at all. To predict a third variable by a linear combination of two others – to "fit a plane" (or a hyperplane, if there are more than two predictors) – is just arithmetic. It did not seem that the coefficients of equation (3.5) were expected to have any particular scientific meaning, nor that they should apply to forecasts for specimens not already included in those sums of squares and cross-products. But the arithmetic cannot circumvent these postulates of direct and indirect causality.

If we change notation so that all the predictors X, Y, etc. are collected in one matrix X, rename Z as the letter Y freed up thereby, and introduce a vector d for the list $d_{Y.X_1}, d_{Y.X_2}, \ldots$ of all the regression coefficients together, we get to write the equations setting derivatives to zero (the *normal equations*, all together), as $(X'X)d = X'Y$, or

$$d = (X'X)^{-1}X'Y, \tag{3.8i}$$

which is where most textbooks anchor their notation. Likewise the predicted value can be written

$$\hat{Y} = Xd = X(X'X)^{-1}X'Y = HY, \tag{3.8ii}$$

where H is the *hat matrix* $X(X'X)^{-1}X'$, projection of the observed dependent variable Y onto the column space of the X's, as in Section 2.5.3. The estimated standard error of prediction is now derived from an equation like (2.30b) where the factor $N - 2$ in the denominator is replaced by $N - p - 1$, where p is the count of predictors. This is why the printed value of 1.955 was called an "an estimated standard error of prediction" back in Section 3.1.1; the actual standard deviation of the residuals from the regression as fitted is a smaller value, 1.897.

3.1.4 Rethinking All Three Versions

We now have seen three different interpretations of the least-squares equation for multiple predictors X_i of a single outcome Y. There were the *normal equations* for fitting a plane (that reduced to $\beta = (X'X)^{-1}X'Y$ and predictions $X(X'X)^{-1}X'Y$), the *counterfactual* adjustment-to-uncorrelated-predictors, and the *path equations*, after Sewall Wright, that arise from chipping apart a joint causal explanation into multiple separate processes each characterized by both direct and indirect paths as sketched in Figure 3.10.

It is mainly owing to this inescapable ambiguity that multiple regression is so often frustrating as part of actual applied statistical practice in biometrics (and everywhere else). In an essay with Hans Zeisel on the relation of the insecticide DDT to birth defects, David Freedman propounded a "parable":

> Some friends are lost in the woods and using a compass to find their way. If the compass is broken, pointing that out is a positive contribution to getting home safely. (Freedman and Zeisel, 1968:46)

To repair the compass (which the parable means to stand for multiple regression) one must closely inspect how its assumptions comport with the data not only for the study in hand but for the entire literature to which it is intended to contribute. (This is hardly a novel point; it was made first by Karl Pearson in the course to his objections to the method that Yule had just introduced with an eye on applications to welfare rates in late nineteenth-century London.) To be an effective example in a textbook like this one, the scientific finding will have to be a simple one: only one variable of interest, with the others serving as distractions from the main message. The student of that context will be helped, in turn, by another witty quote from David Freedman, this one from his 1991 essay "Statistical models and shoe leather":

> A crude four-point scale may be useful:
>
> 1. Regression usually works, although it is (like everything else) imperfect and may sometimes go wrong.
> 2. Regression sometimes works in the hands of skillful practitioners, but it isn't suitable for routine use.
> 3. Regression might work, but it hasn't yet.
> 4. Regression can't work.
>
> Textbooks, courtroom testimony, and newspaper interviews seem to put regression into category 1. Category 4 seems too pessimistic. My own view is bracketed by categories 2 and 3, although good examples are quite hard to find. (page 292)

What follows is an illustration of Freedman's point. Regression might work, but good examples, like those following, are hard to find.

Example 3.1: Passive smoking. Here is a pair of related examples from a current topic of great public health concern.

A paper by Law et al. (1997:978) was explicitly intended (so its authors tell us) to assure readers that the effect of passive smoking on the rate of heart attacks "is a serious environmental hazard, and one that is easily avoided." Part of its argument is the claim that there is "no satisfactory alternative interpretation of the evidence reviewed here than that environmental exposure to tobacco smoke causes an increase in risk of ischaemic heart disease of the order of 25%." This is the claim that one particular direct effect is real and substantial and can be estimated accurately. Let us inspect this claim.

The main study applies the multipath diagram of Figure 3.10 to numbers extracted from the form of literature review known as *meta-analysis*, numerical summary (usually via weighted averaging) of multiple independent studies attempting to estimate very similar quantities. In the present application, there is a clear consensus in the public health literature that the additional risk of heart attacks in nonsmoking wives of smokers is just about 30%. (The puzzle is that this is close to the increase of 39% in risk at even the lowest dose of *active* smoking, one cigarette a day, which in turn is fully half the relative risk increment of 78% for nonsmoking wives of men who smoke a pack a day. The main scientific contribution of the paper is the discovery of a mechanism, platelet aggregation, that careful experimental analyses have shown to mediate exactly this nonlinearity.)

Consider the schematic multiple regression in Figure 3.11, which customizes the middle panel of Figure 3.10 by identifying X with passive smoking, Y with diet, and Z with the rate of heart attacks. There is no mandate that all these quantities be estimated using the same data resources. And so Law and his colleagues have estimated these quantities from a meta-analysis of their own. A single table of theirs cleverly combined estimates from the literature of *both* of the numerical factors that multiply to give the indirect effect: the difference in dietary consumption, smokers versus nonsmokers (and so presumably their spouses), multiplied by the effect of such a difference in consumption on the risk of ischemic heart disease. As these products are not themselves corrected for their own indirect paths via the direct effect of passive smoking, they may be overestimates. But there is no harm to the authors' argument in overcorrecting in this manner, as it results in even more confidence in the final quantity estimated, the (remaining) direct effect of passive smoking per se. Figure 3.11 reproduces two of these computations, one for intake of "fruits" and one for "vegetables," which, of course, are quite highly correlated.

If we were using the third rationale for multiple regression, the optimal-prediction version, we would need to be optimizing over a single coherent data set that measured all of the important quantities involved. However, that is not

Law's logic. We are relying rather on the path-analytic interpretation, in which all the coefficients stand for biologically real processes that can be calibrated using a variety of data sets as long as those retrieved regression analyses are themselves sound. This is a great advantage of the path-analytic jargon, as long as the path coefficients being arrived at are stable over the variety of studies that have estimated them previously. Law et al. attended to this by reporting averages and ranges of slopes from their own meta-analysis, as I mentioned earlier.

It is interesting that by paper's end that unanticipated jump function in the rate of heart attacks (half the rate for one percent of the dose) proves *quantitatively* attributable to an explanation from a wholly different level of measurement, the extent of acceleration of platelet condensation on the occasion of the very lowest levels of exposure to at least one of the components of tobacco smoke. This persuasive numerical match arose from a further meta-analysis of the same evidence that was originally thought to testify to a quantitative mismatch instead.

The same logic, but without the platelets, applies to a companion study (Hackshaw et al., 1997) by some of the same authors in the same issue of the *British Medical Journal*. Hackshaw's team studied the relative risks of a different cause of death, lung cancer, in an otherwise similar design (risks as predicted by exposure to a smoking spouse, along with correlated aspects of diet). The primary literature of lung cancer risks is much more extensive than for heart attack risks, perhaps because of the much higher relative risk of lung cancer within the cohort of smokers per se. There is a clear convergence of the accumulating literature on one single consensual value of about 24% for the increased risk at a standardized level of about a pack a day of smoking by the spouse over an extended period.

Out of concern for the the analogous indirect effect through diet, Hackshaw and colleagues present a similarly explicit table of the known dietary differences between smokers and nonsmokers along with the associations of those dietary differences with lung cancer irrespective of smoking. It is fair to conclude from this literature that one standard deviation of dietary shift alters the risk by about 20%, from one group of studies, and families with smokers differ from families with nonsmokers by about 0.12 of a standard deviation, from another group of studies. There is also an adjustment to be made for the rate at which women who are married to smokers are themselves smokers, or have been, but are lying about that. The net excess risk to nonsmokers of being married to a smoker ends up at an adjusted value (an estimated direct path coefficient) of 26%. The authors point out that this is close to a proportionate reduction by 1:100 of the excess risk of lung cancer in the *active* smoker, who are about twentyfold likelier to get the disease, hence an excess risk of 1900%. And the fraction of 1/100 is roughly the dose of carcinogens in sidestream smoke as a fraction of what the primary smoker actually inhales. Thus the outcome of one multiple regression adjustment is treated as quantitatively consistent with the extrapolation downward of a wholly different sort of study. This is just the kind of cross-design, cross-level comparison that E. O. Wilson (1998) called consilience, about which he said (page 11), "Trust in consilience lies at the foundation of the natural sciences."

Summary of Section 3.1

- A multiple regression is a linear model that accounts for one measured variable, the *dependent variable,* as a linear combination of two or more others, its *predictors,* together with additive noise. The diagram of a regression on two variables is a plane in three dimensions, usually drawn with the dependent variable vertical.
- When the predictors in a multiple regression happen to be uncorrelated, the *beta weights,* coefficients of the predictors in the multiple regression equation, are the same as the slopes of the regression of the dependent variable on each predictor separately.
- Two sorts of slopes are involved in explanations of a multiple linear regression: total effects t and direct effects d.
- When predictors are correlated, the difference between the t's and the d's is due to the *indirect paths* by which change in one predictor affects the dependent variable in addition to any direct effect it may have. To estimate the d's one must take all the indirect effects into account at the same time. The equations that result, one for each predictor, are called the *normal equations.*
- There are three different and equally cogent ways of interpreting the same multiple regression arithmetic: (1) as a counterfactual assertion (what one would find *if* predictors were uncorrelated or if one could change one of their values without affecting any of the others); (2) as the set of paths jointly accounting for all the observed effects causally; (3) as the theory-free least-squares fit of the dependent variable to a linear combination of the predictors. The scientist selects among these rhetorics for scientific, not statistical, reasons.
- The regression coefficients being multiplied to give us the differences $t - d$ need not all have been computed in the same study. These indirect effects can also be estimated from meta-analyses of published literature, by taking products of averaged regression coefficients corresponding to the segments of the indirect paths as published separately.

3.2 Added-Variable Plots

3.2.1 The Problem, the Solution, and the Proofs

Added-variable plots are a robust and straightforward way of getting from a simple regression (one predictor) to a multiple regression (two predictors or more). The textbooks and the web sites all note three properties of this wonderfully useful device. We need some notation, and for our purposes I'll stick to a regression with exactly two predictors (hence, in the following text, x is a single variable, not a whole list on its own). Write $y_{.x}$ for the residual from the prediction of the variable y by the variable x along with a constant term. (In the subscript, the dot means "after regression on.") Similarly, write $z_{.x}$ for the residual of the variable z after the prediction by x and a constant.

Then if we regress $z_{.x}$ on $y_{.x}$, and plot their regression line along with their scatter, we get *the added-variable plot* for y after x has been entered into the regression for z. In this plot,

- the regression line goes through (0,0);
- the coefficient of $y_{.x}$ is the same as the coefficient of y in the regression of z on x, y, and a constant term; and
- the residuals are the same as the residuals from the regression of z on x, y, and a constant term.

This seems almost too good to be true, but the proof that follows (modified from Mosteller and Tukey, 1977) is elementary. Suppose we are fitting z by a multiple linear regression on x and y. Say that the prediction equations for z and y separately as functions of x are $z \sim a + bx$, $y \sim c + dx$:

$$z_{.x} = z - a - bx, \qquad y_{.x} = y - c - dx \qquad (3.9i)$$

And let the least-squares line in the **added-variable plot** of $z_{.x}$ on $y_{.x}$ be

$$z_{.x} \sim e + f y_{.x}. \qquad (3.9ii)$$

(In other words, we have just defined six letters a, b, c, d, e, f by reference to one or another of the three regressions involved here.)

Then the least-squares fit of z to x, y, and a constant will turn out to be

$$z \sim a + bx + f y_{.x} = (a - fc) + (b - df)x + fy. \qquad (3.10)$$

Equation (3.10) says that we just add the new prediction $f y_{.x}$ to the previous equation $z \sim a + bx$ without any further "correction" at this stage. In effect that correction has already been put in place. That coefficient of x in the equation just above is the coefficient adjusted as per our path models: the value b, from the simple regression, minus the indirect effect df, which is the product of the coefficient d for y on x and the coefficient f for z on y.

Proof. We are free to work via any of the three approaches just reviewed in Section 3.1, and it turns out to be simplest to proceed via the normal equations. To show that $z \sim a+bx+fy_{.x}$ is indeed the regression of z on x, y, and a constant term, we show, in order,

$$\Sigma 1(z - a - bx - fy_{.x}) = 0, \tag{3.11a}$$

$$\Sigma x(z - a - bx - fy_{.x}) = 0, \tag{3.11b}$$

$$\Sigma y(z - a - bx - fy_{.x}) = 0, \tag{3.11c}$$

which are the derivatives of the sum of squared residuals with respect to the three unknown parameters a, b, f in equation (3.10).

Normal Equation 1

Because each of the preliminary regressions in equations (3.9) must go through the averages of the variables involved, we have

$$\Sigma(z_{.x}) = \Sigma(y_{.x}) = 0$$

and

$$Ne = \Sigma z_{.x} - f\Sigma y_{.x} = 0.$$

Hence $e = 0$. The regression in the added-variable plot goes through *its* origin $(0,0)$.

Now look at $a+bx+fy_{.x} = a+bx+f(y-c-dx) = (a-fc)+(b-fd)x+fy$. We have $\Sigma z = \Sigma(a + bx) = \Sigma(a + bx) + f\Sigma y_{.x} = \Sigma(a + bx + fy_{.x})$, so

$$\Sigma 1(z - a - bx - fy_{.x}) = 0,$$

which is equation (3.11a) above.

Normal Equation 2

Again: $\Sigma xz = \Sigma x(a + bx)$ (from the second normal equation of that regression) $= \Sigma x(a+bx)+f\Sigma xy_{.x}$ (we have added zero) $= \Sigma x(a+bx+fy_{.x})$, and so

$$\Sigma x(z - (a + bx + fy_{.x})) = 0,$$

which is equation (3.11b) above.

Normal Equation 3

Because $\Sigma y_{.x} = \Sigma x y_{.x} = 0$, by that regression's set of normal equations, we have $\Sigma y_{.x}(a + bx) = 0$ and so

$$\Sigma y_{.x} z_{.x} = \Sigma y_{.x}(z - a - bx) = \Sigma y_{.x} z.$$

But the regression coefficient f was computed so as to make $\Sigma y_{.x}(z_{.x} - f y_{.x}) = 0$, and so

$$\Sigma y(z - a - bx - f y_{.x}) = \Sigma(c + dx + y_{.x})(z - a - bx - f y_{.x})$$
$$= \Sigma(c + dx + y_{.x})(z_{.x} - f y_{.x}) = 0 + 0 + \Sigma y_{.x}(z_{.x} - f y_{.x}) = 0.$$

But this is normal equation (3.11c). We have now confirmed each of the three.

Why are the residuals the same in the two equations? Because, just by moving one parenthesis, the residuals $(z - a - bx - f y_{.x})$ of the multiple regression of z on 1, x, and y are identical with the residuals $(z - a - bx) - f y_{.x}$ of the regression of $z_{.x}$ on $y_{.x}$. See Figure 3.12, which also shows why it doesn't matter which predictor you call x.

Partial correlation. The analysis just reviewed goes in terms of regression coefficients. It is often of interest to report things in terms of correlations of residuals instead (see, for instance, the analysis of persistence of growth for the Vilmann rats in Example 3.6 below). The formula for this conversion is particularly simple if only one variable is being controlled. We have, in fact,

$$r_{XY.Z} = \frac{r_{XY} - r_{XZ}r_{YZ}}{\sqrt{1 - r_{XZ}^2}\sqrt{1 - r_{YZ}^2}}. \tag{3.12a}$$

The numerator in this expression is the covariance of two residuals, that from the regression of Z on X and that from the regression of Z on Y, and the denominator is the square root of the product of their variances. This approach has been expanded into a general tool for causal investigations in the hands of Hubert Blalock (1965), Judea Pearl (2009), and others.

An additional helpful formula. The value of the multiple correlation R can always be computed as the correlation between the dependent variable z and its actual predicted values $d_x x + d_y y + \dots$. For the case of just two predictors, it is convenient as well to have a formula expressing the same quantity in closed form. This is

$$R^2 = \frac{r_{zx}^2 + r_{zy}^2 - 2r_{zx}r_{zy}r_{xy}}{1 - r_{xy}^2}. \tag{3.12b}$$

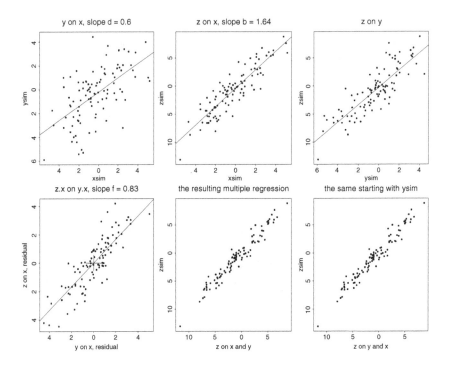

Figure 3.12 Added variable plots for the multiple regression of a simulated measure z on two others x and y. (upper row) Scatterplots of the original variables in pairs, with two of the coefficients used in the analysis. (lower left) If z has already been regressed on x, the added-variable plot for y is the residual of its regression on x plotted against the residual for z's regression on x. (lower center and right) The resulting multiple regression combining the original regression on x with the new added-variable formula as in equation (3.10) gives the correct answer whatever the order in which the multiple predictors are actually entered.

(One minus this expression is the slant height of the parallelopiped expressing the variables x, y, z in terms of their correlations: the fraction

$$\begin{vmatrix} 1 & r_{xy} & r_{xz} \\ r_{xy} & 1 & r_{yz} \\ r_{xz} & r_{yz} & 1 \end{vmatrix} \bigg/ \begin{vmatrix} 1 & r_{xy} \\ r_{xy} & 1 \end{vmatrix}, \text{ its volume divided by the area of its } x, y \text{ face.)}$$

3.2.2 Example 3.2: Prenatal Ultrasound and Birthweight

A regression equation is not only a prediction but a suggestion about the sort of quantity that the prediction formula stands for – the "latent variable," to use the language of a different branch of applied statistics, that is actually carrying the causation. In biometric applications it is often very useful to think through this possibility from the outset. One crucial aspect of this preliminary thinking is to ask what kinds of combinations of the multiple predictors might be argued on a priori grounds to align with sensible explanations of the data even before we have looked at their actual measured values. Here is an example of this kind of reasoning in a data set combining measurements made at two different ages. The task is to forecast a human perinatal measurement, birthweight, by two length measurements, biparietal diameter and abdominal diameter, made on the same fetus at an earlier age. This example was brought to my attention in the book by Andersen and Skovgaard (2010); those authors have posted the full data set on the website `http://publicifsv.sund.ku.dk/` `~linearpredictors/?page=datasets&dataset=Birth` Weight for that book. These data are also included in the online resource for this book.

The paper from which these data were drawn, Secher et al. (1987:2), "Estimation of fetal weight in the third trimester by ultrasound," begins, "An accurate estimation of fetal weight is essential in establishing a plan of obstetric management." We can guess that their job was to find the formula for that "accurate estimation," but also to extend the rhetoric until its implications for "obstetric management" were comprehended fully. Here, that would mean communicating the most powerful warning about low-birthweight babies, and it is that task that our statistical analysis of this data set emphasizes. I will talk only about birthweight, abdominal diameter, and biparietal diameter of the head, variables abbreviated BW, ABD, and BPD, respectively. Figure 3.13 displays the three scatterplots of these variables in pairs, along with an enhancement of one of the three. The sample size for each of these frames is 107.

How do you make a baby? No, that's not what I meant. The question is, how do you *put together* a baby? Head, body, two arms, two legs: a total of six pieces. The data set at hand includes measures of head and body, the two largest compartments of these six. The average density of a baby (or any other human) is just about the density of water, which is 1 g/cc, so birthweight in grams nearly equals volume in cubic centimeters. Then the "true" predictive coefficient for the weight of the head would be something like the volume of the head, which is (very roughly) the cube of BPD, and the "true" predictive coefficient for the weight of the abdomen would, even more roughly, be the cube of ABD. For these regressions, at least, the coefficients would be in the right units: they would be g/cm^3, which *is* a density. Density might be roughly a constant, and so it would be a reasonably realistic metaphor for a regression coefficient.

We check this logic very roughly by looking at some regressions. The raw sum of squares of birthweight around its mean is 50 million. The residual sum of squares from the regression on ABD and BPD is about 10 million; after regressing on ABD^3 and BPD^3, about 9 million. In the code that follows,

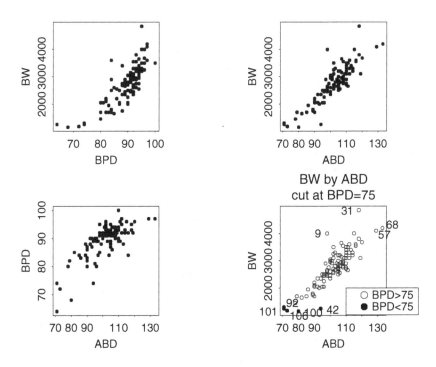

Figure 3.13 The birthweight study data. (upper left, upper right, lower left) The three bivariate scatterplots among the principal measured variables. (lower right) The scatter at upper right, now enhanced by a coding of extreme values on the third variable along with selected case numbers. Ultrasound measurements (in mm): ABD, abdominal diameter; BPD, biparietal diameter. BW, birthweight, in grams.

BW.data[,"BW"] is the variable for birthweight, BW.data[,"BPD"] for biparietal diameter, and BW.data[,"ABD"] for abdominal diameter, and BPD3 and APD3 are the cubes of the latter two.

```
summary(lm(BW.data[,"BW"]~BW.data[,c("ABD","BPD")]))
Coefficients:
Value Std. Error t value
(Intercept) -4628.1181 455.9898 -10.1496
BPD 37.1329 7.6151 4.8762
ABD 39.7631 4.1639 9.549400
Residual standard error: 306.6 on 104 degrees of
  freedom
Multiple R-Squared: 0.8065
```

(3.13)

```
summary(lm(BW.data[,"BW"]~BPD3+ABD3))
Value Std. Error t value
(Intercept) -135.9184 165.9332 -0.8191
BPD3 2.2314 0.3143 7.0991
ABD3 1.1544 0.1213 9.5168
Residual standard error: 294.9 on 104 degrees of
   freedom
Multiple R-Squared: 0.8209
```

$$(3.14)$$

So the dimensionally appropriate regression is actually the better fit, and its coefficients, in units of g/cm^3, are in the range of 1 (abdomen) and 2 (head, for which the biparietal diameter is a relatively short dimension; also, there's a lot of bone around). I will call this the *volumetric regression* in the rest of this section. Notice that every term in either of these regressions is a large multiple of its standard error *except* the intercept for the second regression, the one on the cubes of the ultrasound diameters. That intercept can thus be taken as zero, which is as it should be. (A baby with both diameters zero is a zygote, weighing 0 grams.) See how changing from the silly unit of grams per centimeter to the sensible unit of grams per cubic centimeter makes the scientific task easier? There are now only two coefficients, not three, to understand.

We have thus made considerable progress after we skeptically examined the dimensions of our coefficients. Grams per centimeter – g/cm – doesn't make much sense except for pipes and sausage, but g/cm^3 does. As the weight of the baby is the sum of weights of head, body, arms, and legs, diameters of any of these can be thought of as flawed measures of the cube roots of those component weights. Often such explicitly imperfect measures are called *proxy measures*, e.g., abdominal diameter cubed as a proxy measure for abdominal weight.

But, error or no error, **the situation is obviously causal:** if you give the baby a bigger head, you get a heavier baby; if you give the baby a bigger tummy, you get a heavier baby. (Incidentally, this is the best argument for why *gestational age*, one of the variables in the original publication, isn't worth keeping in the analysis. Its causal role, while indubitable, is solely indirect, via BPD or ABD, the variables that are already being used. In terms of measurement error, I think gestational age is about as error-prone as the ultrasound scores, while birthweight is the only really precise quantity in sight.)

Not only is this situation causal, but the combination of the cranial component and the abdominal component is obviously an additive one. There is no justification for considering an analysis where the dependent variable is the logarithm of volume and in which, therefore, the predicted differential effect of the head measurement and that of the abdomen measurement would be *multiplied* by the grand mean. This is a serious error in the original publication by Secher et al.

We are finally in a position to learn something from a data-based diagram. Please return your attention to Figure 3.13. Now that you have mastered Chapter 2, you will surely have thought of examining the correlations among these three measurements: they are $r_{BW,ABD} = 0.873, r_{BW,BPD} = 0.798, r_{ABD,BPD} = 0.756$. BW is *better predicted* by ABD than by BPD; if you had to pick just one predictor variable, it would be ABD. (This makes sense: the abdomen is the largest component of the finished baby.) Returning to that figure, the lower-right panel improves on the lower-right panel by labeling the small-headed babies (BPD < 75), which also turn out to be those with BW less than 1450 grams. These are the points numbered 101, 92, 106, 100, 42 near the lower left corner. (We also see the case numbers of four interesting points at upper right, to be discussed later.) These interesting black-dotted points are for the really small babies, small on every size measure at the same time. They are worth identifying as a subset because they account for most of the "obstetric management" problems.

Now that they have been numbered by entry line in the data file, one can't help noticing that three of these five are among the last eight babies (sequence numbers 100 through 107) in the data set. So light babies were oversampled at the end of the study? This seems strange. The published paper explains nothing about this, but it sounds like sample inhomogeneity over time, which is often a serious flaw in otherwise sound study designs. In any event, these five light babies are evidently a *separable group* in the upper left panel of Figure 3.13, and they **must** be considered separately. (In the United States, they are officially "low-birthweight babies" and have to be reported to the state.) Figure 3.14 is a plot of predicted versus observed birthweight from this regression, showing how distinct these five small babies actually are.

Filtering the regression using a criterion involving biparietal diameter is perfectly reasonable, since that is measured earlier than the birthweight itself. We omit these five cases and run the volumetric regression again:

```
summary(lm(BW.data[BW.data[,"BPD"]>75,"BW"]~
 BPD3[BW.data[,"BPD"]>75]+ABD3[BW.data[,"BPD"]>75]))
Coefficients:
Value Std. Error t value
(Intercept) -181.1073 224.0813 -0.8082
```

```
BPD3 [BW.data[, "BPD"] > 75] 2.2606 0.3839 5.8883
ABD3 [BW.data[, "BPD"] > 75] 1.1750 0.1238 9.4912
Residual standard error: 295.5 on 99 degrees of
  freedom
Multiple R-Squared: 0.7752
```

$$(3.15)$$

The multiple correlation in this subset of 102 cases, $\sqrt{0.7752} = 0.8804$, is less than $\sqrt{0.8209} = 0.9060$ from the analysis of all 107, consistent with our having restricted the range of one of the predictors. Nevertheless the information content is now more relevant to the declared purpose of the paper (the separation of that subgroup of jointly low BPD and BW). Again the intercept is less than its own standard error, and so can be ignored.

Even with the low-birthweight babies in the analysis, Figure 3.14, the multiple regression on BPD3 and ABD3 is not curved at either end. But it

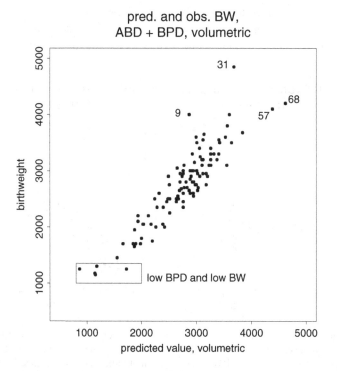

Figure 3.14 Predicted versus observed birthweight from the volumetric regression. There are two subsets of unusually high residuals, corresponding to subsamples of the smallest and the largest babies.

shows considerably greater expected prediction errors there. So the potentially outlying big babies do not alter the interpretation of the regressions; on the average, they lie right on the line of agreement between predicted and observed. It is this volumetric regression, the one on the cubed diameters but no constant term, that sustains a proper biological interpretation. The cases with measured BPD less than 75 mm are clearly the subset of greatest clinical concern. But no regression was needed to flag these – they were obvious as soon as the ultrasound image had been measured and the data scattered as in Figure 3.13.

The usefulness of an added-variable plot. The interpretation of the effect of adding BPD3 to the regression using ABD3 depends on the correlation between these two predictors. The arguments that handle this correctly (i.e., that let you compute the coefficient of the variable you're thinking of adding) are encoded in the added variable plots in Figure 3.15. They are each for 102 cases, omitting the five of lowest BPD/lowest BW.

These plots confirm the logic we had explored prior to any examination of the data at all. A good model will be one that estimates the weight of a baby from its volume, estimates that volume as the sum of the volumes of the

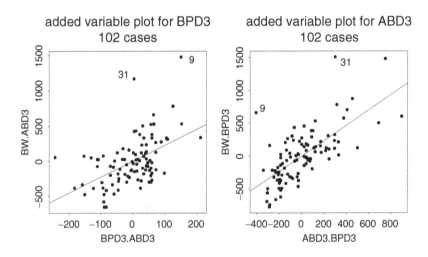

Figure 3.15 Added variable plots for the volumetric regression omitting the five cases of lowest BPD and birthweight. ABD3: biparietal diameter cubed. BPD3: biparietal diameter cubed. BW.ABD3, residual of birthweight after regression on ABD3. BPD3.ABD3, residual of BPD3 after regression on ABD3. BW.BPD3, residual of BW after regression on BPD3. ABD3.BPD3, residual of ABD3 after regression on BPD3. 9, 31: the two cases with the greatest residuals.

parts, and estimates the volumes of the two biggest parts (head and abdomen) as the cubes of the measured diameters of those same parts. The best single predictor of birthweight, we have seen, is the cube of measured abdominal diameter, and the prediction is improved by adding in a multiple of the cube of biparietal diameter. The detection of the clinically fraught cases, those of low birthweight, does not benefit from these or any other regression analysis. It arises instead from the direct observation that all of the babies meeting the legal criterion of low birthweight (BW< 1500g), and no others, were those of BPD less than 75 mm (Figure 3.13 or 3.14). We conclude, then, that while these regressions are instructive about the power and the limits of regression methods, perhaps the clinical context is not benefited by them to anything like the same extent.

Of the two cases of largest positive prediction error in Figure 3.14 or 3.15, one (case 9) has an unusually low ABD for its BPD, while the other, case 31, must be anomalous for other reasons. Remember from the third bullet point near the top of Section 3.2.1 that the residual of the multivariate prediction is not the height of a point above the zero level in these added-variable plots, but its height above the regression line.

3.2.3 A Note on "Optimism" in Model-Fitting

The issue that concerned us in the preceding section – the decision as to whether our scientific understanding is enriched by including an additional predictor in a linear model – exemplifies a protocol for choices among statistical models in the course of the scientific enterprise more generally. For a good introduction to this larger context, see the *Primer on Evidence* by D. R. Anderson (2008). My comment here is limited to introducing and explicating a few central formulas.

Often the same numerical biological data can be imagined to be modeled by a range of different algebraic expressions. Assuming that our data set arose from independent cases, rather than any of the extended structures reviewed in Section 2.6, then when we consider our claims in a probabilistic context (which is the context in which all good quantitative scientists ought to find themselves), each measurement is modeled as the sum of the value predicted by the model together with an additive "error" independent of all the predictors and also of all the other errors. When there are multiple plausible models, our task extends further than merely estimating the values of the parameters from some fixed list. Now the scientific inference must deal as well with uncertainty about the algebraic expression in terms of which actual predicted values are computed. The scientist's choice might be as simple as specifying the list of predictors that go into a multiple linear regression, as when we wondered whether adding information from BPD improved our prediction of birthweight over what was predicted by APD. Or it might deal with the logically prior decision to use the cubes of those ultrasound diameters as predictors instead of the raw diameters themselves, or the even more upstream decision to predict birthweight per se instead of, perhaps, the logarithm of birthweight. Decisions like these, furthermore, may arise in either of two contexts, as the scientist intends to select (or announce) the single best model of some family or instead to assess the comparative merits of multiple models chosen from across the whole family.

Intuitively, the problem posed in all these contexts is rather obvious. Statistical model-fitting incorporates a particularly sophisticated version of "begging the question." Our parametric models are fitted to data by an algorithm (least-squares or maximum likelihood) that takes advantage of chance for the particular data at hand, and so anyone who reads the computer output too literally is too enthusiastic about the precision with which any resulting formulas are likely to apply to new data that was not part of the data used for fitting. In other words, predictions from fits to training data are too optimistic as guides to applications to the test data encountered later. (This is the language of *statistical learning*, as in Hastie et al., 2009, from whom I have borrowed this metaphor of excessive optimism.) We must somehow correct our calculated comparisons of prediction accuracies so as to take account of differences in the number of parameters we were free to adjust in the course of the model-fitting.

One easy way to deal with anxieties of this sort is to turn to the notion of *cross-validation*. In the leave-out-one paradigm, for instance, whatever kind of predictive model one is considering is fitted to the data set leaving out each single case in turn, and then the prediction error is taken as the error of predicting that single case based on fits to the remainder. Stone (1977) showed that "asymptotically" (meaning, in the limit of large samples) the regression model selected as best by this procedure will be the model for which the "corrected likelihood" $-n \log \hat{\sigma} - p$ is the largest, where p is the number of parameters being estimated and $\hat{\sigma}$ is the estimated root-mean-square residual around the best-fitting (maximum-likelihood) version of the usual formula. This subtraction-of-p formula had been introduced a few years earlier to our community as "the Mallows C_p" (after Colin Mallows, who announced it first). If you insist on statistical tests, then assuming that true prediction errors are Gaussian, the test for p *added* parameters is 2 times the difference of likelihoods — that is, $-2n \log(\hat{\sigma}_2/\hat{\sigma}_1)$ — as a χ_p^2, where p is the number of parameters added to the first (less precise) model to get to the second.

If you wish to proceed rationally instead, following the rules of D. R. Anderson (2008), you will treat each model in the candidate set as having a likelihood of its own of $-n \log \hat{\sigma} - p$, where p is the number of parameters relative to the single model of highest such corrected likelihood. This is a version of the celebrated *Akaike information criterion* or *AIC*, named after Hirotugu Akaike, who showed (see Akaike, 1974) that the same formulation applied quite a bit more generally than to just multiple regressions. It is the AIC formalism that Stone (1977) confirmed to be equivalent to the intuitively reasonable cross-validation approach under assumptions some of which are more reasonable (true prediction errors more or less bell-curve-shaped) and others of which are not (to wit, that the true model falls within the class of models under consideration). This latter assumption has the practical effect of taking methods like these out of the domain of the psychological and social sciences, where no models are ever true, but instead sets it squarely in the context of the natural sciences, where some phenomena are indeed pretty nearly lawful. An even more precise formulation, usually named the "corrected AIC" AIC_c, replaces the adjustment p in the AIC formula by the quantity $pn/(n - p - 1)$ In problems of greater generality the expression $-n \log \hat{\sigma}$ here is replaced by $\log L$, the actual likelihood for the data using the parameter estimates that maximize exactly that likelihood.

This same formulary is reviewed in a totally different language in Hastie et al., 2009, sections 7.4–7.5. Their discussion begins with the useful observation that for multiple regression models of the form we analyzed in Section 3.1, we have $\sum_i \text{cov}(\hat{y}_i, y_i) = d\sigma_\varepsilon^2$, where d is the number of parameters estimated and σ_ε^2 is the true error variance of observations around the true model. (The covariances in this expression are taken over replications of the true model with all predictors x fixed.) As Hastie and colleagues explain the centrality of this formulation, our "optimism" is to be calibrated by the extent to which the estimated prediction error underestimates true prediction error, which depends mainly on how strongly each observed dependent variable y_i affects its own prediction. This equation is a variant of one arising in the course of the derivation of the "hat matrix," for the algebra of which see, for instance, Freedman, 2009, section 4.2. Notice here that the concern is not for the uncertainties of the estimated parameters of any prediction formula, which derive from the information matrix approach (Section 4.1), but only for their import for picking or ranking the different prediction models, which is calibrated only by the trace of that matrix times its own inverse, that is, the simple count of parameters involved.

> *Example.* For an example of this sort of computation I anticipate the comparison of Figures 3.39 and 3.51 toward the end of this chapter. Figure 3.39 diagrams the regression of a 0–1 variable (survival of male sparrows) on two linear measurements. Inasmuch as the covariance patterns in the two subgroups are nearly identical (Figure 3.50), the pattern in Figure 3.51 is nearly the same as a refinement of Figure 3.39 that supplements the two linear predictors by three additional ones: their squares and their crossproduct. The sum of squared residuals for the first regression is $59 \cdot 0.3716^2$, and, for the second, 59×0.3665^2. The difference of loglikelihoods is thus $59 \cdot \log(.3716/.3665)$ ~ 0.82, which is to be compared with the difference of 3 in the counts of parameters for the two regressions. Inasmuch as 0.82 is less than 3, there is nothing to be gained by switching to the quadratic computation. (Although the model here cannot involve Gaussian residuals, the formula for corrected likelihood is nevertheless close enough.)

There is a more general discussion of the Akaike approach in Bookstein (2014, section 5.3.2), including a specifically morphometric example more realistic than the mere comparison of two competing multiple regression models.

Summary of Section 3.2

- The *added-variable plot* is an algebraic trick specific to multiple regression. It works to modify an additional predictor so as to be uncorrelated with the predictors that are already there. Then the multiple regression reduces to the sum of simple regressions, as in the left-hand panels of Figures 3.5 and 3.6.
- For a multiple regression to be useful for biological research, the units in which its regression coefficients are computed and reported need to make biological sense. Often one can infer appropriate transforms of predictors just from inspection of their units – for instance, when lengths are predicting volumes or weights, it may be appropriate to represent the lengths by their cubes.
- When a dependent variable is a composite of multiple compartments, often the multiple regression coefficients will correspond to contributions of those compartments one by one.
- The answer to a practical problem based on multiple predictors may end up involving only one of the predictors.
- The deeper issue of model *selection* can often be treated by the AIC (Akaike Information Criterion), according to which models with different

counts p of parameters can be evaluated by treating the diverse values of their "optimism-corrected" loglikelihoods $-p + \log L$ as loglikelihoods of the models themselves with respect to the one that maximizes this expression. For multiple linear regression with Gaussian residuals, these reduce to the Mallows formula $-n \log \hat{\sigma} - p$, where $\hat{\sigma}$ is the regression residual and p the count of predictors.

3.3 Special Case 1: Analysis of Covariance

Section 3.1 introduced three different interpretations of the least-squares equation for multiple predictors X_i of a single outcome Y. The one that is most relevant to the extended context of this section is the path version. Following the logic of Sewall Wright, the path equations represent the net effect of each variable within a causal system as the combination of a *direct effect*, having coefficient equal to the corresponding component of β, together with one *indirect effect* for each of the other predictors.

Exactly this same logic applies to the more general setup where some of the predictors are continuous variables and others are categories. In Figure 3.16, some unnamed outcome is being explained as the effect of some predictor, likewise unnamed, together with two additional shifts of average values that differ from group to group. One of these modifications resets the range of the predictor over the groups, and the other modification resets the height of what would otherwise be a common regression line. In other words, the grouping variable explains the average values of *both* of the continuous variables, the predictor as well as the outcome. The following argument should convince you that the corresponding path equations are still satisfied, so that you can use the same statistical software you are already trained to use as long as you are careful with the role of that grouping variable. This is the case even though the imagery of Figure 3.4 – a plane over a two-dimensional Cartesian chart of predictors – no longer seems to apply.

3.3.1 Group Differences in Regressions as a Path Model

To elaborate on the algebraic relationship here between the path models we already understand and this new kind of bioscientific question, let's turn to the simplest possible situation, two groups (hence one grouping dummy variable) and one single continuous predictor. Figure 3.17 shows one realization of a single model $Y = aG + bX$, in this case without any random errors (i.e., all

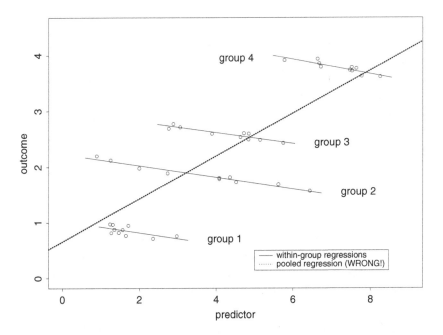

Figure 3.16 Schematic of an analysis of covariance: multiple groups with the same regression slope for the linear fit of an outcome variable by a single predictor, but different averages of both the predictor and the outcome as a function of group. The regression lines within each group are shown, along with the pooled regression (heavy dotted line), the slope of which is the total effect $t_{\text{outcome.predictor}}$, a value that is obviously misleading. In this example, it even has the wrong sign.

residuals zero), where G is a grouping variable taking values $-\frac{1}{2}$ and $\frac{1}{2}$ half the time each. Write X_w for a continuous predictor that is being modeled simply as a uniform distribution from -1.732 to $+1.732$ (so that it has variance 1) within groups. The second predictor X of Y, after G, is this within-group predictor X_w modified by adding some coefficient c times the grouping variable G. That is, $X = X_w + cG$. For this specific figure, a was set to 4, b to 1, and c to 4. In other words, the predictions have a common slope of 1 within group, but the groups differ by 4 in their mean on the predictor X and also on 4 in the intercepts for fixed value of the grouping variable. The net difference in group means on the outcome turns out to be $4 + 4 = 8$.

We can agree that the analysis conveyed by the dashed line, the one that ignores the grouped structure, is wrong. Can we use the path analysis to retrieve the correct analysis (the combination of the solid lines and the locations of their centers) from the available covariances?

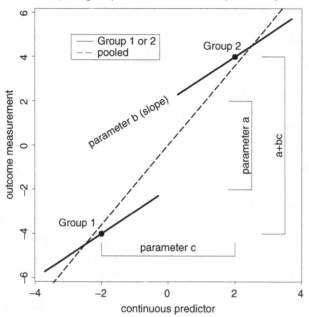

Figure 3.17 Numerical example for verifying the path equations as they apply to an analysis of covariance without error. Dashed line: the wrong regression (total effect of predictor on outcome). Solid lines: correct regressions. Parameters a, b, $a + bc$ of the model are shown as displacements. See text.

Yes, we can. Compute the requisite variances and covariances as follows.

$$\text{var}(X_w) = 1 \text{ (by construction),} \tag{3.16a}$$

$$\text{var}(G) = \tfrac{1}{4} \text{ (flip of one fair coin),} \tag{3.16b}$$

$$\text{cov}(X_w, G) = 0 \text{ (these two are independent), hence} \tag{3.16c}$$

$$\text{var}(X) = \text{var}(X_w + cG) = \text{var}(X_w) + c^2 \text{var}(G) = 1 + \tfrac{c^2}{4}; \tag{3.16d}$$

$$\text{cov}(X, G) = c \, \text{var}(G) = \tfrac{c}{4}, \tag{3.16e}$$

$$\text{cov}(Y, G) = \text{cov}(aG + bX, G) = a \, \text{var}(G) + b \, \text{cov}(X, G) = \tfrac{a+bc}{4}; \text{ and} \tag{3.16f}$$

$$\text{cov}(X, Y) = \text{cov}(X, aG + bX) = a \, \text{cov}(X, G) + b \, \text{var}(X) = \tfrac{ac}{4} + b(1 + \tfrac{c^2}{4}). \tag{3.16g}$$

(And also $\text{var}(Y) = \text{var}(aG + bX) = a^2 \text{var}(G) + b^2 \text{var}(X) + 2ab \, \text{cov}(G, X) = \tfrac{a^2}{4} + b^2(1 + \tfrac{c^2}{4}) + \tfrac{abc}{2}$, although we won't need this.)

The path-equations approach directs us to reconstruct the *direct effects a* and *b* of G and X on Y by decomposing their *total effects* using the associations among the predictors themselves. Here is how this works out in this scenario:

the total effect of G on Y, $\mathrm{cov}(Y, G)/\mathrm{var}(G)$, is $a + bc$, which equals a, the direct effect, plus bc, the *indirect effect*, which in term decomposes as b, the *other* direct effect, times c, the regression of X on G; and,

the total effect of X on Y, $\mathrm{cov}(X, Y)/\mathrm{var}(X)$, is $(\frac{ac}{4} + b(1 + \frac{c^2}{4}))/(1 + \frac{c^2}{4})$, which breaks out as b, the direct effect, plus $(\frac{ac}{4})/(1 + \frac{c^2}{4})$, which is the product of the other direct effect a by the regression $\mathrm{cov}(X, G)/\mathrm{var}(X) = (\frac{c}{4})/(1 + \frac{c^2}{4})$ of G on X.

So the path equations work in this setting of mixed categorical and continuous variables just as they did when the situation involved two continuous variables. In fact, they work out for *any* combination of predictors of *either* type. Continuous or discrete, one single computational engine handles the decomposition of all these joint effects correctly (under the appropriate, stringent assumptions, of course). Ironically, the engine responsible for all this arithmetic has no idea what the scientist is actually going to be doing with the resulting estimates, and hence by itself provides no authority for any reports. For every path in the decomposition just reviewed, there has to be some justification for claiming that it is biologically real.

Example 3.3: Tetrahymena, revisited. Figure 3.18 extends Figure 2.36 to include the second (low-glucose) group from the original publication. Once more the same data is plotted twice: once as measured, once after the log transformations. After the log transformation, the two groups seem to share the same slope of -0.0554 for the linear fit (versus the value of -0.0539 we computed for just the high-glucose group alone).

```
summary(lm(log(tetra.data[,3])~log(tetra.data[,2])
                                      +tetra.data[,1]))
Coefficients:
Value Std. Error t value
(Intercept) 3.7161 0.0263 141.5420
log(tetra.data[, 2]) -0.0554 0.0023 -24.0727
tetra.data[, 1] 0.0650 0.0061 10.6670
Residual standard error: 0.02103 on 48 degrees of
   freedom
Multiple R-Squared: 0.9337
```

$$(3.17)$$

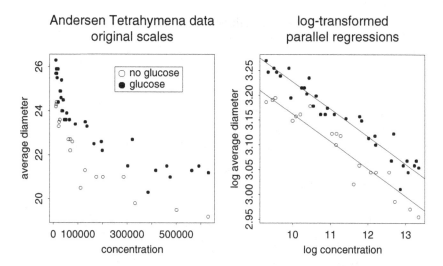

Figure 3.18 The completed *Tetrahymena* data set: two groups for two measurements. (left) The original data as a coded scatterplot. (right) After log-log transformation, the data evidently lie near a model with two parallel regressions.

While the slopes look as if they might be constant, the regression lines for the groups obviously lie at different heights on the plot. (When it is obvious which value of the abscissa we are referring to, these heights are often called *intercepts* – a slightly different use of this word from equation 3.17.) From visual inspection, or from the table, the two lines here differ in elevation by 0.065, on the log plot, which converts to a difference of about 6.7% in the effective diameter at constant concentration, or about 20% in the difference in the cube of this quantity, the per-cell volume at constant concentration.

But we have not discharged our responsibility for the scientific inference until we have checked that our claim of "the same slope" is reasonable in this context. To that end we produce a second analysis that allows for different slopes in the two groups, to see how that changes our interpretation. Figure 3.19 below shows that conditional analysis. It is hardly distinguishable from the earlier version. The two regression lines diverge very slightly toward the right – the lower one (for the low-glucose condition) has a slope of −0.0597, the higher one the same value of −0.0532 we already reported. Also, you see now that that outlying point seventh from the right in the high-glucose condition (Figure 2.36, at the arrow) seems actually to plot right on the low-glucose line. (That is how the suggestion arose, reported already in Chapter 2, that this point is likelier to have arisen from an error in the coding of the glucose variable than from natural within-group variability given the rest of

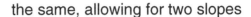

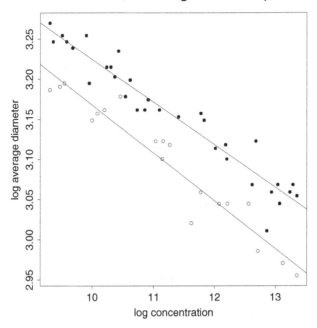

Figure 3.19 Extension of Figure 3.18 to allow for different slopes in the different groups. The slopes differ by only about 12% of their averaged value, which is barely more than the standard error of their difference. They are not worth reporting separately.

the data.) In reading the multiple regression output that follows, please note that the + symbol in the second line of display (3.17) has been replaced by a * symbol in the second line of display (3.18), meaning that an interaction term should be included for the differences of regression slopes across the groups.

```
summary(lm(log(tetra.data[,3])~log(tetra.data[,2])
  *tetra.data[,1]))
Coefficients:
Value Std. Error t value
(Intercept) 3.7642 0.0442 85.1227
log(tetra.data[, 2]) -0.0597 0.0039 -15.2249
tetra.data[, 1] -0.0079 0.0546 -0.1442
log(tetra.data[, 2]):tetra.data[, 1] 0.0065 0.0048
  1.3442
```

```
Residual standard error: 0.02086 on 47 degrees of
    freedom
Multiple R-Squared: 0.9361
```

$$(3.18)$$

How did we configure this analysis as a multiple regression? By creating a **dummy variable** for the difference in slopes. Instead of the previous model, which had two predictors (one for log concentration, one for group number), we use a model with *three* predictors: the same two as before (log concentration and group number) plus a third "predictor," the dummy variable, that represents no new measurement, but instead the change in the question. The dummy variable in question is equal to log concentration *for group 1 only*, otherwise zero. In the resulting three-variable multiple regression, this term is assigned the "path coefficient" of 0.0065 that is the difference between the slopes in the two groups separately.

The reason for partitioning a single computation in this way, instead of, for instance, just computing simple regressions for each of the two groups separately, is that we end up with an additional estimator that is often very useful. You remember from Section 2.2.2 that the simple regression coefficient comes with an error variance that is $\sigma^2/N \, \mathrm{var}(x)$ where σ^2 is the true variance of the data around the linear model and x is the (single) predictor. It is this equation that generalizes to the multiple regression setting.

The regression program lm I am using explicitly reports that the standard error for the interaction term (the difference of slopes) is 0.0048. It is more instructive to arrive at the same result from first principles. We use the propositions from Section 3.2 about added variables in a context where the "added variable" is, in fact, the difference between the slopes in the two groups. Remember that the updated regression for any shared outcome W on a new predictor Z as well as a list of existing predictors $X, Y, \ldots$ is equal to the simple regression of the residual of Z on the previous predictors $X, Y, \ldots$ on the residual of W after regression on that same list of earlier predictors. Here W is the log of average diameter, the new predictor Z is the interaction term we just defined (log of concentration in group 1 only, otherwise 0), and X and Y are the two predictors that already appear in Figure 3.18, namely log concentration and original grouping. The uncertainty of the slope difference, the quantity we wish to calibrate, comes from the formula for the standard error of a regression coefficient that originally appeared in Section 2.2.2. It involves two quantities. One is the standard error of the residual we are trying to improve. In this case, it is the within-group regression in Figure 3.18, the one with the same coefficient for both the groups. The other is the variance of the predictor corresponding to this new effect. This is not the variance of that predictor per se, the interaction term, but rather the variance of its *novelty*, the variance of its residual when predicted by the same X and Y. That variance is 0.3744.

And so the standard error of the regression term for the group difference in slopes is $\sqrt{0.02086^2/(51 \cdot 0.3744)} = 0.0048$. This is only slightly less than the actual slope difference of 0.0065. In other words, the slope difference we computed just about equals its own measurement error given the experimental design at hand. Under the circumstances it is a reasonable scientific decision to consider these slopes as the same (rather than trying, for instance, to find some explanation of why this number should be lower in the one condition than the other).

3.3.2 Example 3.4. Brain Weight – Body Weight Allometry

The techniques here apply to a discussion dear to many potential readers of this book: the evolution of brain size in *Homo sapiens*. One of the important background considerations for speculations on that topic is the understanding of brain size variation in the larger clade of which the primates in general and the hominids in particular are especially interesting subclades. From a variety of published analyses I have extracted three versions that make essentially the same point using somewhat different graphical iconography. The versions share the transformation of all measurements to their logarithms at the outset of each analysis. A regression model $\log y \sim \log b + a \log x$ can be written just as well as $y \sim bx^a$, the *allometric model* of differential growth (Huxley, 1932); hence the slopes a are often referred to as *allometric exponents* in this context.

A first version of our display was published by the comparative neurologist Harry Jerison in his article "Paleoneurology and the evolution of mind" from a 1976 issue of the American semipopular magazine *Scientific American*. Jerison's analysis plotted log brain weight against log body weight for "some 200 species of living vertebrates," coded by class and by order (primate or not) within the mammals. Note, in Figure 3.20a, the representation of our species by a quadrangle "representing the extreme measurements reported for man." There is a clear separation between the upper three groupings (primates, nonprimate mammals, and birds) and the lower two (bony fish and reptiles). According to the caption of this figure, "in both cases the data fall along a line with a slope of 2/3 on log-log coordinates: brain size varies with the 2/3 power (which is the cube root of the square) of body size." Jerison proceeded to compute an "encephalization quotient" (EQ) as the ratio of measured brain size to the expected value for a given animal's body size according to this regression. (Explicitly, the EQ value is 10 to the power of the residual from this regression.) In more conventional terminology, this is just the antilog of

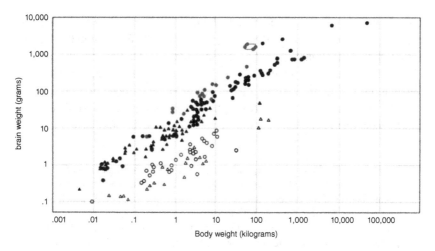

Figure 3.20a Jerison's version, from Jerison (1976). Legend: gray disks, primates; black disks, other mammals; black triangles, birds; open circles, bony fish; open triangles, reptiles. The original caption was: "Brain size is plotted against body size for some 200 species of living vertebrates. The data were collected by George W. Crile and Daniel P. Quiring some years ago. The four gray points connected by a rectangle represent the extreme measurements reported for man, indicating that variation within a species does not loom large in comparison to the distinctions among species. Data fall into two clearly delimited groups, which may be considered to be the lower and the higher vertebrates. In both cases the data fall along a line with a slope of 2/3 on log-log coordinates: brain size varies with the 2/3 power (which is the cube root of the square) of body size." Reproduced with permission. Copyright 1976 Scientific American, a division of Nature America, Inc. All rights reserved.

the regression residual from Figure 3.20a. According to the EQ, there has been a steady increase in relative brain size along the line of hominization from 40 million years ago to the present.

It is remarkable that those claimed lines along which the data purportedly fall are not shown. One can anticipate the critique to come by connecting the points at (.01,1) and (10000,10000) with a straight line. This line has a slope of exactly 2/3 in the log-log plot here, but seems to systematically miss Jerison's data at the left end. A better hand-drawn effort would connect the same upper point at (10000,10000) to the point (.01, .31) halfway (on this log scale) between (.01, .1) and (.01,1) at the lower left. This line seems much better aligned with the filled dots toward the left (the small mammals), and it has a slope of 3/4, corresponding to Martin's claim based on the next figure. So Jerison's caption seems not to match the displayed data very well.

The British anthropologist R. D. Martin took issue with this claim of Jerison's. From the somewhat more detailed presentation of the corresponding regressions[3] that I have excerpted in Figures 3.20b he extracted slopes of approximately 0.58 for birds, 0.54 for reptiles, and 0.76 for mammals. "Hence, for placental mammals, there is no empirical justification for the widely accepted value of 0.67 for the allometric exponent," he noted, nor does that value apply for the birds or reptiles either: in no class does brain size scale with the two-thirds power of body weight (a reasonable proxy for surface area). Martin went on to comment that if his calculations are the more nearly correct, then

> Jerison's use of an allometric exponent value of 0.67 in his calculation of 'encephalization quotients' for individual placental mammal species needs re-examination. If the correct value of the exponent is close to 0.75 [which is still a rational fraction, namely, 3/4], as suggested here for placental mammals, then Jerison's procedure overestimates 'expected' brain size for small-bodied mammals and underestimates them for large-bodied mammals. Secondly, if an allometric exponent of 0.56, rather than 0.67, is appropriate for both birds and reptiles, the converse applies and values for 'expected' brain sizes in large-bodied fossil forms must be revised downwards ... This is directly relevant to discussion of relative brain size in large-bodied dinosaurs. (Martin 1981: 60)

The scatters for birds and for reptiles, in spite of having very nearly the same slope, are nevertheless completely nonoverlapping: brain size in birds differs from that in reptiles by an average factor of 10 at any given body size. This is the sort of difference in intercept we have already seen in connection with Figure 3.18. But when we extend the comparison to the mammals, we encounter a quite different geometry of comparison. A regression line that begins at nearly the same location (0,2) as for the birds ends up at (8,8), a slope of about 0.75, in comparison to the same line for birds, which ends around (6,5), for a slope hardly greater than 1/2.

Martin has thus made his methodological point twice over. A quantity like the EQ can have meaning only in the event of parallel slopes in these log-log plots. This is the case for the comparison of reptiles with birds, but not for the birds or reptiles vis-a-vis the mammals. The mammalian slope of 0.76 closely matches the slope in Max Kleiber's "law" of the 1930s that metabolic rate scales roughly as the 3/4 power of an animal's mass. Martin argues that the fraction 3/4 is likely an expression of the same scaling phenomenon, in view of the mode of reproduction of the placental mammals: fetal brain weight, he suggests, should scale as maternal metabolic turnover, and then the adult

---

[3] Actually, these are "major axis" regressions, in other words the principal components sketched in Figure 2.32, but, as Martin notes, this substitute methodology "does not alter any of the basic conclusions."

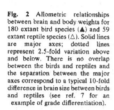

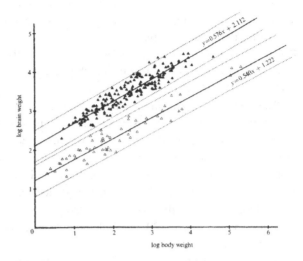

Fig. 2 Allometric relationships between brain and body weights for 180 extant bird species (▲) and 59 extant reptile species (△). Solid lines are major axes; dotted lines represent 2.5-fold variation above and below. There is no overlap between the birds and reptiles and the separation between the major axes corresponds to a typical 10-fold difference in brain size between birds and reptiles (see ref. 7 for an example of grade differentiation).

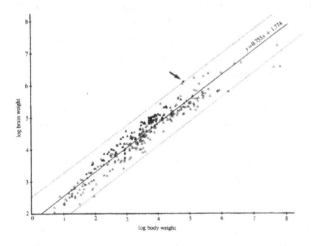

Fig. 1 Allometric relationships between brain and body weights for 309 extant placental mammal species. The solid line is the major axis; dotted lines represent fivefold variation above and below. Primates (▲) are typical of precocial mammals in exhibiting relatively large brains. The closest species to man (arrowed) is not another primate but a cetacean (dolphin).

Figure 3.20b Martin's version, from Martin (1981). (above) Log-log regressions of brain size on body size for reptiles and birds, separately. (below) The same for the mammals. Equations of best-fit regressions are printed on the corresponding lines in both frames. Bordering lines above: factors of 2.5 and 0.4 around the regression estimates. Below: factors of 5 and 0.2 around the estimates. Arrow: the point for *H. sapiens*. See text. Reprinted by permission from Macmillan Publishers Ltd: *Nature* 293:57–60, copyright 1981, https://www.nature.com/articles/293057a0.

brain weight should track the fetal value. Alas, Harvey and Krebs (1990) move the estimated slope to 0.69, most of the way back to Jerison's 0.67, by relying on the method of phylogenetic contrasts reviewed in Section 2.6.3. Further discussion, while fascinating, would evidently fall well outside the bounds of this book. For a late twentieth-century review of this debate, see Schoenemann (1997).

That same Schoenemann source, which is actually a dissertation available on the Web, offers another version of this same presentation (not reproduced here) that copies the regression line from Martin's analysis of the mammals in Figure 3.20b but simplifies the roster of taxa and identifies several more individual species. He can thereby make the point that, while humans have the highest EQ among the primates, a value nearly as high is found in one species of dolphin, the "false killer whale" *(Pseudorca crassidens)* ("a highly social, energetic species," Berta (2015), while among the primates the EQ does *not* rise with grade.

Suzana Herculano-Houzel (2016) takes exception to the focus on brain *weight* in plots like Jerison's or Martin's, arguing instead that an appropriate comparative analysis must involve more detailed aspects of brain architecture, in particular the actual counting of neurons (using a splendid new laboratory technique, "brain soup," that is charmingly described in her book) and that the analysis must be separate by the different components of the brain (specifically, cortex versus cerebellum – an elephant, for instance, has ten times the number of cerebellar neurons predicted from its cortical count, presumably to control the trunk). Figure 3.20c illustrates her argument mostly using the data in table I of Herculano-Houzel et al. (2015) on cortical mass and neuron counts in typical specimens from 40 species of mammals. (I have transcribed her table as one file in this book's online resource.) The allometric scaling of neuron count against cortical mass is different for the primates than for the other mammalian groups: the regression slopes here differ in a ratio of 1.41, comparable to the difference between slopes for mammals and reptiles in Figure 3.20b. Yet once we focus on the cortex alone, the locus of our principal cognitive capacities, *H. sapiens* is adequately close to the allometric regression for primates. The fit is even better if we use an averaged stereological neuron count for the humans (Pakkenberg and Gunderson, 1997), even though Herculano-Houzel deprecates this method as less reliable than the brain soup approach. The elephant, by contrast, in spite of its great cortical mass, falls nearly atop the regression line that pools all the other orders. *Pseudorca*, the species highlighted in Schoenemann's (1997) analysis, may have a large brain mass, but this mass is not characterized by any analogous increase in the cortical neuron count, which remains at a third of the

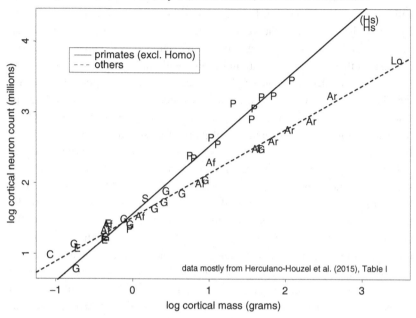

Figure 3.20c A hypothesis regarding "the human advantage": attending to the cortex instead of the whole brain, and counting neurons instead of weighing them. Data from Table I of Herculano-Houzel et al. (2015) on 40 genera of mammals from six orders (P, Primates; E, Eulipotyphla; G, Glires; Af, Afrotheria; S, Scandentia; Ar, Artiodactyla), except for the parenthesized (Hs), for which the neuron count is from Pakkenberg and Gunderson (1997). Two species lie at positions particularly worth noting: Hs, our very own *Homo sapiens*; and Lo, *Loxodonta africana*, the African elephant. Lines are allometric regressions for the nonhuman primates (solid line) and the other orders (dashed line) separately.

human level (Roth and Dicke, 2012) in spite of the whale's much greater body weight (about a metric ton).

"The human advantage," Herculano-Houzel concludes (page 105), "lies in having the largest number of neurons in the cerebral cortex that any animal species has ever managed." The evolutionary trick was to shrink our 16 billion cortical neurons (on the average) in order to fit into our viably small cerebral cortex; but their count is in keeping with the scaling of cortical neuron count against cortical mass over primate brains generally. Thus once again, as if repetition were necessary, we are displaced from the top of the Great Chain of Being: see Kampourakis (2014).

This extended example illustrated all four of the principal organismal applications of simple regression. Figure 3.20a showed how it can be exploited to confirm a slope arrived at theoretically, or, better, to claim such a confirmation (as the slope in question is apparently not the value of 2/3 claimed by Jerison, but instead the value of 3/4 more in keeping with the arguments of West). The figure also included a second application of the method: support for a claim that the point representing a particular specimen or taxon is "on the line" or else above or below. The pair of diagrams in Figure 3.20b showed a third type of rhetoric, the explicit comparison of pairs of these simple regression lines. In the upper panel here, the line for the birds and the line for the reptiles differ only in their intercept – they are parallel but differ by about a factor of 2 on the scale of the original dependent variable, brain weight – while either of these lines differs in slope (scaling of the underlying growth process) from the line for the mammals in the lower panel. Finally, the analysis in Figure 3.20c, produced by Herculano-Houzel quite recently shows a fourth, more radical use of the same technique: to challenge the choice of axes of someone else's analysis. For Jerison, comparing brain weight to body weight, the analysis for primates and that for the other mammals differed mainly in intercept. But when the pair of variables changes to cortical weight vis-á-vis neuron count, that parallelism no longer obtains. On the log scale here, changes in intercept have only arithmetical implications, but changes in slope act exponentially, with steadily greater effects with increasing body size. (In other words, something happened to change the way primates in general scale their neuron counts right from the original branching of the primates away from their mammalian stem.) And yet note that on this regression, in contrast to that reported by Jerison, we *Homo sapiens* fall right on the line of weighted average slope – or perhaps even a little bit below it. Clearly there is plenty of opportunity within the method of analysis of covariance (analogous regressions over multiple groups) for the pursuit of nuanced biological arguments of many different flavors.

The same quartet of rhetorics for regression reportage may be detected in the literatures of several other fields as well, such as the psychological sciences. Note that statistical hypothesis testing (estimation of the probability of a pattern at least this extreme corresponding to some atheoretical or process-free "null hypothesis" inexplicably postulated to govern the data at hand) does not appear on this list of the applications that typically lead to the insights most important for organismal biology, the scientific context within which morphometrics is nested.

3.3.3 A Regression Line Concealed within a Data Model

Sometimes the log-linearity that is called for by some theoretical explanation pertains not to the originally measured data but to some algebraic transform of them. For instance, the *Gompertz law of mortality* states that in typical modern human populations without systematic surges in deaths due to war, plagues, or other natural disasters, the specific death rate (also called "hazard rate") takes the form of an exponential function of age from some age onward. By "specific death rate" here is meant the risk of dying at a particular age after birth, computed as the number of deaths at that age in some standard population divided by the number of persons from that population alive at the start of that year of aging. If the specific death rate is exponential, then its logarithm should be a linear function of age.

Figure 3.21 shows an example using recent data for the United States. The publication cited in the figure caption presents "life tables," which are a combination of enumerated deaths in that year with estimates of the age distribution for the total population as of the beginning of the year (these are estimates because 2003 was not a census year in the United States). There are tables for males and females separately. The hazard rate is computed as the difference between the number surviving to age i and the number surviving to age $i+1$, out of a hypothetical "standard population" of 100,000, divided by the former number. The computations cease at age 100, when counts of observed deaths become too low to be stable. The data for this example are included in this book's online resource.

The Gompertz law (left panel) appears to describe the data remarkably well above an age of 35 or so – the hypothesized linearity of log hazard rate as a function of age seems quite obvious in both sexes. Below that age, there are clear deviations from the model – a nugget effect of about 7 deaths per 1000 during the first year of life, a local peak in death rates for males around age 23 (at which time we are typically at our most foolhardy – the specific death rate for males of that age is nearly three times the rate for females, in spite of the risks of childbirth) – but for the last 65 years of the calculations rates seems to vary not only smoothly but startlingly linearly in both sexes, suggesting a biological, not a sociological, process. There is an entire branch of academic medicine, gerontology, devoted to the modeling of data like these and their possible causal explanations across a wide range of animal species, not just humans: see, e.g., Masoro and Austad (2010) or Finch (2007). The log hazard rate plot is a more effective graphical style for these data than the ordinary survival curves, right panel, as the option of

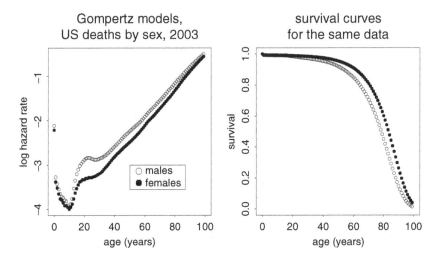

Figure 3.21 Death rates in the United States by sex, for 2003. (left) Graphed as log hazard rates (base 10). These are linear from about age 35 upward, in accordance with a Gompertz model (exponential increase of specific mortality rate with age). The two implied regressions differ between males and females but would apparently converge about age 110. (right) Graphed as survival curves. The visual convenience of linearity is no longer available. Data from Arias (2006), tables 2 and 3.

summarizing by two parameters (an intercept and a slope) is not available for the latter. The survivorship curves are clearer, on the other hand, for presenting the predominance of females in the older age ranges (more than two-thirds of the cohort at every age above 93). Analytically, we have combined the idea of a log regression (this section) with the idea of increments of a temporal process (Section 2.6).

Comparisons of Gompertz curves are often useful in reference to other epochs than the present. For a surprising application, the Black Death as a selective event in the Middle Ages, see Dewitte (2014).

3.3.4 Ecological Regressions and the Ecological Fallacy

None of the figures in the previous analysis have made the mistake noted in the legend of Figure 3.16, the computation of a single regression line in place of what should have been represented as two or more. Nevertheless, this sort of error is quite common, especially among people who tend to forget to display the appropriate data scatters – common enough that it has come to bear its own name, the *ecological fallacy*. Figure 3.18 showed how to translate the basic linear model from Figure 3.4 to match a design with multiple groups but manifestly parallel within-group regressions. The formulas involved three parameters – group predictor mean difference, predictor variance, and intercept mean difference – and worked regardless of their relative magnitudes. But the visual impression of the situation is quite different for different settings of those same magnitudes, and the failure of fit of the regression that failed to take the groups into account is likewise quite different among these various cases.

Figure 3.22 shows the same multiple regression of *Y* on *X* and a binary grouping variable, along with the simple regression that (mistakenly) omits the grouping variable, for a variety of these scenarios. The values of the parameters

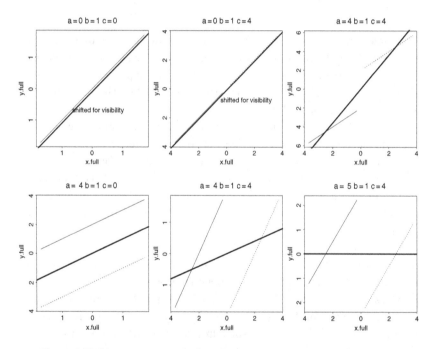

Figure 3.22 Six versions of the ecological fallacy, of which the version in Figure 3.17 is repeated here at upper right. In all panels, the group-specific regressions are drawn in dotted line, and the (inappropriate) pooled regressions in solid line. Upper left and upper center panels, pooled regressions that are the same as the within-group regressions, hence, no apparent fallacy. The situation at lower right leads to a pooled regression that is horizontal, meaning no net correlation, in spite of the obvious structure of nonindependence in this bivariate distribution.

a, b, and c in Figure 3.17 and equations (3.16) are listed across the top of each panel. The example we previously examined in detail falls into this series as the panel at upper right.

The panel at lower right is a very interesting case often encountered all by itself: production of a correlation of zero by cancellation of the two paths (direct and indirect) that it combines. You see how free play with the values of a and c can result in any relation you like between the within-group slope b and this pooled between-group slope for the same pair of variables X, Y as long as the grouping variable alters both of their means. Here I produced an exact zero for that slope by setting $a = -5, b = 1, c = 4$. This also serves as a tantalizing example (different, probably, from what you were shown in your earlier statistics course) of a pair of variables that are uncorrelated but not independent.

A question of a different flavor, answered by the same method. Back in the Berkeley Guidance study data set of Section 2.6, we attend to a previously unexamined variable, strength at ages 9 and 18, that appears to be correlated with the other scores at the same age. (See Figure 3.23.) The sexes differ in average strength by about 13% at age 9 but by nearly 70% at age 18. It would be helpful to build an index of height-adjusted strength, or anything-else-adjusted strength, that corrects for this somewhat invidious difference, which we would prefer not to attribute to pure testosterone. (This situation is familiar enough in the real world of biometrical consulting: a clear dimorphism that discomfits us enough to wish it would go away.) The challenge is to "adjust" the measured difference in strength between the sexes at age 18 for their difference in size at that age.

Whenever you see the word "adjustment" you should be thinking about computing some multiple regression – but also critiquing that regression as earnestly as possible. If we crudely regress ST18 on sex and the other 18-year variables, there is a hint that HT18 and LG18 might be informative. So, recalling the power of the added-variable strategy, we scatter the residual log ST18.sex – the variation of log strength around its sex-specific averages – against the residuals of log HT18, log WT18, and log LG18 similarly centered. The resulting scatters are laid out in Figure 3.24.

These plots seem promising. Each of the three other log size variables seems to correlate with the same within-sex log strength variation. The largest of these, by a smidgen, is LG18. (Remember that LG stands for "leg girth"; probably a lot of that girth is muscle.) Figure 3.25 shows that no further polishing of this prediction is likely to be meaningful.

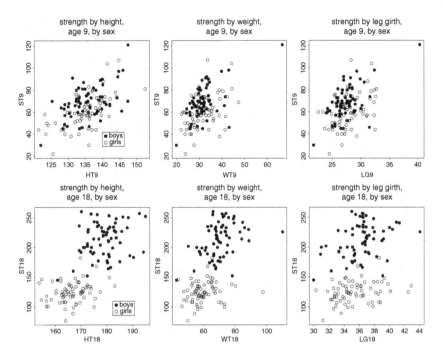

Figure 3.23 Enhancement of earlier displays of data from the Berkeley Guidance Study to include measured "strength" at ages 9 and 18 years. The new measure is scattered against height, weight, and leg girth at both ages. Sex is coded as a solid disk for boys and an open circle for girls.

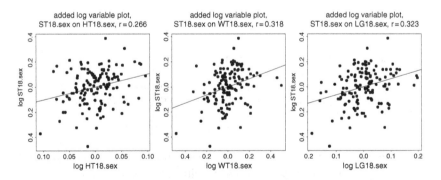

Figure 3.24 Added variable plots for the residual of ST18 (strength at age 18) by three other potential predictors from the Berkeley Guidance Study. The data have been log-transformed per the insights from Figure 2.39.

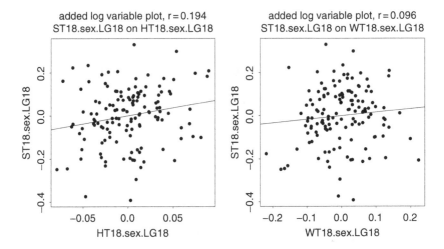

Figure 3.25 Added variable plots for further contributions after Leg Girth has been added to the prediction formula. There is no further meaningful contribution to be had from either height (left panel) or weight (right panel) at this age.

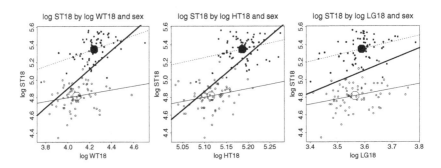

Figure 3.26 A better graphical design: prediction of ST18 by each of the remaining continuous measures, separately by sex. Dotted lines: within-sex regressions. Solid line: pooled (incorrect) regression. Large solid disk: average scattered position for boys. Large open circle: the same for girls. The middle panel is the most informative.

Better, though, to cast this entire investigation into the framework of analysis of covariance we've just been exploiting. See Figure 3.26.

It seems that the presentation by added-variable plots in Figure 3.24 was misleading. In reality, each path combines two different forms of influence: the mean difference between the sexes on the predictor, along with the within-group slope; but the added-variable plots include only the within-group slopes.

The difference between group means of strength at age 18 is apparently not a matter of within-group correlations to any great extent, but instead expresses an irreducible sexual dimorphism: boys are stronger than girls, on average, at every height (and likewise every value of weight, and every value of leg girth), and the pooled regression line comes closest to the sex-specific means for height against strength merely because the difference in heights of the sexes is larger than dimorphism of either weight or leg girth.

In short, the difference between boys' and girls' strength at age 18 does not really adjust away by any combination of the other measures (HT18, WT18, LG18) available at that measurement wave. Yes, the boys are taller on average, but strength is not solely a function of measured height. Ditto weight: the boys are heavier, but their excess strength is far greater than what would be proportional to that increased size. And even the leg girth measure, which would seem to be explicitly related to muscle mass, does not explain the dimorphism (because although it correlates nicely with strength within sex, it does not actually show much of a mean difference between boys and girls). This is a useful demonstration of the limits that actual empirical scientific phenomena place on the power of statistics to (mis)inform. The best presentation of the sexual dimorphism in strength of these Berkeley 18-year-olds is the central panel of Figure 3.26, which shows that most of the difference is irreducible to the other measures taken.

Summary of Section 3.3

- The geometry of Section 3.1 embraces an alternative measurement design in which one of the two predictors is a category name. *Analysis of covariance* is the decomposition of total effects into direct plus indirect when at least one predictor is a category. It works just as well in this setting as in the setting of two continuous predictors.
- When an analysis of covariance is set as a linear model in this way, it is an easy extension to formalize the difference in slopes between two groups as a ratio to its own standard error of estimate.
- One central concern of evolutionary neurology, the scaling of brain weight against body weight over the vertebrates, has been profitably studied and modeled by analysis of covariance for decades. The regression slope for log brain weight against log body weight is shallower for reptiles than for birds and mammals, and the intercept is higher for mammals than for birds. *Homo sapiens* falls well above this regression line, but so does *Pseudorca*.

- Some other data designs reduce to analysis of covariance after a transformation. For instance, the *Gompertz model* for mortality by sex linearizes, at least in the United States, when log survival is converted to its increment, the *log hazard rate.*
- The *ecological fallacy* emerges especially clearly in analysis of covariance when a direct effect and a total effect have opposite signs.
- The stability of a group effect against probes for ecological fallacies over a variety of covariates can be as important a component of data reports as the within-group regressions themselves.

3.4 Special Case 2: Growth Series

Growth series data are size measurements on the same organisms over a list of ages that are the same for every specimen in a data set. There are specialized toolkits for analyzing data of this type, such as growth curve analysis and functional data analysis (Ramsay and Silverman, 2010). But in morphometrics such approaches are less useful than some modest modifications of the techniques we have already introduced – correlation, regression, added-variable plots – so as to apply to variables having just one additional structural facet, the ordering over age. In these simpler approaches, time does not serve as a dimension sustaining the operations of calculus (integration, differentiation), but only the simpler operations of linear statistical theory. In this book, the extension to derivatives is reserved for the *spatial* dimensions introduced as a substrate of the geometric morphometric data bases in the examples of Chapter 4.

In effect, our reasoning here in this book deals with growth as a form of *explanation,* the persistence over time of processes affecting the increments of measured form or function that go unobserved between measurement sessions until subtraction reveals their patterns. We biologists expect constancy of coefficients relating multiple measures of the same quantities over at least small intervals of time, and also we expect (at least for the best-designed samples) commonalities in the numerical aspects of these comparisons across specimens. These explanatory frameworks fit well under the general regression-and-correlation-based tools we have already introduced. Greater abstraction in respect of spatial variations is the topic of the second half of Chapter 4, and deeper digging into the temporal domain is the concern of a good many textbooks that have already been written to cover specific forms of signal analysis for biologists (Kalman filtering, autoregressive and integrated autoregressive processes, and a variety of practical approaches to nonlinear dynamics).

3.4.1 Persistence of Growth: Partial Correlations along Growth Series

Example 3.5: Berkeley lengths, revisited again. We already encountered the Berkeley Guidance Study in connection with the graphical exploration of its trends over time in Section 2.6. Figure 3.27 revisits the height histories of the boys in order to examine individual differences in these trends.

Recall that partial correlations (equation 3.12a) are just correlations between residuals from regressions of different outcome variables on the same predictor list. For this application, we take X to be HT2, Y as HT18, and Z as HT9 – the variables of the growth series, but out of order. The numerator of equation (3.12a) then becomes $(r_{2,18} - r_{2,9}r_{9,18})$ — the difference of the long-term correlation from the product of the short-term correlations. This is just the difference between indirect and total effects in the corresponding path diagram, and so it would estimate the "direct effect" of age-2 height on age-18 height if there were such a direct effect. I will call it a *lagged direct effect* below.

This numerator is then divided by $\sqrt{1 - r_{2,9}^2}\sqrt{1 - r_{9,18}^2}$, the product of the variances of the separate regression residuals, to arrive at the correlation of the two residuals per se (one facing forward in time, one backward). For boys' height, we have $r_{2,9} = 0.703, r_{2,18} = 0.571, r_{9,18} = 0.875$, and the numerator of the partial correlation (the lagged direct effect) evaluates to about -0.044, with a partial correlation of -0.13.

It is worth computing these same lagged direct effects for the other three possible analyses in our little data set: boys' weight, girls' height, and girls' weight. The lagged direct effects are $-0.08, +0.07$, and -0.09 and the partial correlations are $-0.12, 0.17$, and -0.17, respectively. None of these are more

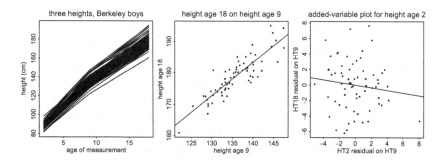

Figure 3.27 A more detailed look at the height histories of the 66 boys in the Berkeley Guidance Study, Figure 2.37. There is a moderately strong regression of the age-18 measurement on the age-9 measurement (center panel), to which the age-2 measurement adds no useful information (right panel, added-variable plot).

than 140% of the corresponding standard error in magnitude, and their signs are inconsistent. If the partial correlation were zero, the prediction of the age-18 score from the age-2 score would be the product of the two paths 2-to-9 and 9-to-18, a so-called *causal chain*. In this circumstance, the two regressions being combined have uncorrelated error terms.

We have already seen this pattern on the quincunx: it is the pattern by which observations of a sample of balls all progressing downward are correlated across any sequence of rows. The situation appears to be the same for the comparisons we just inspected. If any one of these partial correlations were much less than zero, the interpretation would be that the errors of the two predictions are negatively correlated, as, for instance, by some effect of a growth spurt that if observed before age 9 is not available to be observed after age 9. If the one occurrence of a positive partial correlation, height for girls, were more salient, the interpretation would be in terms of a positive correlation of the series of prediction errors, for instance, continuing effects of variations in quality of nutrition (although that finding might be unlikely in an upper-middle-class sample like this one from Berkeley). But it is the case that all the partial correlations reported are within 1.4 standard errors of zero, and thus carry neither positive nor negative implications for growth as observed at these relatively wide intervals of observation.

Example 3.6: The Vilmann rat skull data: areas, revisited. For a more complex growth example, we return to the Vilmann data set of 18 rats at 8 ages, in an attempt to tease out individual-level information. The example is still restricted to measures of extent (distances and areas) only; aspects of shape per se are reserved for later in this book.

Figure 3.28 introduces two successive enhancements of the final panel of Figure 2.42 in Example 2.7. At left, I have altered the vertical axis from octagon area to its logarithm, and replaced Centroid Size along the horizontal by the logarithm of the age-specific average area (in order to straighten out the plot). At right, I have further clarified things by subtracting the columnwise mean from the vertical scores column by column; that subtraction allows the contrasts across animals at the same age to be magnified about fivefold. Several clear features assort our individual animals. For instance, two depart from the litter at the third age – they were large before, but now they are strikingly larger than the third-largest animal, and remain at that relative size advantage through the sixth observation (for one of the two) and right through the end of the study (for the second of the two, an animal whose braincase appears to just keep on growing). Analogously, one animal is lowest at five of our eight observations, in spite of being middling in size at the youngest age.

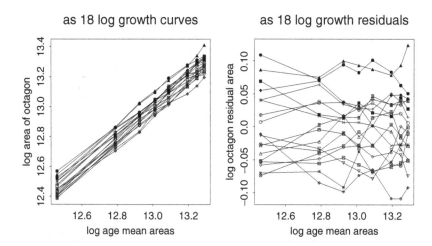

Figure 3.28 When the rodent neurocranial growth curves of Figure 2.42 are spaced according to their own age-by-age averages (left panel), clear patterns emerge in the persistence of deviations by individual animals (right panel). In either plot, each animal is plotted with a different symbol, just to ease the tracing across the vertical milestones.

Can we say more – are some of these age stages, or some of these animals, more labile than others? First, the question of stages. We see the following correlations between log areas at successive stages: 0.821, 0.917, 0.925, 0.924, 0.884, 0.928, 0.923. Five of these are more or less the same value, about 0.92, meaning there is a residual variance of roughly $\sqrt{1 - .92^2} = 0.39$ on this log scale; but between the first two stages the perseveration is far less, with an effective innovation of $\sqrt{1 - .821^2} = .57$. The step from the fifth to the sixth age class is intermediate in this respect. Yet the correlation from beginning to end of these entire series – from the age-7 area to the age-150 area – is a surprisingly large 0.633 (surprising in view of the product of the seven lag-1 correlations, which is only 0.487). So the rodent neural skull's "memory" for whatever it is that sets these changes is quite stable (as we have already seen from the fact that the largest two animals stay largest throughout the 143 days of observation). By comparison, the log area at 30 days predicts this at the end of the series almost perfectly ($r = 0.917$). Change of area in this system is, in the jargon of Conrad Waddington, highly *canalized* over the whole period following weaning. A good report of this pattern is conveyed by the simpler pair of graphics in Figure 3.29: two different predictions of the adult log octagonal area, one from the data at age 7 days, the other the data at age 30 days.

And there is no evidence of random walk (Section 2.6.2). The variance of log area at every age is nearly the same (the range is from 0.0022 to 0.0031

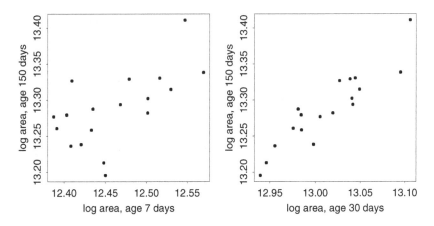

Figure 3.29 Predictions of later area by earlier area. (left) Over the full length of
the data record, age 7 days to 150 days, $r = 0.63$. (right) From age 30 days to the
end of the record, $r = 0.92$.

only), and the actual minimum of these variances is for the data from age
30 days, just about in the middle of the time series. (Once you have noticed
this hint numerically, you can see something that looks like a pinching at this
abscissa in Figure 3.28.) We will see in Section 5.6 that this corresponds to
an apparently real morphometric phenomenon, the canalization of the uniform
component (relative height) of these shapes at that same age.

   This explanation in terms of persistent change, rather than either regression
or random walk, is supported as well by the pattern of partial correlations of
any pair of consecutive measures at ages j and $j + 2$ adjusted for the score at
age $j + 1$. We are in effect assessing the extent to which, as assessed by log
area, these skulls show a "memory" that short-circuits the quincuncial causality
that would otherwise be in place. The partial correlations corresponding to
the nonconsecutive path are $-0.05, 0.37, 0.50, 0.24, 0.03$, and -0.18. Hence
the adolescent triples of these series show persistence, indeed up to quite a
high level for the age 21-30-40 subseries; for the other age intervals, this same
effect is negligible. We can unearth this same persistence without the benefit
of added-variable plots, in the raw correlation structure of the log areas as
well: the correlations among the log areas at ages 21, 30, and 40 days are all
about 0.925. If these were measures from a quincunx, the 21-to-40 correlation
would be instead expected to be the product of the two correlations over shorter
intervals, which is 0.855 only. The pairwise plots in Figure 3.29 show that
much of this stability is due to the stubbornly large area of the largest animal.
As Figure 3.28 hints, there is an additional animal whose large size was stable
over the last five measures but not before that.

3.4.2 Uncertainties of Correlations

Equation (2.10) set out the standard error of a computed regression slope. It is equally helpful to have a formula for the standard errors of correlations. For true values of r near zero, the standard error of the estimated r is $1/\sqrt{N-3}$, which is our usual inverse-square-root formula in N modified by the fact that we have estimated three parameters (the covariance and the two standard deviations). A useful formula from R. A. Fisher is that in the absence of a true correlation in samples from a bivariate Gaussian distribution (e.g., a situation like that in Figure 2.28), the *Fisher's z*, the formula

$$z = \frac{1}{2} \log \frac{1+r}{1-r} \tag{3.19}$$

is distributed around 0 with a standard error of $1/\sqrt{N-3}$ *everywhere*. The formula assigns the same standard error of $1/\sqrt{N-3}$ for correlations very near 0 with N large, but accommodates the shrinkage of the range with respect to a Gaussian as the correlation moves closer to 1 or -1. If the true population correlation is a value ρ, zero or not, the same evaluate $\frac{1}{2} \log \frac{1+r}{1-r}$ is distributed around $\frac{1}{2} \log \frac{1+\rho}{1-\rho}$ with the same standard error of $1/\sqrt{N-3}$. This corresponds to

$$\sigma_\rho \cong \frac{1-\rho^2}{\sqrt{n}} \tag{3.20}$$

as long as ρ falls short of 1 by at least a few multiples of this standard error. It is this version that was published first: it is from Pearson and Filon (1898), which is a remarkably early date.[4] The Pearson-Filon paper declared formula (3.20) "novel" at the time. I return to the general nature and provenance of formulas like these at the beginning of the next chapter, where I show precisely how (3.20) was derived.

> Here is how the z-transform follows directly from equation (3.20): If the standard error of ρ is proportional to $1 - \rho^2$, then the error variance of the function $z = \int_0^r \frac{1}{1-s^2} ds$, the so-called *stabilizing transformation*, is constant. But $\int_0^r \frac{1}{1-s^2} ds = \int_0^r \frac{1}{2} \left(\frac{1}{1+s} + \frac{1}{1-s} \right) ds = \frac{1}{2} (\log(1+r) - \log(1-r))$, which is z. This remarkably succinct derivation is from Kendall (1953).

Figure 3.30 may help clarify this. The figure reports the result of nine different simulations of 2000 correlations of 2000 random Gaussian pairs. The simulations correspond to values of the correlation set (by the technique

---

[4] Although this item is even older than Pearson and Lee (1903), the source of the data for Figure 2.28, nevertheless it is likewise available on the Web via the scholarly journal archive JSTOR.

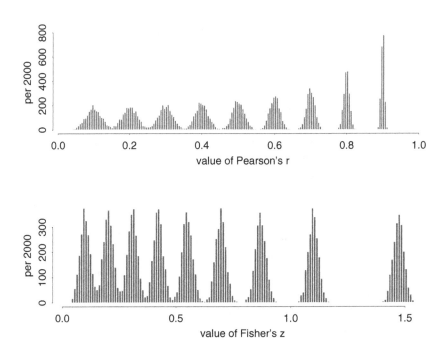

Figure 3.30 Distributions of repeated random samples of correlations (upper row) and their Fisher's z transforms (lower row) for 2000 simulations each of 2000 cases of Gaussian data with true correlations $0.1, 0.2, \ldots, 0.9$.

of Figure 2.23) at values evenly spaced from 0.1 to 0.9. The top row shows the distribution of the correlation coefficients on the usual scale. You see that these distributions become steadily narrower with increasing r – the variance of the same 2000 r's, the quantity approximated by the formula $(1 - r^2)^2/2000$, falls with r. Inspected more closely, the distributions of r toward the right of the diagram are detectably skew, with longer tails to the left than to the right. The bottom row shows exactly the same 18,000 simulations now expressed as $\frac{1}{2} \log \frac{1+r}{1-r}$, the Fisher z-transformation. The distribution of each of the nine correlation classes now looks the same, but the effect of the transformation is to spread out the nine separate correlation classes toward the right, corresponding to the fact that the difference between an r of 0.1 and one of 0.2 is much less important than the difference between 0.8 and 0.9. (Indeed, the difference of z's for $r = 0.1$ vs 0.2 is 0.13, versus 0.37 for $r = 0.8$ vs 0.9.)

We apply this approach to put some inferential force behind our question about persistence by attending to the partial correlations

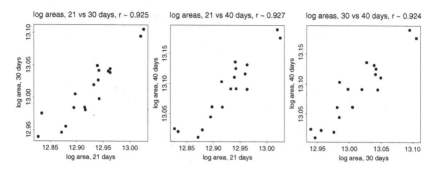

Figure 3.31 Three lagged correlations of the log octagonal area for Vilmann's rodent skulls. The correlation between ages 21 and 40 is much higher than it would be if these data arose as a causal chain without persistence.

$r\left(\left((\log A_j)|\log A_{j-1}\right),\left((\log A_{j-2})|\log A_{j-1}\right)\right)$ of rodent neurocranial octagonal area just computed above. The largest partial correlation we observed was 0.50. On the present sample of N=18 rats, we find $\frac{1}{2}\log\frac{1+r}{1-r} = 0.55$ with a standard error of $1/\sqrt{15} = 0.26$. So the partial correlation for persistence of midsagittal area around the time of the fourth age measurement in this sample is a bit more than twice its standard error. (In conventional terms, $p = 0.035$.) In other words, this may be a serious finding, not a toy. The situation is as depicted in Figure 3.31. We will return to this issue of persistence in Section 5.6 when we reexamine the data of this example at a greater level of spatial detail, and confirm it by production of the explicit growth-gradient, *partial warp 1*, that drives it.

3.4.3 Predicting a Summary Growth Measure from Its Components

We have thus far represented the neurocranial octagon of landmarks in Figure 2.41 by just one quantity, its area. It is remarkable how tightly integrated this summary is with a wide range of other descriptors. To demonstrate this proposition, even before introducing the morphometric techniques that describe that pattern, I show how easy it is to predict this areal measure from two distance measures across this form, as long as I get to select the pair of distances. Based on the fact that they give the best regression R^2, I suggest choosing the two in Figure 3.32: the segment from SES to Opisthion, and the segment from ISS to Bregma. The transect from SES to Opisthion is the longest diameter of this octagon; the segment from ISS to Bregma cuts it at roughly 90 degrees, a phenomenon that is not at all accidental, as we shall

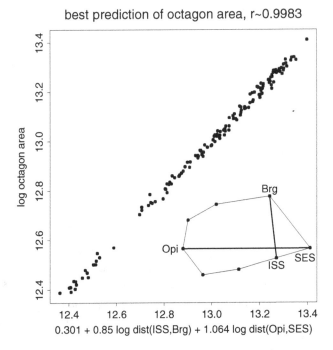

Figure 3.32 Multiple regression of the log area of our neurocranial octagon on the logs of two selected interlandmark distances. The high multiple correlation is remarkable, as is the fact that the coefficients of the two logged distances are strikingly distinct.

see in Section 5.2. This pair of single distances, using only four points of the octagon and only two quantities out of the eight coordinates needed for those four points, predicts the net area of the octagon delimited by all eight of the points with a correlation of 0.9983. Undoing the log transformations, the actual prediction equation is

$$\text{octagon.area} \sim 1.3512 \times |\text{Brg–ISS}|^{0.8504} \times |\text{Opi–SES}|^{1.0639} \qquad (3.21)$$

where $|\cdot|$ means "the length of [the segment between the two named landmarks inside the bars]" and the landmark abbreviations are as in Figure 2.41. The two distance measures involved are those sketched in the inset to the figure here. Here is the regression output:

```
summary(lm(log(vilmann.area)~log(vilmann.dists.
  complete[,5,7])+log(vilmann.dists.complete[,2,6])))
(Intercept) 0.3011 0.1396 2.1567
```

```
log(vilmann.dists.complete[, 5, 7]) 0.8504 0.0360
  23.6298
log(vilmann.dists.complete[, 2, 6]) 1.0639 0.0148
  71.8368
Residual standard error: 0.01514 on 141 degrees of
  freedom
Multiple R-Squared: 0.9967
```

$$(3.22)$$

Notice that the exponents of the two distances are different. We will see in Section 5.6 that the dominance of the horizontal transect over the vertical in the formula is related to the geometry of the first principal component (relative warp) of this set of landmarked forms. The horizontal diameter scales faster with size than the vertical diameter (the difference is almost five times the standard error of this difference), and (to the log scale) the formula takes on the general format of a weighted average as in Section 2.2. The standard error of this prediction, on the log scale, is about 1.5% of the area being predicted. Back at the scale of the original data, without the logging, this is a prediction standard error of about 7000 square units over a range of 240,000 to 677,000 square units, which is an unusually high prediction accuracy for a composite measure over so great a growth range. Note, finally, that the units of equation (3.21) almost work out: $cm^{0.85} \times cm^{1.06} = cm^{1.91} \sim cm^2$, the appropriate units for an area.

Summary of Section 3.4

- While there is a substantial toolkit of advanced techniques for handling data that come as series measured on the same organisms at different ages, often the questions of greatest biological interest can be answered by simple modifications of the linear modeling tools we have already encountered.

- One simple exploration of whether a growth series data set shows evidence for "memory" examines estimates of the magnitude of the indirect paths spanning two intervals between measurements. When these partial correlations are all small, the progression of scores can be modeled as a *causal chain* corresponding to balls falling down successive aggregates of rows of a quincunx.

- Large partial correlations instead indicate patterns of persistent change possibly arising from longer-term variability in hidden system parameters. Such data often fail to show regression to the mean.

- The comparison of correlations that are not close to zero is made feasible by *Fisher's z-transformation*, their conversion by the formula $z = \frac{1}{2}\log\frac{1+r}{1-r}$. After a z-transformation, correlations around different true slopes have the same standard error of sampling, $1/\sqrt{N-3}$, making it much easier to compare their values.
- In growth studies, summary measures such as area often can be predicted well by loglinear models using just two of their components. In the example here, Vilmann's growing rodent skulls, the multiple regression of the logarithm of the area of the octagon on the logs of a particular pair of its diameters predicts its value with a multiple correlation of 0.9983.

3.5 Special Case 3a: Linear Discriminant Analysis

3.5.1 Classification via a Likelihood Ratio Loglinear in the Data

Let us return to the contemplation of the Gaussian distribution, equation (2.16). Suppose that we have two of these distributions, with the same variance but different means, as in the left panel of Figure 3.33. To be precise, the means

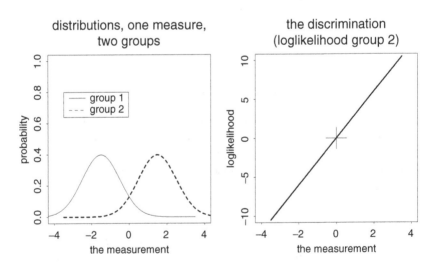

Figure 3.33 The simplest context of a linear discriminant analysis: one single measurement with a Gaussian distribution of the same standard deviation in each of two groups. (left) The data distributions. (right) The corresponding loglikelihood in favor of group 2 for a new specimen. This is a straight line whose height is zero (the log of 1) at the measurement where the two group-specific bell curves intersect. This point is an example of the *measurement value locus of indifference* explained in the text.

are ± 1.5, and the variance of either bell curve is 1.0 – these are just left and right shifts of the standard variance-1 curve. Now imagine that a new specimen arrives with a new measurement – call it x – and that we want to *classify* this specimen as to the group that it likely came from.

This is a perfect setting for the evocation of Laplace's Principle from Section 2.1.4. We have two *hypotheses:* either x came from the first group, or it came from the second. The probability that it came from the first group is $\frac{1}{\sqrt{2\pi}}e^{-(x+1.5)^2/2}$; from the second group, $\frac{1}{\sqrt{2\pi}}e^{-(x-1.5)^2/2}$. The ratio of these is $e^{-((x-1.5)^2-(x+1.5)^2)/2} = e^{3x}$ — the π's and the quadratic terms cancel, leaving only the linear part. Thus the loglikelihood for the hypothesis that x was a measure coming from the second group, vis-á-vis the first, is just $3x$. This is the line that is drawn in the right-hand panel of Figure 3.33. We assign cases with $x < 0$ to group 1, and cases with $x > 0$ to group 2, and the odds ratio supporting our assignments would be just e^{3x} in favor of group 2, or e^{-3x} in favor of group 1, whichever quantity is greater than 1. The line drawn here goes through the point $(0, 0)$ of this plot, at the plus sign, because at that point, just halfway between the group means, the probabilities of membership in the two groups are the same (i.e., the bell curves on the left cross there), and so the log-odds ratio is the log of 1, which is zero. This point is called the *locus of indifference*, as the corresponding data are equivocal (indifferent) with respect to the choice between the two hypotheses. (When the variances differ between the groups, the locus has more than one point. Discussion of this situation is deferred to Section 3.6.)

Now consider the diagram in Figure 3.34, where there are two predictors instead of just one. At left, we see two circles of the same radius around different centers that, just to ease the visualization, are further apart than the diameter of the circle. The diagram is meant to suggest the following task: given *two* measurements of each of the cases in a labeled sample (a "training set"), to assign a new specimen with measures (x, y), say, to one of the two groups. The circles cannot draw the entire probability distribution in this space, the way they did (via the bell-curve icon) in the one-dimensional situation. By convention we set them to trace the locus of points exactly one standard deviation away from the group mean in their direction (a sort of "belt" around the bell).

On the left side of Figure 3.34, the variable y is completely uninformative about the grouping, so the problem reduces to that of the preceding figure. There are still two hypotheses, (x, y) arising from group 1 or from group 2, and the likelihood ratio favors group 1 for points (x, y) with their x-value nearer the group-1 average and group 2 for points with x nearer *that* average. The heavy line in the figure (the locus of indifference in this two-predictor setting) separates these two classes, and the likelihood of the likelier hypothesis will be constant on lines parallel to this one at even spacings in the log odds. Do

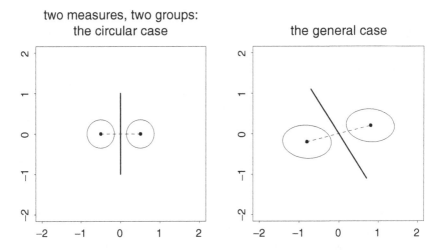

Figure 3.34 The symmetry of the univariate setting (Figure 3.33) is copied over unchanged to the general case by postulating an uncorrelated second variable and then ignoring it (left panel). Here the locus of indifference (heavy line) is just the extension of the point in Figure 3.33 by that second, irrelevant coordinate. (right panel) In reality, most pairs of predictors are correlated. In that case, transform the entire diagram by the appropriate shear, rotation, and scaling (here it is done graphically) until those covariance ellipses become circles. The line of indifference of the original problem is the result of shearing the obvious line *back* to the diagram of ellipses with which we started. It is no longer the perpendicular bisector of the segment connecting the group centers, but instead cuts that segment at its midpoint in the direction along the tangents to the covariance ellipse at either point where this segment intercepts those ellipses. A construction like this one is an analysis in terms of *affine geometry*, unchanging over uniform shears of the type to be analyzed in Section 5.5.3.

not think of this line's direction as "perpendicular to the line between the group centers"; think of it instead as parallel to the tangent direction of either concentration ellipse where it is cut by that intercenter segment.

The right-hand panel takes the figure on the left and gives it a shear and a twist, so that the circles turn into ellipses of general shape in general position. But the logic of our assigned task remains exactly the same. The locus of indifference continues to be the line through the midpoint of the group centers in the direction of the tangent to either ellipse where the segment joining the centers cuts it. Points on one side of this line are likelier to have come from group 1, points on the other side from group 2, and the loglikelihood is constant on lines parallel to this line and evenly spaced in the log odds. In other words, the entire diagram participated in that shearing and twisting: the whole linear discrimination, not just the data.

This is a general theorem: scaling, shearing, shifting, or rotating of a diagram like that one does not change the likelihood ratios driving the classifications in this approach. (The reason is that probability goes as an integral over tiny elements of area, and under the given list of transformations – these are the *affine* transformations that leave parallel lines parallel – all ratios of areas remain unchanged.) So regardless of shears, rotations, etc., the previous logic applies verbatim.

The efficiency of the classification – the steepness of that gradient of log odds – varies as the orientation of the group mean separation varies with respect to the axis of greatest variability of the within-group covariance structure. Notice, please, that in the general case (the right-hand panel of Figure 3.34), the discrimination is **not** equivalent to any sort of projection on the line between the group means. The gradient of the discriminant function need not align with this direction. The situation is the same in Figure 3.35. When the within-group covariance matrix is not circular (Figure 3.35), the

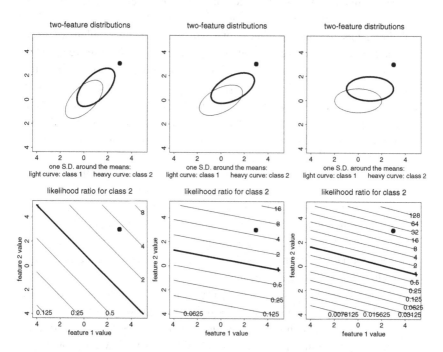

Figure 3.35 The efficiency of a classification rises as the long axis of the within-group scatter matrix rotates away from the line connecting the group means. Small numbers: likelihood ratios line by line. The group centroids are unchanging across the three panels here; only the covariance structures are rotating. Lines of constant loglikelihood in all three lower panels are spaced uniformly in increments of log 2.

direction of the line of indifference can rotate arbitrarily far from perpendicularity to the direction joining the group means, according to the shear matrix Σ^{-1} to be derived in equation (3.23).

3.5.2 Why This Works: The Algebra of Linear Discrimination

(This subsection may be skipped on a first reading.) To prove all the preceding assertions, we will need a formula from standard matrix algebra. If I_p is the $p \times p$ identity matrix and B is any p-vector, then, as one checks just by multiplying things out,

$$(I_p + BB')^{-1} = I_p - BB'/(1 + B'B). \tag{3.23}$$

Here BB' is a rank-1 matrix, and $B'B$ is just a decimal number, the squared length of B. In the simplest case, when B itself is just a number, equation (3.23) turns into $1/(1 + x^2) = 1 - \left(x^2/(1 + x^2)\right)$, which is true.

Holding this formula in reserve, we will consider the problem of *linear discrimination* that we have just been posing informally. Suppose we have two groups of specimens (call them A and B) and a set of one or more quantitative measurements – a *vector* $X = (X_1, X_2, \ldots)$ of observations on every specimen. A new specimen shows up, with measurement vector Z, say, and we want to *classify it* – to assign it to one or the other of the groups, A or B. We also want to specify the degree of confidence that we have in the resulting classification.

The linear machinery already introduced in this chapter is sufficient for us to proceed rationally toward this goal. To say the unknown specimen belongs to group A is one hypothesis, that it belongs to group B, a contrary hypothesis. Each of these hypotheses will have a likelihood given the data. We want to assign every new specimen to the group for which its membership is the hypothesis with the larger likelihood, and we want a formula for the confidence we should attach to that assignment.

We can proceed with this task as soon as we have a model for the likelihood of either hypothesis given the data. For this algebra to work out in the nicest possible way it is enough to assume, along with everybody else's textbook, that within each group the measurements of the p-vector X are Gaussianly distributed according to some mean vector μ_1 or μ_2 with the same covariance matrix Σ regardless of group. We further simplify by assuming that the grand mean across the two groups is the zero vector, and that the groups are the same size N. Write $\mu_1 = -\mu_2 = \mu$, say.

At the outset, we will consider only the special case $\Sigma = I$, a covariance structure that is the identity matrix, so that the general formula

$$N(X|\mu_i, \Sigma) = \frac{1}{\sqrt{\det(2\pi\Sigma)}}\exp(-(X - \mu_i)'\Sigma^{-1}(X - \mu_i)/2) \qquad (3.24)$$

for the probability density function of group i at location X simplifies to

$$N(X|\mu_i, I) = (2\pi)^{-p/2}\exp(-(X - \mu_i)'(X - \mu_i)/2). \qquad (3.25)$$

To classify a new measurement vector Z that happens along, we need the likelihood ratio for the hypothesis that Z's group is A rather than B – that the appropriate group mean is μ rather than $-\mu$. It is enough to examine the logarithm of that ratio, which is the difference of two copies of equation (3.25) with different means. Because that factor in front of the exponential cancels, the log of this ratio is

$$(-(Z - \mu_1)'(Z - \mu_1)/2) - (-(Z - \mu_2)'(Z - \mu_2)/2) = 2\mu'Z, \qquad (3.26)$$

the projection of the measurement vector Z on the segment 2μ between the group averages, because $\mu_1 = -\mu_2$.

Now, seemingly starting over, let us set up the ordinary (apparently nonsensical) multiple regression problem that regresses *group number* on the same vector X of predictors. (The regression is nonsense because it is group number that predicts the measured features, not vice versa.) I am free to decide how to encode the group name (A or B) as a number, and I choose to use the coding $y = -1$ or 1 (again to simplify the notation to follow). We are predicting y, the group membership score, from the measured variables (e.g., lengths) X. The prediction function for group Y, evaluated at Z, is $\hat{Y} = Z(X'X)^{-1}X'Y$, where Y is the vector of all the sample group numbers, probably a list of $+1$'s followed by a list of -1's, and now $X'X/2N$ is the covariance structure of the data set *as pooled over group*. We recall from the very first theorems about least-squares that in this setting of groups with within-group covariance structure I and group means $\pm\mu$, we have $X'X/2N = I + \mu\mu'$, the sum of the within-group covariance matrix plus the expected outer product of the mean shift vector by itself, averaged over the groups (the choice of which group is scored 1 makes no difference here, as $\mu\mu'$ and $(-\mu)(-\mu')$ are the same).

The regression (which, remember, makes no scientific sense) of group number on the measurement vector then has coefficients that are the entries of the vector that premultiplies the covariance of X with Y by the inverse of the covariance matrix of the X's, likewise pooled over the full data set of $2N$ cases. That covariance is the expected value of XY, but XY averages μ in group A and

$-1 \cdot (-\mu)$ in group B, which is the same vector; so the covariance $\overline{XY}$ is just μ. Then the regression coefficient vector is

$$(I + \mu\mu')^{-1}\mu = (I - \mu\mu'/(1 + \mu'\mu))\mu = \mu/(1 + \mu'\mu). \qquad (3.27)$$

The line through $(0, 0)$ with this slope does *not* go through the group means.– it shows its version of "regression to the mean" (zero) just as it should.

Applying this to a single new case with observation vector Z, this is the prediction $(\mu'/(1 + \mu'\mu))Z$, which differs from the log likelihood ratio formula only by two times that scalar attenuation factor $1 + \mu'\mu$. Hence: assuming that each within-group covariance matrix is the identity, the optimal (maximum-likelihood) solution to the *classification problem,* the assignment of a new specimen to a group, is the assignment based on the sign of the regression predictor from the *(apparently nonsensical)* regression of a group dummy variable, -1 or $+1$, on the vector of available measurements for this purpose, and, the loglikelihood for the hypothesis of membership in one group or the other is strictly proportional to that regression predictor.

> One can think about the inferences that follow here in a slightly different way. Suppose that the measured value for the new specimen we are trying to classify is exactly equal to the average for one of the existing groups – say that what we measured was exactly μ. Then, from formula (3.26), the log of the likelihood ratio in favor of the group whose mean that is is $2\mu'\mu = 2|\mu|^2$, twice the squared length of μ. From formula (3.27), the "predicted group" for this case is the regression prediction $y = b'z$ for $b = \mu/(1 + \mu'\mu)$; this evaluates to $\mu'\mu/(1 + \mu'\mu)$. With respect to the group whose group code is 1, the regression thus entails a residual of $1 - \mu'\mu/(1 + \mu'\mu) = 1/(1 + \mu'\mu)$. With respect to the other group, of group code -1, the residual is instead $-\left(1 + \mu'\mu/(1 + \mu'\mu)\right) = -(1 + 2\mu'\mu)/(1 + \mu'\mu)$. Now assume that we are careful enough to actually examine the regression residuals within group. We discover that their actual variance is 1 (the variance of the original bell curves in Figure 3.33). Then the loglikelihood supporting a classification to group 2 given these residuals is $\frac{1}{2}\left(((1 + 2\mu'\mu)/(1 + \mu'\mu))^2 - (1/(1 + \mu'\mu))^2\right)$. This rearranges to $2\mu'\mu/(1 + \mu'\mu)$, which is an attenuation of the correct assessment $2\mu'\mu$ by a factor $1 + |\mu|^2$ that is close to 1 when μ is small relative to the standard deviation of the assumed Gaussian within-group distributions but that falls toward zero (i.e., that systematically understates the actual strength of the data-based inference more and more) as μ grows.

To generalize from the stringent assumption of an identity covariance matrix within group, we argue from invariances. Because likelihood ratios do not change under affine transformation, the likelihood ratio in the preceding exegesis applies whenever we can transform the within-group covariance structure to the identity, which is to say, whenever it is of full rank (since we can always rotate to the principal axes of this structure [if this concept is new to you, see Section 4.2.2] and then divide each by the standard deviation of the corresponding principal component score). The coefficient vector μ and the observed vector Z have both been transformed right along with this covariance structure, so the loglikelihood is now the more general expression $2\mu\Sigma^{-1}Z$. Similarly, nothing has changed about the least-squares fit to the "dependent" variable Y, the group number, except that both predictor and predictand now have to be re-expressed in terms of the new basis set of variables so that what was $\mu'Z$ is now

$$\mu'\Sigma^{-1}Z, \tag{3.28}$$

now divided by an attenuation factor $1 + \mu'\Sigma^{-1}\mu$. Thus the strict proportionality of loglikelihood to regression predictor is true in the general case of any invertible within-group covariance structure.

3.5.3 Example 3.7: Bumpus's Snow-Beset Sparrows

We apply this logic of classification to a celebrated nineteenth-century data set: measurements by Hermon Bumpus of a total of 136 sparrows that did or did not survive a sudden snowstorm in Rhode Island in February 1898. (Section 3.1 has already exploited some of the data for 35 of these birds, the surviving adult males.) The data are online in a transcription by Peter Lowther of the Field Museum, Chicago. Writing before the turn of the twentieth century, Bumpus lived when the truth of natural selection was still uncertain:

> We are so in the habit of referring carelessly to the process of natural selection, and of invoking its aid whenever some pet theory seems a little feeble, that we forget we are really using a hypothesis that still remains unproved, and that specific examples of the destruction of animals of known physical disability are very infrequent. Even if the theory of natural selection were as firmly established as Newton's theory of the attraction of gravity, scientific method would still require frequent examination of its claims, and scientific honesty should welcome such examination and insist on its thoroughness.
>
> A possible instance of the operation of natural selection, through the process of the elimination of the unfit, was brought to our notice on February 1 of the present year [1898], when, after an uncommonly severe storm of snow, rain, and sleet, a number of English sparrows were brought to the Anatomical Laboratory of Brown University. Seventy-two of these birds revived; sixty-four perished; and it is the purpose of this lecture to show that the birds which perished, perished not through accident, but because they were physically disqualified, and that the birds which survived, survived because they possessed certain physical characters. (Bumpus, 1898:209)

I incorporate his listing as one of the files in this book's online resource.

Bumpus's professorship preceded the time of biometrics. He could only report averages of his measures within his two groups, and instead of multiple regression he was restricted to statements about individual variables and, sometimes, their contrast with other variables. We can do much better. The following discussion deals with the 59 adult male birds in this data set; there were also 28 male juveniles and 49 females. Figure 3.36 shows the cumulative distribution functions (areas to the left of a vertical threshold in a histogram) for these nine measurements separately. At lower center is the single curve that these are all approximating in spite of their different means and variances. This is the *cumulative Gaussian distribution* $(\sqrt{2\pi})^{-1} \int_{-\infty}^{x} e^{-t^2/2} dt$. The scientific usefulness of these curves, also called *ogives*, had not been recognized yet at the time of Bumpus's work.

For these males, the correlations of survival with the nine measured variables in Figure 3.36 are -0.48, 0.09, -0.29, -0.05, 0.23, 0.23, 0.20, -0.04, and 0.16. So the obvious first predictor of survival is total length, abbreviated totL (for "total length") or totLAM (for "total length, adult males"), corresponding to the upper left panel in Figure 3.36. The surviving males are substantially shorter than the nonsurvivors, about 3 mm on average, which is a substantial shift for a variable that has a full range of only 13 mm. This mean difference is more than four times its own standard error – there is no doubt at all about the scientific meaningfulness of this first observation. For purposes of the comparisons to follow, it is helpful to represent this correlation in terms of the corresponding linear prediction equation for the dependent variable, male survival (coded 0:1):

$$\text{survival} \sim 13.378 - 0.0798 \times \text{total length},$$

where the coefficient of total length has a value more than four times its standard error.

Following the advice in Section 3.2, consider the added-variable plot (Figure 3.37), for each additional variable after this first measure is regressed out.

The largest of these partial correlations is 0.502, for the panel in the middle of the plot, the contribution of femoral length. The rational procedure is thus to pass to a second regression equation that includes both predictors, total length (which we had acknowledged previously) and femoral length (which is new at this step). The resulting equation is

$$\text{survival} \sim 10.3566 - 0.1080 \times \text{total length} + 10.5842 \times \text{femoral length} \quad (3.29)$$

The two-variable prediction definitely is an improvement over the predictor using total length alone. Now the multiple correlation is 0.65, versus 0.48

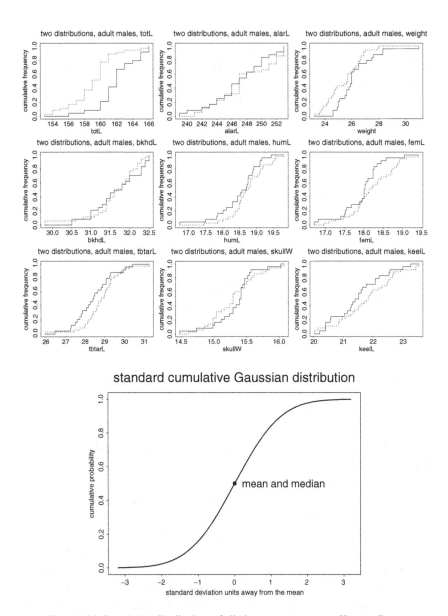

Figure 3.36 Cumulative distributions of all nine measurements on Hermon Bumpus's 59 adult male sparrows as found in the snow in Providence, Rhode Island, one day in February 1898. Dotted line: birds that could not be revived. Solid line: birds that recovered. Bottom: the *ogive* (cumulative Gaussian distribution) that all these curves are echoing.

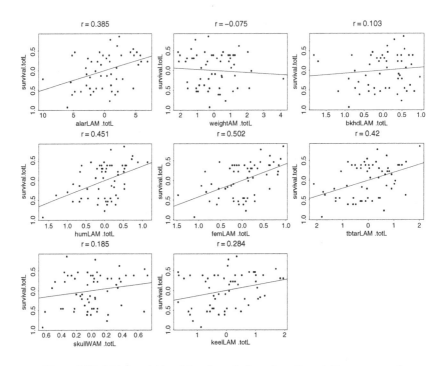

Figure 3.37 Added-variable plots of survival on the other eight measures of Bumpus's sparrows, adjusting for total length.

before. The coefficient of total length is now six times its standard error, not four times, and the new coefficient for femoral length is more than four times *its* standard error. The sign of this new coefficient is *positive*, the opposite of the sign for total length. This implies that survival is predicted by a *contrast* of these variables, smaller total length but larger femur length. Furthermore, when normalized for the ranges of the predictors, these coefficients are nearly commensurate – 0.1080 times the range of total length is 1.404, 10.58 times the range of femoral length is 1.132. This means that in the discriminant plot to come in Figure 3.39 the line of indifference will lie very nearly along one main diagonal and the prediction gradient along the other main diagonal: the two measures we are using are equally informative about survival. This is the case even though their correlations separately with survival, 0.48 and 0.23, are strikingly different.

One reasonable guess is that (1) smaller birds survive, but also (2) birds survive better with stronger legs because that lets them hold on longer to the branches on which they ride out the storm. Today this is called "directional

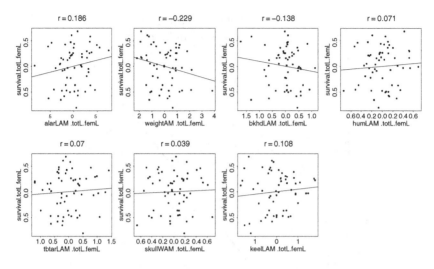

Figure 3.38 Further added-variable plots for the seven remaining Bumpus measures after both total length and femur length are regressed out.

selection," as discussed in endless detail for birds of another genus in the splendid book by Weiner (1995).

Proceeding with the next round of added-variable plots (Figure 3.38), we find no further variables worth adding (no correlations much larger than their standard errors) – note that the correlation for weight, the panel second from the left in the upper row, is contaminated by an outlier at lower right (a bird much heavier than it should have been given its total length and leg length – perhaps this is a measurement error?). In a regression that augments the previous pair of predictors, total length and femoral length, by this third candidate, animal weight, the coefficient for weight is less than two times its standard error and thus would be ignored even if we had not selected it as the best of seven. But when that case is sequestered from the computation, this weight "effect" is hardly more than its own standard error, and so there is no reason for the evolutionary ornithologist to take it seriously.

The analysis is completed, then, by producing the appropriate discriminant plot, following the logic of the preceding exposition, whereupon we abandon all talk of paths and regressions and simply interpret the points as they fall on the linearized likelihood surface. The analysis here is reasonably powerful, with a total of 12 classification errors out of the 59 birds, and all but one of those errors falls in the first band to either side of the line of indifference. In passing we can inspect the extent to which these data comport with the model of identical covariance structures that justifies our recourse to this method of

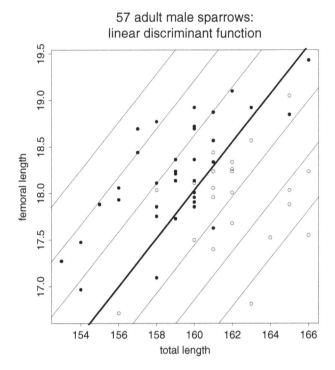

Figure 3.39 Two-dimensional discriminant function for log odds of survival, Bumpus's male sparrows. The heavy line is the line of equal odds of surviving or not according to the multiple regression of group on the pair of variables along the Cartesian axes here (total length and femoral length). Note that the contours of constant odds ratio run from lower left to upper right – the discriminant function is a *contrast*, the composite of lower total length but higher femoral length. Heavy line: the line of indifference (odds ratio 1:1).

multiple regression in the first place. Variances for total length are 5.8 and 7.9 in the two survival groups; for femoral length, 0.00041 and 0.00051. Neither of these is intriguing, but the comparison of the within-group correlations is: 0.30 for the deceased sparrows, but 0.69 for the survivors, suggesting a functional constraint. Fisher's z-test can easily be modified to help us think about this difference. The two z-transforms are 0.314 and 0.856. Their standard errors are $1/\sqrt{N-3} = 0.177$ and 0.218, respectively, so that of their difference (recall the discussion following equation 2.8b) is $\sqrt{0.177^2 + 0.218^2} = 0.281$. The difference of z's is nearly twice this standard error; it is worth taking seriously. We will return to these data in Section 3.6, and a more sophisticated approach to comparing pairs of covariance matrices will be introduced in Section 4.3.6.

We can return to the initial graphical icon, the paired cumulative distribution function, by displaying the formula at which we have arrived. The linear

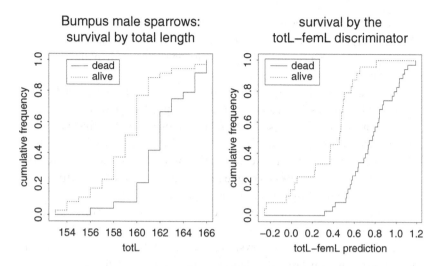

Figure 3.40 A comparison of the cumulative distribution function of total length by survival (left) to that of the "prediction formula" from equation (3.29) or Figure 3.39 shows the increased signal strength afforded by the incorporation of a second measurement of these birds.

discriminator indeed shows more shift than any of the separate curves for the males (Figure 3.40), just as it was designed to do. More importantly, *it has generated a new hypothesis,* the biomechanics of gripping the perch in a snowstorm, and thus would lead to further studies should Bumpus's successors still be interested.

Notice how irrelevant the conventional statistician's distinction is between "independent" and "dependent" variables here. Survival is a grouping variable for the cumulative distribution plots (i.e., "independent"), but is instead an outcome variable for the classification analysis or the regression that underlies it (i.e., "dependent"). We grapple with this same issue in more depth in Chapter 4. Note also that formal statistical analysis is a relatively small part of the scientific exposition here. We relied overwhelmingly on graphics, not on formulas.

Summary of Section 3.5

- *Linear discriminant analysis* is the computation of a log-odds ratio between two hypotheses (membership of an unknown specimen in one group versus membership in another) by manipulation of the linear regression of the grouping variable on one or more measurements.

- The computation makes no sense as a path analysis after the logic of Section 3.1, but, nevertheless, results in correct (though mislabeled) contours of likelihood ratio for the comparison of the two hypotheses under certain assumptions.
- The diagrams for this analysis exemplify *affine geometry*, the geometry of lines and tangencies, not distances. The line or plane of predictors is divided into two regions: specimens falling on one side of the line are assigned to the first group, and on the other side, to the second.
- When there are two or more predictors, the information content of a linear discriminant formula depends on the relation of the difference of group averages to the within-group covariance structure.
- Added-variable plots apply to the regressions driving a linear discriminant analysis. An example manipulated Hermon Bumpus's measurements of adult male sparrows after a snowstorm so as to yield a summary in terms of one single ratio of measured distances, femur length to total length, two variables whose relationship within the subsample of surviving adult males we have already examined in Section 3.1.

3.6 Special Case 3b: Quadratic Discrimination

3.6.1 Classification When Variances Are Not the Same

The preceding exegesis has relied on a hidden axiom that is almost certainly false as the number of dimensions rises: that both groups had the same variances and covariances. This was just barely plausible in the Bumpus example, but is quite unlikely in general. What happens to this simple, elegant methodology when that assumption must be waived?

We start, as before, with the case of one single measurement. If we remain in the context of a Gaussian model, the formalism is quite similar to what you already saw in Section 3.5 for the case of two groups of the same variance but different means. Equation (3.26) showed how the form of the Gaussian, the exponential of a (negative) multiple of x^2 around some center, reduced to a linear term for the loglikelihood around a locus of indifference halfway between the two group means. When we free the covariance structure to vary, the loglikelihood is still the difference between the two exponents in the two Gaussian models (plus one more term, a constant, for the log of the ratio of their standard deviations).

But the odds ratio as a function of the predictor value now is no longer a straight line. The difference term in the log-odds formula now may incorporate the difference between two *different* multiples of x^2, and so it can be any parabola at all, centered anywhere and pointing upward or downward with any curvature. If the center is far from the data, it will resemble the straight lines we have already encountered; but it does not have to do so. This parabola will always cut the horizontal axis in two points, not one, so in the presence of different variances the locus of indifference of a quadratic classifier divides the predictor axis into three segments, not two. The middle segment is classified into the group of lower variance, and both outer intervals are classified into the other group, the group of higher variance.

Figure 3.41 summarizes all of the possibilities here. The pair of panels at upper left corresponds to the situation we already considered in Section 3.5, where the variances in the two groups are equal. (In the real world, where variances are never equal, this corresponds to a situation where one point in the locus of indifference is within the range of the data and the other locus is unrealistically far outside that range.) The other three pairs of panels pertain to the much more common situation where groups differ in variance as well. At upper right, they have the same mean. In the lower row are two examples of a situation where the groups have both different means *and* different variances. The loglikelihood is still always a parabolic curve, perhaps centered outside the interval between the group means or perhaps inside. Measures sufficiently

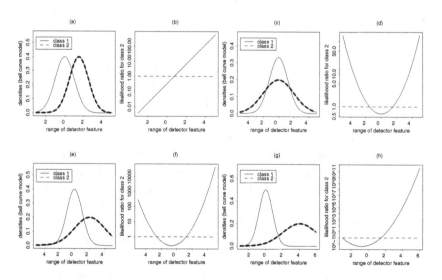

Figure 3.41 Quadratic discrimination for one measurement. The panels of this diagram come in pairs. (a,b) The classic linear discrimination of Figure 3.33. (c,d) The same mean but different variances. (e,f) Different means and variances; the region classified into group 2 is disconnected. (g,h) The same with a larger mean shift.

far from the grand mean will be assigned to the group of larger variance, with steadily increasing log odds. Notice that the absolute value of this curve is bounded from below but unbounded above – some specimens can be assigned much more confidently to the group of higher variance than any specimen could have been assigned to the group of lower variance.

3.6.2 Classification When Covariances Are Not the Same

That was for the case of one single measurement. The general case can be understood adequately just by examining the simplest possible generalization, from one predictor to two. When we free the covariance structure of two or more measurements to vary, the loglikelihood is still the difference between the two exponents in the two Gaussian models (plus one more term, a constant, for the log of the ratio of their determinants). But now that difference term can be any difference of two positive-definite quadratic forms, which is to say, it can be any quadratic surface at all. In two dimensions, while a covariance model itself has to look like an ellipse (see Section 4.1), the logarithm of the ratio of two of the corresponding Gaussian probability densities can look like an ellipse, a parabola, a hyperbola, or two parallel lines. In three dimensions or more, the possibilities are an ellipsoid, a paraboloid, a hyperboloid of any signature,[5] a cylinder, a hyperbolic paraboloid, or any of a range of other relatively unlikely possibilities.

To each of these surfaces there corresponds a locus of indifference where the surface crosses the horizontal plane in the diagram, the plane where the odds of the two hypotheses are equal. Figure 3.42 exemplifies some of the interesting cases encountered in practice. The figure should be read as a series of four pairs of plots, corresponding to four different situations (out of a total of seventeen essentially different mathematical possibilities). Each pair has a diagram on the left showing two covariance matrices, drawn as two ellipses in different line weights, and a diagram on the right showing contours of loglikelihood. In the scenario at upper left, the two groups have the same mean, and one of the two groups always has the greater variance, regardless of direction. The likelihood contours are then ellipses centered near the center of the group with the smaller variances, and the locus of indifference is a third ellipse in-between

---

[5] The *signature* of a quadratic form is, imprecisely speaking, the count of plus signs when it is diagonalized as $(a_1'x)^2 \pm (a_2'x)^2 \pm \ldots \pm (a_k'x)^2 = 1$, where x is a measurement vector and the a's are orthogonal vectors of loadings. For $p = 3$ there are two types of hyperboloids, for instance, with formulas $(a_1'x)^2 + (a_2'x)^2 - (a_3'x)^2 = 1$ — the hyperboloids of two sheets, having signature 2 — and $(a_1'x)^2 - (a_2'x)^2 - (a_3'x)^2 = 1$, the hyperboloids of one sheet, having signature 1. See Bookstein, 2014, figure 6.2.

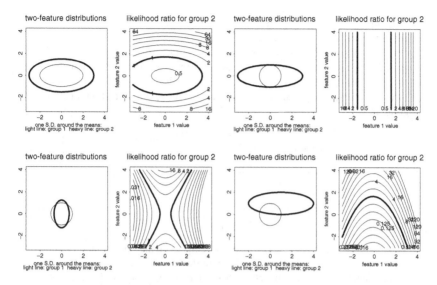

Figure 3.42 Four examples of a quadratic discrimination on two variables. First and third columns: the two covariance structures by group. Second and fourth columns: contours of loglikelihood, spaced roughly evenly. The locus of indifference (odds 1:1, log odds = 0) is the heavy curve in these two columns. Upper left pair: one group consistently dominant in variance, likelihood contours elliptical. Upper right pair: one group has the larger variance except in one single direction, group means the same, indifference contours a pair of parallel lines. Lower left pair: sign of the variance difference inconsistent as a function of direction, loglikelihood contours hyperbolas. Formula (3.32) covers this and the previous two cases. Lower right pair: one group has the larger variance except in one single direction, group means not the same, loglikelihood contours are parabolas. For this situation a formula complementing (3.32) would be an expression in x^2 and y instead of x^2 and y^2.

the first two. At upper right is one of the special cases: the plot pair for a situation of identical group means where the variances are the same in one direction and otherwise always larger in one group. The likelihood contours are now straight lines parallel to the direction of equal variances. It remains the case that, as in one dimension, the support that the data can offer to the hypothesis of membership in the group of smaller variance is limited, but for the other hypothesis it is unlimited. At lower left we see the case of variance dominance that divides the compass into two sets of directions, in each of which group 1 or group 2 consistently has the larger variance; the discriminant contours are hyperbolas. Finally, at lower right is another of the special cases, one group having the larger variance in every direction except one, but with different group means. The loglikelihood contours now are parabolas.

Some of my readers may appreciate a sketch of the algebraic notation corresponding to one of these cases, for instance, the one at upper left, where a discriminant analysis is possible even though the two groups have exactly the same average measurements. The situation is of two uncorrelated Gaussians in each group with one group's variance always less than the other's. Write these variances as $\sigma_{1x} < \sigma_{2x}$ and $\sigma_{1y} < \sigma_{2y}$. Then the distribution function for the ith group is

$$\frac{1}{2\pi \sigma_{ix}\sigma_{iy}} e^{-\frac{1}{2}\left((x^2/\sigma_{ix}^2)+(y^2/\sigma_{iy}^2)\right)}, \quad i = 1, 2, \tag{3.30}$$

so, taking logs and subtracting, the loglikelihood is

$$\log\left(\frac{\sigma_{1x}\sigma_{1y}}{\sigma_{2x}\sigma_{2y}}\right) - \frac{1}{2}\left(\frac{x^2(\sigma_{2x}^2 - \sigma_{1x}^2)}{\sigma_{1x}^2\sigma_{2x}^2} + \frac{y^2(\sigma_{2y}^2 - \sigma_{1y}^2)}{\sigma_{1y}^2\sigma_{2y}^2}\right), \tag{3.31}$$

the isolines of which are just another set of ellipses on the same center. For the situation at lower left, reverse the polarity of the σ_2's. The scenarios in the right column involve equal σ_2's, which alters the algebra. The locus of indifference in all these scenes except the one at lower right has the equation

$$\log\left(\frac{\sigma_{1x}\sigma_{1y}}{\sigma_{2x}\sigma_{2y}}\right) - \frac{1}{2}\left(\frac{x^2(\sigma_{2x}^2 - \sigma_{1x}^2)}{\sigma_{1x}^2\sigma_{2x}^2} + \frac{y^2(\sigma_{2y}^2 - \sigma_{1y}^2)}{\sigma_{1y}^2\sigma_{2y}^2}\right) = 0, \tag{3.32}$$

which, depending on the values of the coefficients of x^2, xy, and y^2, is an ellipse, a hyperbola (meaning it has two branches, not one), or a pair of straight lines.

3.6.3 Example 3.8: An Adult Fetal Alcohol Brain Study

This example combines the scenarios of the lower left and lower right panel pairs in Figure 3.42. The structure of interest is the callosal midcurve, the curve of greatest local symmetry up the "middle" of the corpus callosum near the midline of the human brain. I was part of a Seattle collaboration that published a group of papers in 2001–2002 about the form of this curve in a sample combining the brains of 60 normal Seattle citizens with the brains of 120 subjects who already had been diagnosed with what we now call a fetal alcohol spectrum disorder, or FASD. (Back then they were called either FAS [fetal alcohol syndrome] or FAE [fetal-alcohol-affected], and even though it turns out that that distinction was of little use, the plots will be labeled that way.) The 180 subjects formed a balanced design, 15 each of normals, FAE, and FAS within four subsamples of adolescent (aged 14–17) males, adolescent females, adult (aged 18–50) males, and adult females. The analysis to follow is for the 45 adult males (15 normals, 30 FASDs). It has been previously reported in several venues including Bookstein et al. (2001, 2002a, 2002b), Bookstein and Kowell (2010), Mardia et al. (2013), and Bookstein (2014, 2019). The brains were imaged by magnetic resonance (a procedure that requires the subject to hold his head still in a very noisy and confined tube for about ten minutes) and were then measured by the careful computer-aided procedure described in Bookstein et al. (2001, 2002a, 2002b).

Figure 3.43 shows one particularly interesting part of the resulting data: a two-dimensional vector (hence, two measured variables) representing a transect of this structure that had previously been reported to be of interest in studies of smaller samples from the decade of the 1990s. From the scatter you can see how the points representing this vector in the patients (the + and × symbols) fall mostly outside the limits of the distribution of the normal

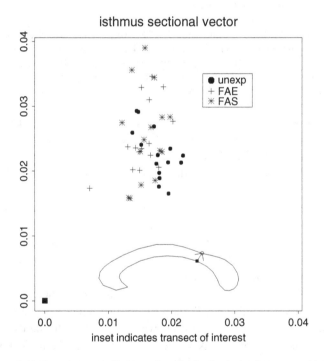

Figure 3.43 Data for an application of quadratic discrimination to a problem in neuroteratology. Large solid square: registration of the transects on their anterior-caudad (lower left) endpoint. Scatter for the Seattle sample of 45 adult males: registered location of the posterior-craniad (upper right) endpoint, with syndromal group coded as in the legend. (inset) 40-point schematic of the callosal midcurve (corpus callosum midline, projected from three dimensions down to two), with the transect of interest indicated. Subject is facing left.

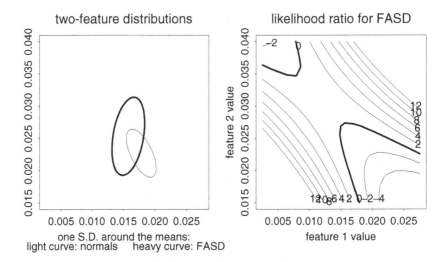

Figure 3.44 Quadratic discrimination of FASD versus unexposed Seattle adult male subsamples by the technique of Figure 3.42. (left) Covariance structures of the two groups. (right) The corresponding likelihood contours. Heavy curves: the locus of indifference, which in this example takes the form of the two branches of a hyperbola (of which only one is relevant to the data at hand).

subjects (the • symbols) in two directions, strongly suggesting that a quadratic discrimination might be useful. Note that this really is two variables – not one single measurement, like "thickness," but a vector combining that thickness with a directionality (within a coordinate system standardized as explained in Section 5.4).

Following the methodology just reviewed, Figure 3.44 distills the situation down to a two-group Gaussian model. At left, in light line is the 1-standard-deviation ellipse for the 15 normal adult males, and, in heavy line, the same for the 30 FASDs. This is the situation of the lower row of scenarios in Figure 3.42, the situation where the group dominating the directional variance varies from direction to direction. At right in Figure 3.44 is the corresponding plot of contours of loglikelihood. The locus of indifference (equal likelihood for the two groups) is the hyperbola shown in heavy line. Inside its arms are the regions where vectors are likelier to have arisen from the normal group – this region is disconnected – and between its arms, extending indefinitely outward toward the "northeast," is the single region where likelihood is higher for the hypothesis of FASD. The two coordinates underlying this example are included as one of the files in this book's online resource.

Figure 3.45 redraws these contours over the scatter of the actual data, together with an additional point for subject "XX" (actually a convicted

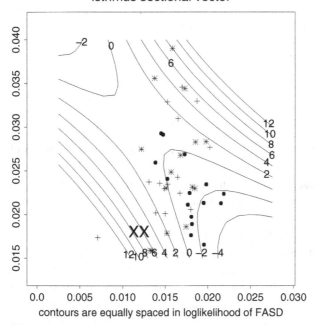

Figure 3.45 Results of the quadratic discrimination for the data in Figure 3.43 together with one additional case, "XX." Most of the FASD patients are found outside the heavy curve of indifference toward the lower right in Figure 3.44. Mr. XX lies on an interpolated contour at 6.7 on this scoring, and thus has odds of some 800:1 of having arisen from the FASD group.

murderer; not his real initials), who is being used as a probe. You will notice that the subsample of cases classified as "normal" is not actually disconnected; no subject can be found in the sector toward the "northwest" in Figure 3.44. As you see, Mr. XX falls in the region of the plot where the FASD hypothesis is the likelier one. In fact, it is *very much* the likelier for him. Reading from the levels of the contour lines, we see that his particular classification has a log-odds of about 6.7, corresponding to chances of about 800:1 of an FASD origin.

Using the formula

$$\operatorname{var}\left(\frac{X}{Y}\right) \sim \frac{\bar{X}^2}{\bar{Y}^2}\left(\frac{\operatorname{var}(X)}{\bar{X}^2} + \frac{\operatorname{var}(Y)}{\bar{Y}^2}\right) \qquad (3.33)$$

for the variance of a ratio of uncorrelated quantities X and Y with Y far from zero (Stuart and Ord, 1994, section 10.6), and anticipating the formula $\operatorname{var}(\sigma^2) = \left(\sigma^2\sqrt{2/n}\right)^2$ from Section 4.1, one can verify that, in this situation where one group has both the more distant mean and the smaller variance, the coefficient of variation of that loglikelihood of 6.7 – its standard deviation divided by its mean – is approximately $\sqrt{2/15} \sim 0.365$, where 15 is the count of that less likely group. The central 50% confidence interval of this odds ratio $e^{6.7}$ is thus, even more approximately, the range $e^{6.7(1\pm0.675\times0.365)}$, 155 to 4250.

3.6.4 Example 3.9: The Same for Infants

The preceding exegesis counted as an actual discovery – one could classify adults suspected of fetal alcohol damage by a relatively simple measurement of one clearly visible brain structure, and the classification could often be informative enough to affect an actual social decision process (a death sentence imposed or withheld; see Bookstein and Kowell 2010). It would be good to know if comparable discriminations were possible in early infancy, a time when the FASD subject has not yet been exposed to the social pressures that aggravate the effects of the actual neuroanatomical damage (see Streissguth et al., 2004). My same Seattle group set out, therefore, to explore the discriminatory information content of the analogous structure in the brains of very young babies, aged from birth through four months only. At that age, while the babies cannot easily hold still for a magnetic resonance image, their skulls still have an aperture toward the front, the *fontanelle,* through which an ultrasound image can be formed. The study reported here, previously published as Bookstein et al. (2007) and elaborated in Bookstein and Mitteroecker (2014) and Bookstein (2014), compared 21 normal infants to 23 whose mothers reported them to have been exposed to high levels of alcohol before birth.

The images are of a baby being followed by a handheld transducer touching the head through the fontanelle (the open membrane above the forehead where the skull has not fused into a bony sheet yet) through a blob of cold jelly. Babies don't like being treated this way, so they squirm, making the ultrasound images noisy. They needed to be averaged, as in Figure 3.46, before being measured. (The images, not the babies!) Here we show one such average image, for an alcohol-exposed infant. The figure shows the locations of the four points that together supply a total of eight Cartesian coordinates according to the rules of Procrustes morphometrics to be introduced in Chapter 5.

The standard statistical analysis of data like these is the scatter of *Procrustes shape coordinates* that will be introduced in detail in Section 5.4. Their display, shown in Figure 3.47, is read as a series of four coordinate pairs, one pair for each original data location, all plotted together in one carefully concocted

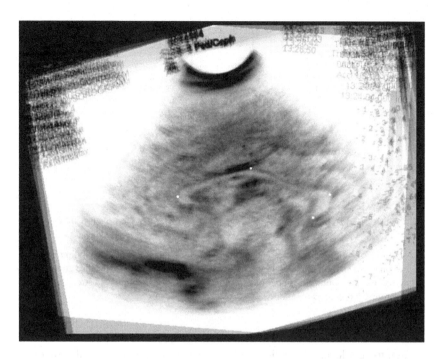

Figure 3.46 Averaged midsagittal transfontanelle ultrasound for one infant subject in the FASD baby brain study (infant 4, alcohol-exposed, the one at farthest
right in Figure 3.48). The multiple text blocks arise from the individual video
frames that have been averaged here via the positions of the four landmark points
indicated. This infant's callosal form is the most extreme of all 23 exposed babies
in the direction of the exposure signal per se. For a listing of this small data set,
consult this book's online resources.

coordinate system. While the distributions of three of these points appear
uninformative for the distinction of interest, the fourth point, uppermost at the
right, appears to offer the possibility of a discrimination.

That possibility was the theme of the paper arising from this study,
(Bookstein et al., 2007). For a listing of this small data set, consult this book's
online resource. The summary finding from that paper is in Figure 3.48. It
is a univariate discrimination (after the fashion of Figure 3.33) based on
a conveniently round numerical threshold (90°) for the angle between the
horizontal connection between the lowest two landmarks and the vertical
through the rightmost pair of landmarks in this quadrangular configuration.
Thresholding this angle at 90° detected 13 cases of greater angle, of whom 12
were in fact highly exposed to alcohol. The distinction here ought to be strong

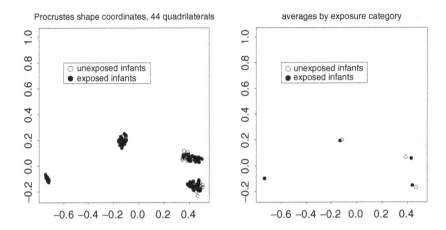

Figure 3.47 (left) Procrustes shape coordinates for the four landmark points of
Figure 3.46 in the sample of 44 infant brains. (right) Averages by exposure group.
One landmark point, the upper one toward the right, hints particularly strongly at
a promising group separation.

enough to be relevant in applied contexts such as adoption or qualification for
special services, although we have not yet been able to raise the research funds
to see this possibility through. On this specific issue, see Bookstein 2019.

That was as much new technology as the peer reviewers of 2006 could
tolerate. But the methods of this section apply nevertheless to produce a
much better discrimination criterion from the same data. The coordinates of
Figure 3.47 conduce to an analysis in four dimensions (not two), which begins
by considering a version of one of the frames of Figure 3.42 (the pair at upper
left, one group dominating the other in variance in all directions) that takes a
special form. A relative eigenanalysis (see Section 4.3.6) shows that variance
in the alcohol-exposed infants strongly dominates that of the unexposed in
two directions, not just one, and that the ratio of FASD variance to normal
variance in these two directions is the same. By reducing the data set to that
pair of dimensions (Figure 3.49), we generate a diagram in which the locus of
indifference is not just any ellipse but an actual *circle*.

This immediately affords us access to a much more powerful narrative
language. Instead of talking about the conceptually complex quantity that
is loglikelihood, we can refer instead to the visually obvious criterion of
distance from the center of the circles. The forms closer to this point are
overwhelmingly from the unexposed infants. Those farther away are more
likely to have arisen from the exposed infants, those who (if the adult study is of

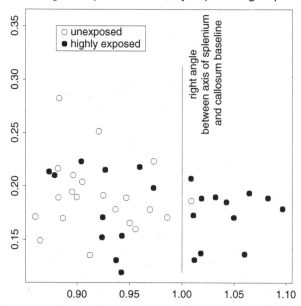

Figure 3.48 Enhancement of the information conveyed by the single landmark above at right from Figure 3.47. The vertical line is the line directly above the landmark at the lower right in a superposition corresponding to the Bookstein shape coordinates on the lower pair as baseline (see Section 5.3). Twelve of the 13 points to the right of this line arose from the subgroup of alcohol-exposed infants.

any use as a prophecy) are going to end up quite often with an FASD diagnosis of their own. The role of the form at the center of the circles is thus that of an "ideal" form: not the average unexposed configuration, but the configuration likeliest to be classified as normal (this is a different criterion). Furthermore, the two axes of the plot can each be interpreted in potentially biological terms. As shown by the little grids aligned with the axes in the margin, the horizontal stands for the systematic shift in the position of that upper-right landmark we already noted in Figure 3.48. The grid for the vertical dimension is nearly aligned with a vertical stretch: forms that are either much higher or much lower than average are likelier to have been damaged by alcohol. This neatly matches the spirit of the findings for the adult form of this curve already hinted at in Example 3.8, and thus the hermeneutic circle is closed. Yes, we can interpret the fragmentary infant findings in terms of well-established adult characterizations.

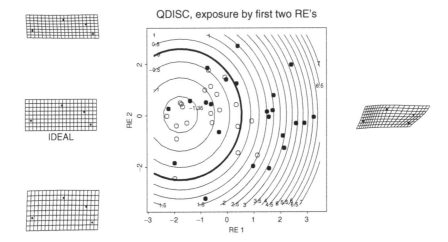

Figure 3.49 Elaboration of Figure 3.48 into a quadratic discrimination in the plane of greatest variance for the exposed infant subsample vis-à-vis the others. The variance ratio, exposed to unexposed infants, is nearly the same in every direction of this plane. Hence the contours of likelihood ratio are circles around a center plotted as the "ideal" in the margin. The heavy circle is the curve of indifference (log odds ratio 0). Also plotted in the margin are depictions of the axes of this plot as thin-plate splines separately. Vertical: a nearly uniform term, interpretable as the *aspect ratio* (height-to-width ratio) for the quadrilateral as a whole. Horizontal: displacement of the landmark toward the upper right, showing both a mean shift and a variance shift – the same shape feature as in Figure 3.48.

3.6.5 Back to Bumpus's Birds

The scatter of numerator versus denominator of that discriminatory ratio for survival among Bumpus's birds (Figure 3.39), shows different correlations between the two groups. Figure 3.50 indicates this a bit more accessibly by drawing the *convex hulls* around each of the distributions, survivors or nonsurvivors, for the scatter in Figure 3.39. The distribution for the survivors apparently has a little more variation along the main diagonal and a little less variation along the minor diagonal. Then indeed a discriminant analysis *might* be improved by stepping up from the linear to the quadratic domain.

There results the diagram in Figure 3.51, revising the contours of loglikelihood while leaving the underlying scatter of total length against femur length alone. The locus of indifference appears to curve gently around a central alignment that agrees with the heavy line in the simpler (linear) analysis. In either version, the longer birds with shorter legs died, and the shorter birds with longer legs survived. Compared to that earlier figure, misclassifications

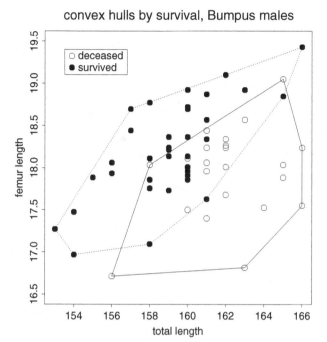

Figure 3.50 Annotation of the scatter in Figure 3.39 by the convex hulls of the two survivorship groups. These look different enough to suggest the quadratic discrimination in the next figure.

appear to be closer to this locus, which also seems to do better at separating nearby pairs of opposite color (the pair near (157,17), for instance, or the pair near (165,19).) In a larger sample of organisms or in the presence of a properly controlled experiment (instead of the spatial randomness of a snowstorm) one might expect to see more substantial changes in the quality of such a discrimination.

3.6.6 Changing One Group's Covariance Can Change a Likelihood Ratio by a Lot

Still in this context of classification (discrimination, forensic detection), let us explore a paradox inherent in the approach we have just been reviewing. It hinges on the discrepancy between what the scientist considers to be the information content of a data set and how the applied statistician construes the same phrase. This paradox actually arose in the course of one of my own

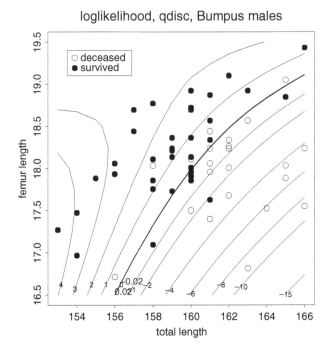

Figure 3.51 Analysis of the Bumpus survival discriminant plane by the quadratic method of this section results in a slightly different analysis from that in Figure 3.39, with the same total number of classification errors but a more realistic indifference curve.

forensic tasks, and it took quite a while to convince myself that it was not just a programming error.

Let us begin by taking a closer look at formula (3.30) in Section 3.6.2. This is the net probability for the combination of two measurements x and y when they are independent Gaussians with mean 0 and two different standard deviations. Setting aside the 2π, we see that this net probability takes the form of the product of two terms. The e-to-the part is the product of the terms $e^{-x^2/2\sigma^2}$ for the two single-variable Gaussians separately. Preceding it in the formula is a factor that puts the product of the two standard deviations into the *denominator*, meaning that, roughly speaking, the higher the standard deviation of a bell curve that gave you a scaled score of x/σ, the lower the probability assigned to a small interval around that value of x. We will rely on both of these observations to make sense of the next example.

Assume, for the moment, that we have two groups of cases (specimens, skulls, people), "Group 1" and "Group 2," and two measurements of them, "Variable 1" and "Variable 2." Each measurement is to have unit variance in each group, but the means will differ by 2.0 (that is, by double the standard deviation in either group separately). For convenience, set the means to 0 and 3. Then for each variable separately, the situation is as in panel (a) of Figure 3.52. A case scoring 1.5 on Variable 1 is 1.5σ above the Group 1 mean but the same 1.5σ below the Group 2 mean, and so lies in equipoise with respect to the classification task. Consider instead a case scoring 2 on this measure. This is 2σ above the Group 1 mean but only 1σ below the Group 2 mean, and so has a

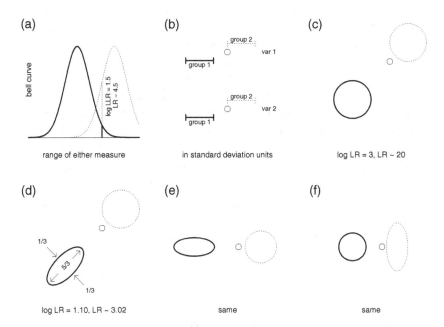

Figure 3.52 Sketch of a paradox in quadratic discrimination. (a) If a variable has the same variance in two groups, a probe closer to one center than the other is assigned to the group with the closer center. (b, c) The same is the case in the two-dimensional case if the covariance structures are circular. The net loglikelihood of the classification hypothesis is double what it would be for either variable alone. (d) Altering the covariance of one group can substantially alter the support afforded by the data for classifying the probe we are considering even if the positions of the group means are not changed. The ellipse here follows the model of those in Figure 2.23 with $a = \sqrt{5}$. As the text explains, the loglikelihood for the open circle is now *less* than it was at panel (c) – less, in fact, than it was in panel (a). Numbers along the axes of this ellipse are variances, not standard deviations. (e) Another view, rotated to line of centers horizontal. Neither this transformation nor the one in (f) alters likelihood ratios. (f) Yet another view, vertically expanded by a factor of $\sqrt{5}$. In any of the figures of the lower row, evidence supporting assignment to the group that had been the likelier is substantially weakened by the evident implausibility of its appearance so close to the mean on one of the two coordinates.

loglikelihood of $(2^2 - 1^2)/2 = 1.5$ for the hypothesis that it arose from Group 2. Exponentiating, this is a likelihood ratio of about 4.5 to 1, as shown in the figure by the pair of ordinates of the two bell curves we are comparing. The ratio of their heights is just $e^{1.5}$, as you can check with a ruler.

Suppose now that a second measurement (call it Variable 2) is at hand that has the same means, the same standard deviations, and, by chance, the same value of 2 for the case at hand. Now that we have to draw a second measurement, it is good to simplify panel (a) into panel (b). The horizontal bars now indicate intervals of $\pm\sigma$ around the group means, and the big open circle shows the values of the two variables we measured. As hypothesized, Variable 1 and Variable 2 appear to be completely redundant for our purposes. For each, we find ourselves at $+2\sigma$ with respect to Group 1 and at -1σ with respect to Group 2, for a loglikelihood of $e^{1.5}$ each.

The scientist *may* have arranged things so that these measurements are independent within each group separately. That is the situation in the upper right panel. (To check this condition, of course, you have to compute those correlations within group. The pooled correlation here, the correlation ignoring the group structure, is $\sqrt{\frac{9}{13}} \sim 0.83$; but this number has nothing much to do with the task at hand.) In this scenario, the likelihood ratios multiply over the variables, so their logarithms add. The net loglikelihood for the assignment of the case to Group 2 vis-à-vis Group 1 is $1.5 + 1.5 = 3$, corresponding to an odds ratio of about 20 to 1. Having the additional information of that second measurement, *in this case of uncorrelated characters*, considerably increases our confidence in the group assignment – it has, in fact, doubled our loglikelihood.

But it is easy to make this computation go haywire. Just inject a correlation between the measurements that appears in one group but not the other. Panel (d) diagrams such a situation. Our two variables remain uncorrelated in Group 2 but now correlate 0.667 in Group 1. In this situation, the availability of that second measurement, far from doubling our confidence as in the preceding scenario, has actually *lowered* it. Instead of the loglikelihood of 1.5 we had for the first measurement taken alone, we now have a loglikelihood of $1.4 - 0.5 \log(9/5) = 1.106$, which is odds of 3.02 to 1. (For the arithmetic, see below.) Remember that in panel (c) the same computation gave us a likelihood ratio of 20 to 1. So when the two predictors are strongly correlated, a classification into Group 2 can have become a great deal *less* secure, and our assignment of the specimen to Group 2 correspondingly less confident, especially if the cost of an error in this direction is high.

What happened to blow up our intuition in this situation? One way of understanding the difficulty takes advantage of the fact (already mentioned in Section 3.5) that a likelihood ratio, because it is a ratio of probability densities, is invariant under affine transformations of the data, which alter that density by exactly the same factor everywhere in the domain.[6] We can exploit this to clarify the situation in two ways. Panel (e) of Figure 3.52 is a copy of panel (d) that has been rotated to the principal axes of that elliptical scatter in Group 1. The rotated variables are now independent within groups, and so the loglikelihoods add just as your intuition wanted them to do all along. Along the horizontal, the open circle is now at a distance $\sqrt{2}$ from the center of Group 2, and so continues to have loglikelihood e^{-1} with respect to that distribution. But as regards Group 1, things have changed. The observed score of $\sqrt{2^2 + 2^2} = \sqrt{8}$ now pertains to a dimension having a variance of 5/3, which is more than the variance of 1 it had in panel (c). So the exponential in the likelihood formula is now not $e^{-4/2} \times e^{-4/2} = e^{-8/2}$ but $e^{-(8/(2(5/3)))} = e^{-2.4}$. Because the variables are correlated, their joint likelihood has *risen* past the product of the two marginal likelihoods taken separately – there is less information in the combination of correlated variables than in the combination of independent scores. This information is further attenuated just a bit by the additional correction for the product of the standard errors along the two axes of this ellipse. That product, $\sqrt{5/3} \times \sqrt{1/3} = \sqrt{5/9}$, appears in the denominator of equation (3.30), the one we just reviewed, and so it is divided out of the likelihood ratio we are investigating, which thus ends up equal to $e^{2.4-1} \times \sqrt{5/9} \sim 3.02$, the value you have already encountered.

If one affine transformation leaves the likelihood ratio and its logarithm unaltered, so does the composite of two. We can render the same forensic task in a coordinate system where it is the *first* group's covariance structure, not the second's, that is circular. This transformation, which expands the vertical axis of the lower central panel by a factor of $\sqrt{5}$, is the one shown in panel (f). Group 1 is now distributed as a circular Gaussian with variance 5/3 in every direction. The relation of the case (the little open circle) to Group 1 is now exactly the same as we saw in panel (e). It is displaced from the bivariate mean by $\sqrt{8}$ along an axis with a variance of 5/3, and so has a likelihood that goes as $e^{-2.4}/\sqrt{5/3}$, times a likelihood of $e^0/\sqrt{5/3}$ on the other, independent axis, for a net of $e^{-2.4}/(5/3)$. Likewise in this new coordinate system, the likelihood of coming from Group 2 goes as $e^{-2/2}$ along one of the pair of axes and e^0 along the other. One of these axes has a variance of 1, the other, of 5; so the net likelihood, up to that factor of 2π, is $e^{-1}/\sqrt{5}$. The resulting ratio looks like $e^{1.4}\sqrt{5}/3$, as before. The thinning of the ellipse in panel (d) had the effect of

---

[6] See Bookstein and Mitteroecker (2014). The idea of hinging the pedagogy on this invariance was suggested by Michael Karcher of the University of Washington.

increasing the likelihood of being found right at the mean of the Gaussian in that direction, and, conversely, the effect of stretching the circle in panel (e) into the ellipse in panel (f) is to *decrease* the likelihood of being found right at the mean. A bit of numerical exploration shows that for the particular value of $r = 0.9385$ the loglikelihood of the two hypotheses is precisely zero – on the bivariate Gaussian assumption the probabilities of the point at $(2, 2)$ coming from the two groups are *equal* in spite of the "obvious" affinity to Group 2.

In this way, inconsistency of variance-covariance matrices between two groups can destroy every bit of the intuitive interpretation of position on a scatterplot that would otherwise lead to a superficially sensible but actually inappropriate guess in place of the formal likelihood ratio method. When covariance structures are discordant, the optimal classifier is diagrammed as a quadratic or quadric form, not a plane, and the curve of indifference is a function of both within-group covariance structures in a way that requires close inspection.

Summary of Section 3.6

- The method of linear discriminant analysis requires an assumption that the variances and covariances of the "predictors" (classifiers) are the same between the groups. When this assumption is obviously false, an analogous method, *quadratic discriminant analysis,* can sometimes be effective.
- For one predictor, a quadratic discriminant analysis assigns a central segment of the predictor interval to one group and the remainder, both outer tails, to the other. For two predictors, the locus of indifference is a *conic section* (an ellipse, parabola, hyperbola, or pair of lines).
- In organismal applications it is frequently helpful to reduce the complexity of the data by careful winnowing of the available information *before* proceeding with one of these analyses. Two examples are presented from the author's work with a human birth defect, fetal alcohol damage.
- The report of a quadratic discrimination is particularly straightforward when the locus of indifference is a circle. One can then report the discriminant function as the distance of the specimen's values on the plot from some ideal type that often can be identified with a particular feasible region of the actual data.
- When covariance structures are different, a quadratic classifier can appear to be arbitrarily counterintuitive if the investigator does not explicitly diagram the within-group covariance structures as ellipses.

4

Transition to Multivariate Analysis

The preceding two chapters explored diverse uses of one common formula, linear regression, and the kinds of biological explanations they afford. These techniques ramify in many different directions that are the subject of extended treatments in other textbooks. For instance, the multiple linear regressions that mapped so neatly onto the geometry of Sewall Wright's path models in Figure 3.10 generalize to nonadditive regression and analysis of response surfaces (Draper and Smith, 1998, chapter 24; Seber and Wild, 2003). Similarly, the linear and quadratic discriminant functions we reviewed in Sections 3.5 and 3.6 generalize to the whole toolkit of statistical learning theory, including neural nets and support vector machines (Hastie, Tibshirani, and Friedman, 2009).

Such approaches center on one particular measurement or grouping at a time as the principal focus of attention. And, yes, we have seen many good examples of the ways that arithmetic is turned into understanding for a variety of biological explanatory purposes that involve explaining one particular variable at a time. But there is a more general and powerful formulation of how multiple measures on the same organism can relate to each other. It is time to switch languages and introduce the tools that let us ask *explicitly* about the existence and magnitude of the patterns that we have inspected only indirectly through our careful examination of the dozens of diagrams preceding. This contrasting approach, not regression but *multivariate statistical analysis*, occupies the core of the geometric morphometric toolkit for analysis of landmark locations. Think of it, if you like, as an intentional refusal to focus on one or another single measurement.

Such a recentering is consistent with a fundamental change in the role of statistics within biology that follows from how expeditiously the massively parallel data sets like images or whole genomes have turned into cheap and widespread data sources. The processes we study remain those that have interested quantitative biologists all along – morphogenesis, growth, physiology, locomotion, evolution. But in these huge, redundant new data sets the distinction between "independent" and "dependent" variables no longer makes much scientific sense. The central concern is no longer the values of particular *individual* variables (log height, octagon area, disease, species) but the patterns of *relationships among multiple measurements* of the same organism.

We begin to change the focus of biometrics by shifting our concern from the description of averages or the prediction of individual values to the geometry of those multivariate ellipses per se: not their centers (averages of data) but their sizes and shapes, and especially the variation among those sizes and shapes in different subgroups. The biologist is used to talking about these ellipses in terms of single numerical summaries. For instance, a regression coefficient is (ideally) the calibration of one single validated causal process highlighted via careful measurements of these complex organized systems. But beyond the simple formulas for variance and correlation we need a language for the logical ties among these concepts and particularly among their variations as they are revealed in nature or in well-designed experimental or observational studies. Multivariate analysis supplies most of the pattern language that we need in a quantitatively comprehensible way that can be made intuitively accessible if we work hard enough on the design of our diagrams.

4.1 Aspects of Covariance Structure: An Introduction

4.1.1 The Three Dimensions of a Bivariate Covariance Ellipse

We can prototype concerns in this spirit by continuing to learn from the seminal reference by Pearson and Filon (1898) cited earlier. Section 3.4 mentioned their formula

$$\sigma_r = (1 - r^2)/\sqrt{n} \qquad (3.20)$$

for the standard error of a correlation that led to Fisher's z-transform and thereafter every modern protocol for comparing correlations. Another formula there sets out the standard error of the standard error, a formula $\sigma_\sigma = \sigma/\sqrt{2n}$, along with a corresponding formula for the variance of the variance. We will confirm all three of these presently. This same Pearson-Filon paper introduced two other formulas that do not involve a factor of $1/\sqrt{n}$ and so do not tend to zero even for arbitrarily large sample sizes. The first formula deals with the correlation of the error estimates of σ_1 and σ_2, the standard deviations of any two measured variables on the same specimens. This correlation is r^2, the square of the correlation between the two measurements in question, and thus is independent of n as long as the data are Gaussian and n is large. Analogously, the correlation of the sampling errors of either σ with the sampling error of the correlation is $r/\sqrt{2}$, again independent of the sample size n for large n. In this way the formulas link the value of what would appear to be *univariate* statistics – those σ's – to the correlations of the variable in question with other variables.

The design of a study matters. If the σ's are known to much greater accuracy than r is, then the standard error of r from formula (3.20) is reduced by a factor $\sqrt{1 + r^2}$, as the contribution of the uncertainties in the σ's no longer applies. This is the situation when, for instance, we have a large sample of arms, and a large sample of legs, but only a small sample of specimens possessing both limbs. Or, as another instance, it can be shown that from a change $\Delta\sigma$ in a standard deviation we expect a corresponding change $\Delta r = r(1 - r^2)\Delta\sigma/\sigma$ in the corresponding estimated correlation. That prefactor ranges up to 0.385 (for $r = \sqrt{1/3}$). Such links between the sampling properties of quantities that are not necessarily related in biological theory are essential if we are to apprehend the biological import of the best data sets. Nevertheless, the source of all these formulas is the same old bell surface we have already encountered, with its same five parameters (two means, two variances, one covariance). For p variables, the count is $p(p + 3)/2$. However algebraically convenient this model of biometric variation is, that count of parameters grows faster than the complexity of the measurements themselves. We need to pay attention to all these parameters, not only averages, if our reports of research findings are to be robust and trustworthy.

This new level of analysis applies to all of the dimensions of variability of the covariance structure, as shown in Figure 4.1 for the simplest case, just a pair of measurements. In this situation, covariance structure per se has three dimensions. The horizontal axis in the figure corresponds to increases or decreases in σ_1, the vertical to increases or decreases in σ_2, and the third axis, "out of the page," the interesting one, alters the independence of these two original axes to either a positive or a negative correlation. The core technique to be introduced in Section 4.3 is the *Wishart distribution*, which is the generalization of this to the description of variation in patterns of the $p(p+1)/2$ variances and covariances among measures that number, in total, p, where p need not be small.

In this way, the statistician's concerns for the formalities of error estimation are no longer just of academic interest, but instead have become a crucial part of any exploration of multiple measures of the same organism. When such maneuvers touch on advanced mathematics from time to time, as with the diffusion equation in Section 2.3.5 or the geometry of the Wishart distribution and its metrics in Section 4.3, it is not because the mathematics is elegant (although it is) but because the properties of the formal structures under consideration (the location and halfwidth of the bell curve, the probability or improbability of a particular pattern of covariances, etc.) are inseparable from the theorems. In the same way that geometry explains the behavior of rulers (i.e., putting them end-to-end gives you addition, putting them at 90° gives you multiplication), these theorems likewise underlie the properties that, like correlation itself, supply the names for the patterns that, in turn, bear the possibility of biological understanding.

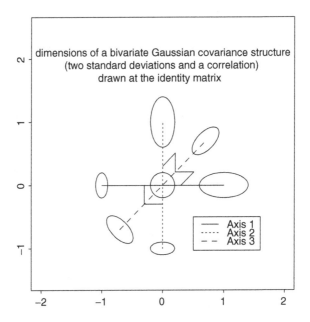

Figure 4.1 (above) Schematic of the three dimensions of variation for a 2×2 covariance structure as referred to a true matrix parameter that is circular (i.e., independent Gaussians of the same variance). Horizontal: Axis 1, variation of σ_1. Vertical: Axis 2, variation of σ_2. Into the page (drawn obliquely in this projection but not foreshortened in the rendering): Axis 3, variation of the magnitude of r, from negative (lower left) to positive (upper right), leaving variances of both x and y unchanged. (below) On the Wishart model of Section 4.3.3, the likelihood of a covariance matrix is spherical in this coordinate system if the scaling along Axis 3 is larger than that along Axis 1 or Axis 2 by a factor of $\sqrt{2}$. This figure panel shows the central section of this sphere by the (s_x, r) plane. Other central sections are identical. Negative integers: offsets of the loglikelihood contours with respect to their maximum at the center of the graph (the identity matrix, $\begin{pmatrix} 1 & 0 \\ 0 & 1 \end{pmatrix}$).

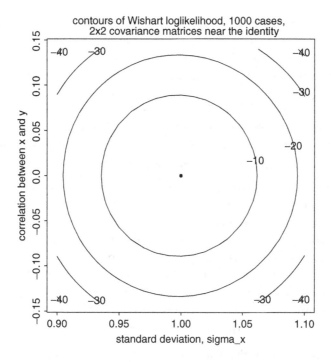

Figure 4.1 *(Cont.)*

Where do formulas like Pearson's come from? Formula (3.20) and others like it arise as generalizations of the simplest such computation, the approach that was already demonstrated in Section 2.1. There we were talking about why the ordinary arithmetic average of a set of quantities is maximum-likelihood for the value of their mean on a Gaussian model. Recall the equation (2.4) at which we finally arrived: on a Gaussian hypothesis, the net likelihood of the data set (a series of n x's) as a whole is $e^{-\sum(x_i-\mu)^2/2\sigma^2}$ up to multiplication by a function of σ that does not yet concern us (it will in a moment). The *loglikelihood* of this expression, again ignoring that function of σ (which now, on the log scale, is a matter of addition, not multiplication), is just the exponent, $-\sum(x_i-\mu)^2/2\sigma^2$. In the Pearson–Fisher method, which extends the Laplace Principle, the negative reciprocal of the second derivative of this quantity with respect to the parameter of interest (here, μ, the theoretical mean) is a good estimate of the sampling variance of the maximum-likelihood estimate of the corresponding parameter μ. By the usual formulas for taking derivatives, this second derivative with respect to μ is just $-\sum \frac{1}{\sigma^2} = -n/\sigma^2$. Hence the uncertainty of that estimated mean is $1/\sqrt{n/\sigma^2} = \sigma/\sqrt{n}$, the formula at which we had already arrived early in Chapter 2 without calculus.

A more general turn-of-the-twentieth-century method, now universally accepted, extends this approach to models that involve *any number* of parameters, for instance, the list that supplements the μ we were just talking about by an estimate of σ as well. Using the same expression for the loglikelihood, and no longer ignoring the term in $\log(1/\sigma) = -\log\sigma$ in the scaling prefactor of equation (2.16), the first derivative with respect to σ is $-n/\sigma + \sum(x_i - \mu)^2\sigma^{-3}$, and the second derivative is $n/\sigma^2 - 3\sum(x_i - \mu)^2\sigma^{-4}$. But $\sum(x_i - \mu)^2 = n\sigma^2$ at the maximum, so this formula condenses to $-2n\sigma^{-2}$. The estimated standard error of the standard deviation is therefore $\sqrt{1/(2n\sigma^{-2})} = \sigma/\sqrt{2n}$, which is the usual formula from the textbooks. Also, the mixed second derivative $\frac{\partial^2}{\partial\mu\,\partial\sigma}\left(-\sum(x_i - \mu)^2/2\sigma^2\right) = 2\sum(x_i - \mu)/\sigma^3 = 0$, since the x's average μ. This means that for large Gaussian samples our estimates of the mean and the variance are independent, which, again, has already been mentioned.

This approach also covers changes of parameters. For instance, suppose that you wanted to write out the formula for the Gaussian using σ^2, the variance, as the parameter of interest instead of σ, the standard deviation. Notate this decision as a new parameter $\nu = \sigma^2$. The density that was $\frac{1}{\sigma\sqrt{2\pi}}e^{-(x-\mu)^2/2\sigma^2}$ is now $\frac{1}{\sqrt{\nu}\sqrt{2\pi}}e^{-(x-\mu)^2/2\nu}$. The log of this is $-\frac{1}{2}\log 2\pi - \frac{1}{2}\log\nu - \frac{1}{2}(x-\mu)^2/\nu$. The first derivative of this with respect to ν is $-\frac{1}{2\nu} + \frac{1}{2}(x-\mu)^2/\nu^2$ and the second derivative is $\frac{1}{2\nu^2} - (x-\mu)^2/\nu^3$. Summed over all n cases, this is $\frac{n}{2\nu^2} - \sum(x-\mu)^2/\nu^3$. But at the estimate, $\sum(x-\mu)^2 = n\sigma^2 = n\nu$. So this second derivative simplifies to $-n/2\nu^2$. The negative reciprocal of that expression is $2\nu^2/n$, and the estimated standard deviation of the estimated variance is the square root of that, which is $\nu\sqrt{\frac{2}{n}} = \sigma^2\sqrt{\frac{2}{n}}$, which, again, is the standard textbook formula. Notice that the ratio $\sigma_{\sigma^2}/\sigma^2$ is exactly double the ratio σ_σ/σ.

The formula for the variance of the variance is actually a special case of the general formula for the *variance of a covariance*: the variance of the sample-based estimate $r_{XY}\sigma_X\sigma_Y$ of the covariance between X and Y is

$$(1 + r_{XY}^2)(\sigma_X\sigma_Y)^2/n. \tag{4.1}$$

(But this formula is not from Pearson. It is problem 3.1 of Muirhead, 1982, which reduces to formula 2.8(d) if $r = 0$.)

For other distributions than the univariate Gaussian, or for other combinations of parameters than mean and variance, the mixed partial derivatives that we computed for μ vis-à-vis σ (or ν) are not identically zero, meaning that the parameter estimates driving the covariance model are correlated. The Pearson-Filon (1898) formulas dealt with the three independent entries in the covariance matrix in the Gaussian distribution for two variables – what we have been calling the bell surface – written as a formula in the three parameters σ_x, σ_y, r. The formula one starts with is the formula for the *bivariate Gaussian*, the probability distribution $p(x, y)$ at a point (x, y) for a Gaussian on two variables x and y that have mean zero and correlation r:

$$p_{\text{general}}(x, y) = \frac{1}{2\pi\sigma_x\sigma_y\sqrt{1-r^2}}\, e^{-\frac{1}{2}\left(\frac{x^2}{\sigma_x^2(1-r^2)} - \frac{2xyr}{\sigma_x\sigma_y(1-r^2)} + \frac{y^2}{\sigma_y^2(1-r^2)}\right)}. \quad (4.2a)$$

In connection with our development of the Wishart distribution in Section 4.3, it will also be helpful to have the explicit form of this distribution for a multivariable Gaussian on any arbitrary list of measurements $(x_1, x_2, \ldots, x_p)$, **assuming the x's to be uncorrelated Gaussians all of mean zero and variance 1:**

$$p_{\text{standard}}(x_1, x_2, \ldots, x_p) = \frac{1}{(2\pi)^{p/2}}\, e^{-\frac{1}{2}(x_1^2 + x_2^2 + \cdots + x_p^2)}. \quad (4.2b)$$

Note that the prefactor that was $\frac{1}{\sqrt{2\pi}\sigma}$ in one dimension, equation (2.16), has turned into $\frac{1}{2\pi\sigma_x\sigma_y\sqrt{1-r^2}}$ in two dimensions and into $\frac{1}{(2\pi\sigma^2)^{p/2}}$ for uncorrelated Gaussians all of variance σ^2 in p dimensions, as for the Wishart distribution around the identity matrix to be introduced in Section 4.3.2. In the case of a general covariance structure, the prefactor takes the form $\frac{1}{(2\pi)^{p/2}|\Sigma|^{p/2}}$ where Σ is the covariance matrix of all p of the measured variables and $|\cdot|$ means the determinant (equivalently, the product of the eigenvalues; see Section 4.2) of whatever matrix is between the vertical lines. This factor multiplies the exponential of minus one-half of a term that generalizes Pearson's expression $\left(\frac{x^2}{\sigma_x^2(1-r^2)} - \frac{2xyr}{\sigma_x\sigma_y(1-r^2)} + \frac{y^2}{\sigma_y^2(1-r^2)}\right)$ above. The result is

$$p_{\text{general}}(x_1, x_2, \ldots, x_p) = \frac{1}{(2\pi)^{p/2}|\Sigma|^{p/2}}\, e^{-\frac{1}{2}\left((\mathbf{x}-\mu)'\Sigma^{-1}(\mathbf{x}-\mu)\right)} \quad (4.2c)$$

where μ is the mean of the vector $\mathbf{x} = (x_1, x_2, \ldots, x_p)$. Formula (4.2a) is the special case of this with $\Sigma = \begin{pmatrix} \sigma_x^2 & r\sigma_x\sigma_y \\ r\sigma_x\sigma_y & \sigma_y^2 \end{pmatrix}$, $|\Sigma| = \sigma_x^2\sigma_y^2 - (r\sigma_x\sigma_y)^2 = \sigma_x^2\sigma_y^2(1-r^2)$, $\Sigma^{-1} = \begin{pmatrix} \sigma_y^2 & -r\sigma_x\sigma_y \\ -r\sigma_x\sigma_y & \sigma_x^2 \end{pmatrix}/|\Sigma|$.

When there is more than one parameter in this way, the second derivative required for the evaluation of the information approach turns into a square matrix, which we multiply by -1, invert (Section 4.1.3), divide by sample size n, and interpret element by element, first its diagonal, then the rest. In complete detail, the matrix of second derivatives Pearson and Filon computed for this case of the three-parameter (σ_x, σ_y, r) bivariate Gaussian is the negative of

$$\begin{pmatrix} \frac{1}{\sigma_x^2}\frac{2-r^2}{1-r^2} & -\frac{r^2}{\sigma_x\sigma_y(1-r^2)} & -\frac{r}{\sigma_x(1-r^2)} \\ -\frac{r^2}{\sigma_x\sigma_y(1-r^2)} & \frac{1}{\sigma_y^2}\frac{2-r^2}{1-r^2} & -\frac{r}{\sigma_y(1-r^2)} \\ -\frac{r}{\sigma_x(1-r^2)} & -\frac{r}{\sigma_y(1-r^2)} & \frac{1+r^2}{(1-r^2)^2} \end{pmatrix} \quad (4.3a)$$

of which the matrix inverse (which Pearson computed symbolically, by hand!) is

$$
\begin{pmatrix}
\frac{\sigma_x^2}{2} & \frac{r^2\sigma_x\sigma_y}{2} & \frac{r\sigma_x(1-r^2)}{2} \\
\frac{r^2\sigma_x\sigma_y}{2} & \frac{\sigma_y^2}{2} & \frac{r\sigma_y(1-r^2)}{2} \\
\frac{r\sigma_x(1-r^2)}{2} & \frac{r\sigma_y(1-r^2)}{2} & (1-r^2)^2
\end{pmatrix}
\tag{4.3b}
$$

The diagonal elements here, divided by sample size, are the squares of the imputed standard errors of the parameters σ_x, σ_y, r separately, and each off-diagonal term, divided by the square-root of the product of the two diagonal terms in its row and column, is the correlation of the sampling errors of the pair of parameters in question. For instance, the standard error of the correlation r is the square root of the (3,3) cell of this matrix, divided by $\sqrt{n}$. This yields $(1-r^2)/\sqrt{n}$, the result already copied in from equation (3.20). The correlation of the two σ's, rows and columns 1 and 2, is $(r^2\sigma_x\sigma_y/2) \Big/ \sqrt{(\sigma_x^2/2)(\sigma_y^2/2)} = r^2$, as the σ's, $\sqrt{n}$'s, and 2's all cancel.

Example. For Pearson's family data, Figure 2.28, presume $\sigma_x = \sigma_y = 2.5$, $r = 0.5$, and (to ease the arithmetic) 1000 cases instead of the actual 1375. Then the matrix in equation (4.3a) is

$$
\begin{pmatrix}
0.3733 & -0.0533 & -0.2667 \\
-0.0533 & 0.3733 & -0.2667 \\
-0.2667 & -0.2667 & 2.2222
\end{pmatrix}
\tag{4.4}
$$

with inverse

$$
\begin{pmatrix}
3.12500 & 0.78125 & 0.46875 \\
0.78125 & 3.12500 & 0.46875 \\
0.46875 & 0.46875 & 0.56250
\end{pmatrix}
\tag{4.5}
$$

and so $\sigma_r = .5625/\sqrt{1000} = 0.0178$, $\sigma_{\sigma_x} = \sigma_{\sigma_y} = \sqrt{.003125} = 0.0559$, the correlation between the two σ's is $0.7825/\sqrt{3.125 \times 3.125} = 0.25$ (which equals r^2 as we just verified symbolically), and the correlation between either σ and r is $.46875/\sqrt{3.125 \times 0.5625} \sim 0.3535 = r/\sqrt{2}$.

There is a lovely shortcut formula (Mardia and Marshall, 1984 – this is surprisingly recent) for arriving at the symbolic matrix (4.3a). For a general Gaussian model (4.2c) where the mean vector has parameters that do not overlap with the parameters θ_i of the covariance term Σ, the matrix to be multiplied by n and then inverted to yield the asymptotic standard errors of the covariance parameters has (i,j)th entry

$$
\frac{1}{2}\mathrm{tr}\left(\Sigma^{-1}\frac{\partial\Sigma}{\partial\theta_i}\Sigma^{-1}\frac{\partial\Sigma}{\partial\theta_j}\right).
\tag{4.6}
$$

where the partialling of the matrix Σ with respect to each of its parameters in turn is componentwise, and tr$(\cdot)$ means the trace (sum of the diagonal entries) of whatever square matrix lies between the parentheses.

For instance, for the Pearson-Filon example, writing the covariance matrix as $\Sigma = \begin{pmatrix} \sigma_1^2 & \sigma_1\sigma_2 r \\ \sigma_1\sigma_2 r & \sigma_2^2 \end{pmatrix}$, listing the parameters in the order (σ_1, σ_2, r),

and keeping in mind that $\Sigma^{-1} = \begin{pmatrix} \sigma_2^2 & -\sigma_1\sigma_2 r \\ -\sigma_1\sigma_2 r & \sigma_1^2 \end{pmatrix} / \sigma_1^2 \sigma_2^2 (1 - r^2)$, the

$(3, 3)$ cell of the matrix above is

$$
\frac{1}{2} \text{tr} \left(\Sigma^{-1} \frac{\partial \Sigma}{\partial r} \Sigma^{-1} \frac{\partial \Sigma}{\partial r} \right)
$$

$$
= \frac{1}{2} \left(\sigma_1^2 \sigma_2^2 (1 - r^2) \right)^{-2} \text{tr} \left(\left(\begin{pmatrix} \sigma_2^2 & -\sigma_1\sigma_2 r \\ -\sigma_1\sigma_2 r & \sigma_1^2 \end{pmatrix} \begin{pmatrix} 0 & \sigma_1\sigma_2 \\ \sigma_1\sigma_2 & 0 \end{pmatrix} \right)^2 \right)
$$

$$
= \frac{1}{2} \left(\sigma_1^2 \sigma_2^2 (1 - r^2) \right)^{-2} \text{tr} \left(\begin{pmatrix} -\sigma_1^2 \sigma_2^2 r & \sigma_1\sigma_2^3 \\ \sigma_1^3\sigma_2 & -\sigma_1^2\sigma_2^2 r \end{pmatrix}^2 \right)
$$

$$
= \frac{1}{2} \left(\sigma_1^2 \sigma_2^2 (1 - r^2) \right)^{-2} \left(2\sigma_1^4\sigma_2^4 + 2\sigma_1^4\sigma_2^4 r^2 \right)
$$

$$
= (1 + r^2)/(1 - r^2)^2, \tag{4.7}
$$

just as Pearson had it in equation (4.2). The matrix of all 3×3 of these still has to be inverted to arrive at the individual standard errors and their correlations.

4.1.2 The Centrality of Multivariate Analysis for Studies of Complex Organized Systems

The examples analyzed in Chapters 2 and 3 dealt mainly with measures of size – lengths, areas, weights. Even when we considered an explicit ratio index (the BMI, Section 2.6), we ended up using it as an aid to interpretation instead of an actual quantity: as isolines on a scatterplot, not as a predictor or predictand in any regression. In contrast, geometric morphometrics (GMM) is the extension of all the preceding approaches to the study of one explicit set of measurements of shape as well as size (the domain that, as a composite, is usually called *form*). Its techniques will not necessarily apply to just any ratio in arbitrary units: not, for instance, to BMI with its weird ad hoc formula in units of pressure. Nevertheless, GMM suits most of the biometrical problems that arise in data sets of *landmark locations* (Section 5.1) or the extended notion of *semilandmark locations* (Section 5.5.3). We will return to the topic of index construction for data sets of this type in Section 5.4.

Before one encounters landmark data sets, one should first explore the statistical approaches that are competent to handle them. As they will be taught here, these mostly newer tools, all dependent on the availability of fast distributed computation and flexible (often playful) visualization, are based on several aspects of multivariate statistics that do not much resemble the variable-by-variable least-squares approaches of my previous chapters or your previous courses. The reason is mainly that morphometrics organizes your *measurements* in a disciplined but unusual way irrevocably altering the meaning of every subsequent pattern analysis. The following subsections explore the possibilities and pitfalls of this situation, beginning with the underlying multivariate algebra and geometry and ending with a variety of tools for generating biological hypotheses from morphometric data summaries comporting with these inference styles.

Collectively this content comprises the missing component of the morphometrics curriculum nearly everywhere that it is taught. If the art of morphometrics is one of *selection* – choosing the most suggestive pattern descriptions from a huge range of possibilities – then the underlying toolkit needs to devote a good deal of attention to the rules governing those selections. Generally speaking, the reported patterns fall into two classes: usually, the pattern of interest is either (1) a *profile* (a set of coefficients applying to an explanatory task set in advance) or else (2) an *extremum* (a descriptor that picks one element out of some geometrical manifold to stand for the "best" or "most powerful" summary of a data set in some sense). Either approach might be exploited once and then reported as if the remainder of the signal in the data is mere noise, or else repeated recursively in order that we might renew our consideration of whatever biometrical information remains after the earlier description has been computed, considered from a biological point of view, and then set aside (or constrained experimentally).

The GMM protocols overseeing analyses of this flavor typically refer to a *covariance structure* that summarizes numerical relationships among multiple measures of the organisms you measured. With the help of tools like principal components analysis or likelihood ratio analysis, that covariance structure is transformed into summaries of the relative plausibility of diverse pattern descriptions and their persuasive power for the biological context under study. The rest of this chapter reviews the statistical approach to patterns of covariance (an approach that is not itself particularly biological), introduces some of the biological extensions of this notion, and thereby sets the stage for their joint application (in Chapter 5) to the measurements that arise in manipulations of landmark or semilandmark locations, which is the formalism by which GMM arrives at an understanding of shape or form.

Considered one by one, the covariances we reviewed in Section 2.1 incorporate hardly any biometrical meaning. A covariance coefficient $\sigma_x \sigma_y r$ of 50 could arise as a correlation of 0.005 between two measures of standard deviation 50 and 200 or instead as a correlation of 0.50 between measures both having standard deviation 10. Section 2.4.4 showed how the computation of a particularly interesting pair of contrasts among two variables, the pair that was orthogonal both geometrically and biometrically, required that attention be paid to both of the variances as well as that covariance. As soon as we broaden our vision to consider these coefficients in organized sets – all the covariances among pairs drawn from a set of variables, together with all of their variances separately – we gain a tremendous quantitative leverage that more than compensates for the cost of the additional axioms required (the human effort involved in stating them, I mean; not the possibly greater cost of verifying them). GMM is driven by a rhetoric for *patterns of covariances*, not for their values one at a time.

4.1.3 Inverses versus Eigenanalysis: The Two Roles of the Matrix

This subsection, building on the simpler examples introduced before, characterizes the algebra and geometry behind both of the two principal approaches. Matrix inversion methods are for situations where variables are clearly distinct from one another, and eigenanalysis (principal component) methods are for contexts where individual measures are not as important as the pleiotropic genes or diffuse functional factors that plausibly account for them.

From time to time the preceding chapters mentioned *matrices,* rectangular arrays of numbers, and even set out formulas where some of the letters (perhaps X, perhaps Σ) stand for matrices. You encountered matrices, for instance, in the discussion of the "hat matrix" in Section 2.4, in the general discussion of Sewall Wright's path coefficients d for direct effects in Section 3.1, and in the exegeses of discriminant analysis in Sections 3.5 and 3.6. There they were a simple way of keeping track of least-squares arithmetic on the data. In morphometrics, however, their role is much deeper: they explicitly generate the patterns that intervene between arithmetic and biological interpretatios or explanations.

I have been careful not to claim any biological reality a priori for these constructions. The plain meaning of any derived result based on algebraic manipulation of some matrix is overwhelmingly likely to remain a mere notational convenience, not a coherent biological finding, unless and until it is identified and independently validated with developmental or evolutionary features of the organismal physiology under study. (See the various examples in Figure 5.9 of Bookstein, 2014.) In truth, a matrix, specifically the covariance matrix that is our main concern in this section, is not a biological quantity but only a hint of one: the substrate for disciplined algorithmic arithmetic calling attention to one or another numerical aspect of an organism under study that might calibrate a known process or suggest other networks for further exploration. For instance, it is not rational to claim that a "data matrix," the array with rows for specimens and columns for variables, has any biological reality (although a particular abstraction from it, the singular-value decomposition, can be very suggestive; Section 4.2); nor does a covariance matrix exist in any organismal sense; nor does the information matrix of Section 4.1.1, or its negative inverse. The organism knows as little about these constructs as it does about its own scientific name or its origins in the Burgess Shale. Still, if causal relations between multiple measured variables are real, there should be a real biological foundation to the ways that we typically *interpret* descriptive or analytic matrices in practice. It is in geometric morphometrics, the focal applications area of this book, that these techniques have their highest and best justification: the domain where the actual measured variables (which will be landmark and semilandmark coordinates) have the strongest biological organization of their own.

Before Chapter 5 introduces and justifies the *shape coordinates*, a structure of measured variables specialized for biological shape per se, it is helpful to survey the numerical rhetoric by which they can sometimes be attached to biometrical analyses. As Figure 4.2 notes, sometimes it is the approach by matrix *inversion* that leads to this interpretability, and sometimes the approach by matrix *eigenanalysis*. Even though there are algebraic relationships between these two formalisms, they tap entirely different domains of biometrical interpretation. In short:

• Matrix inversion drives prediction technologies that accommodate the measured variables one at a time. Applications relying on matrix inversion implicitly presume that each measured variable is individuated in some sense: different enough from all the other variables that the analytic task of isolating its specific information content has a chance of leading to enlightenment. Random sampling, in this context, applies mainly to getting the *specimens* that are to be treated as representative of their original biological population(s). Wright-style path analysis for predictions of one specific outcome score (Section 3.1) is one canonical example of this context. Another is the construction of a linear discriminant function for classification of an unknown organism into one of two predefined groups (Section 3.5); yet another is the re-expression of a Gaussian probability model for any data set in terms of the sampling error variances and covariances of all its parameters via the Pearson–Fisher information matrix in Section 4.1.

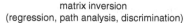

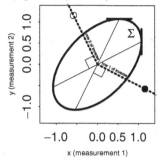

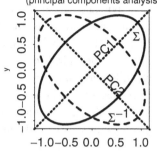

the same in a different geometry

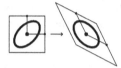

Figure 4.2 Matrix inversion versus eigenanalysis for the matrix $\begin{pmatrix} 2 & 1 \\ 1 & 2 \end{pmatrix}/\sqrt{3}$:
schematic of the two main thrusts of covariance structure analysis, here applied
to a simple 2×2 covariance matrix Σ with $r = \frac{1}{2}$ as previously discussed in the
context of regression analysis. Each version is drawn in the lines with the closely
spaced dots. Solid curve: the "belt of the bell" – the isoline, elliptical in form,
corresponding to probability density $1/2\pi\sqrt{e}$. Each point of this ellipse is at a
distance from the center equal to the standard deviation of the linear combination
of unit length in its direction. For instance, the horizontal line through the center
cuts the ellipse at a distance 1.075 on this scale, because the variance of the
linear combination that is just x is $2/\sqrt{3}$, the square root of which is 1.075.
(upper left) Rows of the *inverse matrix* $\Sigma^{-1} = \begin{pmatrix} 2 & -1 \\ -1 & 2 \end{pmatrix}/\sqrt{3}$, dotted lines,
lie along perpendiculars to the regression lines characterizing Σ; they specify the
linear combinations of the measured variables that correlate precisely zero with
all of the original measurements except one, with which they have a covariance
of precisely 1. Filled circle, the linear combination $(2x - y)/\sqrt{3}$, first row of
the inverse matrix. Open circle, the linear combination $(2y - x)/\sqrt{3}$, second
row of the inverse. (upper right) The *eigenanalysis* of Σ instead involves the
construction of composite measurements (here, $x+y$ and $x-y$) that are consistent
with their own role as pattern summaries for Σ – the directions that are left
unchanged when expressed as their own separate profiles of covariance with the
list of measured variables. Dashed curve: expressing the inverse matrix Σ^{-1} by
its own elliptical isoline instead of by its rows. Σ and its inverse have the same
principal directions but eigenvalues that are reciprocals of one another. Here those
eigenvalues are $\sqrt{3}$ and $\frac{1}{\sqrt{3}}$, and the semiaxes at right in Figure 4.2, which go as
the square roots of these, have lengths in the ratio of $\sqrt{3}$:1. These directions are

- Applications relying on matrix *eigenanalysis*, in contrast, treat variables not as individuated but as themselves arbitrary samples of a universe of possible measurements. Eigenanalysis is more concerned with this type of sampling than with the sampling of specimens, which could very well represent the entirety of some population, not necessarily a random sample at all. In place of assumptions about samples of specimens, the formalisms of eigenanalysis substitute stringent assumptions about the biometrical nature of the descriptions at which we are aiming. Arbitrary linear combinations $\Sigma a_i x_i$ of the measured variables x_i must be potentially meaningful regardless of the values of the coefficients a_i, *which may be positive or negative,* and variances of such linear combinations must be commensurate across directions a_i. Such assumptions about what it means to add and multiply variables demand considerably more sophistication on the part of any biologist who wishes to exploit these techniques. In my view, out of all the application domains, morphometrics is the one where those assumptions are the least unreasonable.

Other literatures have highlighted this distinction before. Perhaps the most congenial phrasing is the contrast delineated in structural equation models (and their cousins, partial least-squares models) between *reflective* and *formative* indicator sets. Formative indicators are combined in accordance with the rules in Section 3.1 for the optimal least-squares prediction of some exogenous quantity, while reflective indicators are combined using coefficients that are proportional to the separate covariances or correlations of the constituent indicators with respect to some endogenous or exogenous causal process. Put more simply: in a formative setting, the indicators cause the construct (their linear combination); in a reflective setting, the more appropriate when indicators are highly intercorrelated, the construct causes the indicators. See, in general, Bollen (1989), and, for the partial least squares context, Fornell and Bookstein (1982).

---

perpendicular in the geometry of these figures and also are uncorrelated in the geometry of the data (another interpretation of the statement that they are "self-predictive" in terms of the covariance structure they are designed to summarize). For the justification of this construction, see footnote 10. (lower left) Alternative construal of the oblique directions in the panel above left: images of the original x- and y-axes when the ellipse representing Σ is sheared into the ellipse representing Σ^{-1}.

The two great strategies of matrix algebra that concern us can now be characterized as follows. Both begin with a *covariance matrix,* which is the pattern of covariances between every variable of some list of p variables and every other variable of that list. More generally, it is the pattern of covariances between every variable of one list and every variable of another list measured on the same sample that probably involves a different machine and a different count of measurements. If your data come in the form of a "data matrix," that notion is relevant here by reason of the easier notation it affords for this covariance structure. Let X be that data matrix, rows for specimens, columns for variables, and assume the measures in X have been mean-centered (set to average 0 one by one). Then the covariance matrix of the X's with themselves is $X'X/n$, where n is the sample size, and the covariance vector of the X's with any predictand y is the vector $X'y/n$. The matrix $X'X/n$ is a symmetrical square of numbers, $p \times p$, one for each pair of measurements from the data matrix X, and the expression $X'y/n$ is a vector of p numbers, one for each of the p measures of the data matrix X. Section 3.1 noted that for any task of least-squares linear prediction of a single measurement y, the vector of direct effects is the matrix product $(X'X)^{-1}X'y$, the product of the covariance vector $X'y/n$ by the inverse of the covariance matrix $X'X/n$ of the measured predictors X_i. (The n's cancelled.) In these formulas, the prime (') means "transpose," switch of rows and columns. This is just a shortcut to what would otherwise be a clumsier way of indicating which numbers multiply and divide which others.

Matrix inversion. In this setting, matrix inversion is the construction of a new list of variables, of the same count p as the original set of variables. Each of the new variables is a linear combination of the same list of p original variables, and they are computed all at once, such that the kth new variable has covariance 1 with the kth original variable and covariance 0 with all of the others.[1] This manipulation will thereby permit us to separate the

---

[1] This is an elementary consequence of the other interpretation of the matrix inverse operation – that it results in a multiplicative inverse [hence the name] under the operation of matrix multiplication. This is the property $\Sigma_{XX}\Sigma_{XX}^{-1} = I_p$, where I_p, a matrix with 1's down the diagonal and 0's everywhere else, is the multiplicative identity for the square matrices of size $p \times p$. In the interpretation of the text, the rows of the inverse matrix $(X'X)^{-1}$ stand for linear combinations $X(X'X)^{-1}$ that have covariance 1 with the corresponding original X-variable and zero with every other original measure; this is just another interpretation of the identity $X'X(X'X)^{-1} = I_p$. In other words, I_p is reinterpreted as a covariance matrix in its own right, the pattern of covariances equal to 1 for the first, second, ... pairs of variables and 0's for every other pair. Hence the result: the covariance $X'(X\Sigma_{XX}^{-1})$ of any vector X of measurements with

information relevant to predicting or accounting for each original quantity in turn. If the covariances are among measured variables, the context is of prediction; if they deal with model parameters, as in equations (4.4) and (4.5), the concern is with the precision of those parameters and their combinations instead.

The left-hand side of Figure 4.2 shows this construction for the covariance matrix $\begin{pmatrix} 2 & 1 \\ 1 & 2 \end{pmatrix} / \sqrt{3}$, a multiple of a matrix that previously appeared in Figure 2.21. (The factor of $\sqrt{3}$ is there so that it has determinant 1, whereupon the two matrices can be drawn together in the second panel.) With the same scaling, the inverse matrix is $\begin{pmatrix} 2 & -1 \\ -1 & 2 \end{pmatrix} / \sqrt{3}$. This means that the derived variable $(2x - y)/\sqrt{3}$ (solid circle) is uncorrelated with y and has covariance 1 with x, while the derived variable $(-x + 2y)/\sqrt{3}$ (open circle) is uncorrelated with x and has covariance 1 with y. (In both cases this is because $r = \frac{1}{2}$ – this noncorrelation between predictor and regression residuals was already mentioned in the text of Section 2.1.) These two rows of Σ^{-1} are symbolized by the two dots in the figure along the lines orthogonal to the two regressions of the original matrix Σ.

This concern for the individuality of the separate rows or columns of a covariance structure is even clearer in the analysis of the Pearson–Fisher information matrix just introduced in Section 4.1. The matrix of parameter covariances we are seeking is itself the negative inverse of the second derivatives of the loglikelihood. Whereas the sample of specimens itself is presumed homogeneous, the bivariate Gaussian model converts the pair of measured variables into *three* separate parameters that have heterogeneous biological interpretations. Two are the standard deviations of the original measurements, which could have been computed separately measure by measure, but the third is the correlation between them, which is a function of every datum in the entire data set. None of the entries in the information matrix are measureable properties of individual specimens. They pertain only to the sample of specimens as a whole, and in order for any parameters to be meaningful, that sample must itself be homogeneous.[2] The inverse matrix in

---

the new vector $X\Sigma_{XX}^{-1}$ of derived linear combinations is $\Sigma_{XX}\Sigma_{XX}^{-1} = I_p$, the identity matrix of rank p.

[2] In the present context this means: without any recognizable subgroupings that might inherit different values of the parameters in question but that have been fixed at arbitrary fractions of the pooled sample by some subjective decision of the analyst or her predecessors, e.g., "all the intact fossils in the Natural History Museum." Other contexts for biometric inference entail other definitions of homogeneity. For a comment, see Bookstein (2014), and for a general discussion, see Elsasser (1975).

equation (4.3) or (4.5) is interpreted as the covariance matrix of these same parameters, including all of their own individual sampling errors. They are thus, explicitly, measurements on the sample per se, not on the individual specimens in any biometrically meaningful sense.

It would be remiss of a book like this not to give the actual formula for checking a matrix inversion. It rests on the formula for matrix multiplication, which is easy to write down. For two matrices $A = (a_{ij})$, $m \times n$, and $B = (b_{kl})$, $n \times p$, the matrix product AB is defined as $(\sum_{q=1}^{n} a_{iq}b_{qj})$, $m \times p$. Even if $m = p$, this is usually not the same as BA. For numbers, multiplying by 1 leaves them unchanged. For matrices, there is an equivalent, the *identity matrix*, a square matrix with 1's down the diagonal and 0's everywhere else. Write this (as in footnote 1) as I_p where p is the count of rows. Then it is easy to check that for the matrix A above, $m \times n$, multiplying it by I_m on the *left* leaves it unchanged, as does multiplying it by I_n on the *right*. If $m = n$ (the case of A a square matrix), these two I's are the same. Just as the inverse of an ordinary number b is the number $1/b$ that, when you multiply by b, gives you back the multiplicative identity 1, likewise the *inverse* of a square matrix $A = (a_{ij})$, $n \times n$, is the square matrix $B = (b_{kl})$ for which $AB = BA = I_n$ (if there is such a matrix B, otherwise A is called *noninvertible*; such A's have determinant 0). This is really n^2 different equations: $\sum_{q=1}^{n} a_{iq}b_{qi} = 1$ for every i, and also $\sum_{q=1}^{n} a_{iq}b_{qj} = 0$ whenever $i \neq j$. There will be another approach, simpler to explain once we have access to the machinery of principal components, in Figure 4.2 (right) and footnote 10.

Using these formulas we can check Pearson's important assertion that the matrices in Section 4.1 are inverses. *Numerically*, equations (4.4) and (4.5), we must have[3]

$$.3733 \times 3.125 - .0533 \times .78125 - .2667 \times .46875 = 0.9999063 \sim 1,$$

$$- .0533 \times 3.125 + .3733 \times .78125 - .2667 \times .46875$$

$$= .0000625 \sim 0, \quad \text{etc.}$$

Symbolically, which is the way Pearson actually computed this, equations (4.2) and (4.3), we have

---

[3] In practice, one relies on a computational statistical package for operations of these sort – the only time one computes a numerical inverse by hand is as homework for the lecture that introduces the matrix inverse in the first place. For the very patient person, and for the computer programmer, there are a variety of good numerical algorithms for these computations, beginning with one invented by Gauss before the turn of the eighteenth century. For the 3×3 case, Pearson used some special formulas based on the vector crossproduct.

$$\frac{1}{\sigma_x^2} \frac{2-r^2}{1-r^2} \times \frac{\sigma_x^2}{2} - \frac{r^2}{\sigma_x \sigma_y (1-r^2)} \times \frac{r^2 \sigma_x \sigma_y}{2} - \frac{r}{\sigma_x (1-r^2)} \times \frac{r \sigma_x (1-r^2)}{2}$$

$$= \frac{1}{2(1-r^2)} \left(2 - r^2 - r^4 - r^2(1-r^2) \right) = \frac{2 - 2r^2}{2(1-r^2)} = 1,$$

$$\frac{1}{\sigma_x^2} \frac{2-r^2}{1-r^2} \times \frac{r^2 \sigma_x \sigma_y}{2} - \frac{r^2}{\sigma_x \sigma_y (1-r^2)} \times \frac{\sigma_y^2}{2} - \frac{r}{\sigma_x (1-r^2)} \times \frac{r \sigma_y (1-r^2)}{2}$$

$$= \frac{1}{2(1-r^2)} \left((2 - r^2)r^2 - r^2 - r^2(1-r^2) \right)$$

$$= \frac{r^2}{2(1-r^2)} (2 - r^2 - 2 + r^2) = 0, \quad \text{etc.} \tag{4.8}$$

Sometimes it is enough to just inspect a matrix inverse, without computing anything else. The inverse of a correlation matrix has a surprising special property: when it is normalized by dividing each element $(\Sigma^{-1})_{ij}$ by the square root of the product $(\Sigma^{-1})_{ii}(\Sigma^{-1})_{jj}$ of the two relevant diagonal entries, each offdiagonal entry is the negative of the partial correlation of that pair of variables *holding all of the others constant*. (For a proof of this elementary but rarely taught theorem, see Bookstein, 2014, section 5.2.3.3.) We apply this insight to the correlation matrix of Sewall Wright's six chicken measurements, equation (2.21). The inverse is

$$R^{-1} = \begin{pmatrix} 1.886 & -0.620 & -0.140 & -0.376 & -0.341 & -0.273 \\ -0.620 & 1.803 & 0.275 & -0.523 & -1.235 & 0.824 \\ 0.140 & 0.276 & 8.402 & -5.861 & -2.513 & 0.496 \\ -0.376 & -0.523 & -5.861 & 9.986 & 0.283 & -3.628 \\ -0.341 & -1.235 & -2.513 & 0.283 & 11.675 & -8.222 \\ -0.273 & 0.824 & 0.496 & -3.628 & -8.222 & 11.731 \end{pmatrix},$$

so that the matrix with those completely partialled correlations off the diagonal is

$$\begin{pmatrix} 1.000 & 0.336 & -0.035 & 0.087 & 0.073 & 0.058 \\ 0.336 & 1.000 & -0.071 & 0.123 & 0.269 & -0.179 \\ -0.035 & -0.071 & 1.000 & 0.640 & 0.254 & -0.005 \\ 0.087 & 0.123 & 0.640 & 1.000 & -0.026 & 0.335 \\ 0.073 & -0.269 & 0.254 & -0.026 & 1.000 & 0.705 \\ 0.058 & -0.179 & -0.005 & 0.335 & 0.705 & 1.000 \end{pmatrix}$$

in which the largest entries are evidently in the [1,2] and [2,1] cells, the [3,4] and [4,3] cells, and the [5,6] and [6,5] cells. But these are just the cells for the correlations of the measures of the same structure – skull with skull, wing with wing, leg with leg. We have thus reconstituted Wright's original observations about modularity by an antirely automatic procedure, applied to an extremely carefully designed measurement scheme where every special factor was probed exactly twice. This manipulation does not preclude the existence of a general factor against which all of these increments of selected bivariate correlations constitute "special factors," but it shows how manipulations based on matrix inverses can help us focus on properties of pairs of variables in a way different from the path analyses of Section 3.1.

Matrix eigenanalysis. Whereas matrix inversion is founded on a presumption that the measured variables have well-defined and biologically individuated interpretations variable by variable, eigenanalysis is based on the opposite assumption: that the measured variables individually have no special meaning, but instead it is what they have in common that matters for biological interpretation. Instead of constructed linear combinations that uniquely predict just one original measure, eigenanalysis seeks constructs that uniquely predict only themselves. The matrix inversion approach privileges individuality of each measured variable x; the eigenanalysis approach privileges meaningfulness of the pattern analysis per se. To be precise, we seek new variables $Xw_1, \ldots, Xw_p$, each one a linear combination of the original measured x's, such that the regression of any Xw on the others is zero, meaning that there are no overlaps of information among them via either covariances or angles in the picture – that is, that they are both *orthogonal* (geometrically perpendicular) and *uncorrelated*. There are two alternative characterizations of the same formulas that are often useful components of a potential explanation. First, these new linear combinations w are *reproduced* by the covariance matrix of the x's – each one satisfies an equation $\Sigma_{XX} w_i = \lambda_i w_i$ for some positive number λ_i, its *eigenvalue*.[4] Second, when the Xw's are ordered by these λ's, the first of them, Xw_1, has the largest variance of any linear combination of the x's with coefficients summing in square to 1.0; the second, Xw_2, has the largest variance of any linear combination with coefficients summing in square to 1.0 that is uncorrelated with the linear combination Xw_1; and so forth through all p of them. It is also helpful to note two properties we will explicitly demonstrate for the case of 2×2 matrices in Section 4.2 and exploit extensively in Section 4.3: the product of all the eigenvalues is the determinant of the matrix, and their sum is its trace (the sum of the diagonal elements). The w's are called the *eigenvectors* of Σ_{XX}.

At the right in Figure 4.2 is the graph of this version of the analysis for the same matrix $\Sigma = \begin{pmatrix} 2 & 1 \\ 1 & 2 \end{pmatrix} / \sqrt{3}$ that we already inspected in the left panel.

---

[4] This is why the particle "eigen" is there in the name of the technique: it is the German word for "of one's own" or "distinct." Cf. *Eigenschaft*, characteristic, property. (λ is the Greek letter "lambda.")

The inverse matrix Σ^{-1} has the same eigenvectors (principal directions) as Σ but eigenvalues that are the reciprocals of those of Σ (so that its eigenvectors w come in the opposite order from those of Σ). In this example, because the eigenvalues of the original covariance structure Σ have product 1, so do their reciprocals – the axes have simply swapped lengths. In this case of two measured variables only, of the same variance, the eigenvectors are just the diagonal axes of the ellipses in figures like this.[5]

The natural tie between these two diagrams is sketched in the little demonstration at lower left in Figure 4.2, where the the actual *drawing* of Σ is altered so as to overlie the actual drawing of Σ^{-1}. One arranges for this by shrinking distances in the direction of PC1 by the ratio of λ_2 to λ_1, and vice versa: in other words, by replacing the scale along every principal axis by its reciprocal. Here that means shrinking the SW–NE diagonal by a factor of $\sqrt{3}$ and expanding the perpendicular diagonal by the same factor. When this shear is applied to the entire original diagram of Σ, the Cartesian axes there are transformed into the two rows of the inverse matrix that were drawn at upper left.

In three dimensions, the linear combinations that stand for the rows of the inverse matrix (Figure 4.2, left) are proportional to the vector cross products[6] of the lines from the origin through the touching points of tangent planes normal to the coordinate axes, and the corresponding covariance structure itself (Figure 4.2, right) is the ellipsoid on the same axes with axis lengths that are the inverses of those of the original covariance matrix. The situation in higher dimensions is closely analogous but can no longer be visualized by diagrams on paper. The construction at lower left in Figure 4.2, the rows of the inverse as sheared versions of the original Cartesian axes when the covariance matrix is squashed or stretched into its inverse axis by axis, is the same in any number of dimensions.

In spite of this overlap of pedagogy, to claim that an eigenanalysis is meaningful makes demands on any biological investigation that are much more strenuous than those for the matrix inversion approach were. In the matrix

---

[5] Even more than for matrix inverses, the computation of these useful decompositions is best left to publicly tested and certified statistical software except for the 2×2 case that is illustrated here and that I am about to demonstrate in Section 4.2. The 2×2 setting, because it reduces to the quadratic formula, is the only one susceptible nowadays to error-free computation by hand in a reasonable amount of time. As it was for the matrix inverse, the first algorithms for computing matrix eigenanalyses by hand are ancient by today's standards, requiring the solution of an algebraic equation of degree p (the number of variables) instead of iterating to the intended diagonal form or any of its re-expressions. When was the last time you found the roots of a cubic polynomial by hand using the formula?

[6] For two vectors X_1, X_2 in three dimensions, the vector crossproduct $X_1 \times X_2$ is a vector perpendicular to both X_1 and X_2 with length equal to the product of the lengths of X_1 and X_2 times the sine of the angle between them.

inversion approach, the rows of the inverse functioned only as coefficients of a predictor. In the eigenanalysis, the coefficients specify new linear combinations that have to be meaningful in their own right. This demands, in particular, that combinations should make sense even when their coefficients vary in sign. The inevitability of this is the content of the Perron–Frobenius Theorem, which guarantees that in a matrix of all positive covariances, such as typically describes our suites of measured lengths within a single homogeneous sample, only the first eigenvector of those covariances can have all coefficients positive so as to be interpretable as a "pattern of allometric growth." Every other eigenvector must have coefficients that vary in sign, and thus must be interpreted as a "contrast" (recall the analysis of Bumpus's sparrows, Section 3.5.3). But not every linear combination of mixed sign on a set of measured variables *can* formally make sense as a contrast – the equivalent notion of weighted averages (Section 2.1), after all, offers no role for a negative "weight." We will see in Chapter 5 how the milieu of geometric morphometrics circumvents this otherwise often crippling limitation by replacing the sign of a scalar coefficient by a circle of potential coefficient *pairs* – shift vectors – that no longer has any natural reference orientation. In place of a profile of coefficients there is a grid of suggested deformation gradients, a metaphor quite a bit more effective as the generator of developmental or evolutionary hypotheses.

Any general methodological concern for making quantitative organismal bioscience coherent must come to terms with these two fundamentally different ways of analyzing the information implicit in a suite of multiple measurements and the import of that multiplicity per se for the scientific inference motivating the original investment in collecting and collating the data. In a sound study involving multiple measurements, either the original measures were designed to be kept separate for explanatory purposes, or they were designed not to be kept separate. The rules for computation are completely different in the two situations. The third possibility, "I don't know," is ruled out by the definition of soundness in such studies.

For a set of p variables, matrix inversion and eigenextraction both involve the generation of a new set likewise of p variables having properties defined in terms of noncorrelation. But the rhetoric of those properties is quite different one from the other, and different, too, from the underlying language of biological explanation in its properly causal or experimental setting. The matrix inverse specifies the property of noncorrelation with *all but one of the original p variables*. This notation is meaningful to the extent that the set of p variables was assembled with the goal of linearly predicting some $(p + 1)$st mensurand, as we reviewed in the context of Sewall Wright's method of path analysis in the preceding chapter. The calculation evidently becomes biologically meaningful just to the extent that those separate paths are, in fact, separable processes of an underlying causal plexus – separable, for instance, via the construal of interventions "other things being equal," interventions on one single predictor variable at a time with the others clamped. For instance, in Figure 3.16 the estimated slopes of the lines represent the "independent" contribution of variation in the horizontal measurement presuming invariance of subgroup membership, even though in actuality subgroup varies with that very same measured predictor.

In contrast, an eigenanalysis specifies uncorrelated patterns from among these same p variables, this time without reference to any exogenous $(p + 1)$st quantity. Here it is the patterns, not the predictions, that are required to be uncorrelated. Prediction comes in when we think of the patterns as themselves undergoing prediction by the same measured p variables; then the requirement is that these predictions be self-consistent, each coefficient proportional to its own covariance with the underlying pattern. Under this assumption, it turns out that each pattern predicts only itself, not any of the others. Here, too, there is no automatic guarantee of biological meaningfulness. The known biological processes underlying these observations – for instance, the common dependence on a shorter list of pleiotropic genes – are not necessarily uncorrelated; genes, after all, are not independently distributed. Orthogonality is a property of explanations, not of data.[7] For instance, the *single-factor allometric models* that will be introduced in Section 4.3.5 presume an absence of subgroupings within the sample by such criteria as taxonomic identification. If those subgroups are present, they distort the information criteria driving the eigenanalysis. In this circumstance the standard computed pattern representations can represent allometry correctly only if the corresponding process of differential growth is empirically uncorrelated with the pattern of size dependence embodied in the pattern analysis (i.e., only in the presence of strict *heterochrony*; see Mitteroecker et al., 2004). Otherwise the principal components confound two biologically distinct processes, allometry and phylogeny, in a way that can be disentangled only by additional data collection.

A similar critique applies to the technique of singular-value decomposition introduced in the next section. For data that have not been mean-centered, the first right singular vector typically is quite close to the sample average,

---

[7] This point is far from new. Its importance was first emphasized to me by Richard Reyment's books on quantitative paleobiology, e.g., Reyment (1991), but in the more general context it dates back to the invention of "rotation to simple structure" in the psychometric methodology of L. L. Thurstone around the middle of the twentieth century.

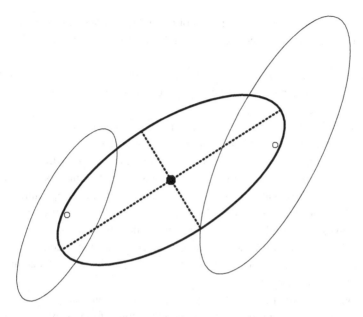

Figure 4.3 Diagram of a fallacious principal components analysis. Light ellipses: schematic of a Gaussianly distributed pair of variables in each of two subpopulations (open circles, means of the subpopulations separately). Heavy ellipse: the corresponding locus of points at one standard deviation's distance from the grand mean (the big black dot). Heavy dotted lines: the corresponding pooled principal components, having no particular relationship either to the within-group principal components here (the axes of the two ellipses separately) or to the vector between their means. Compare Figure 3.22, which displays the corresponding ecological fallacy in the context of analysis of covariance (regression over multiple groups).

and the second singular vector is thus constrained to have zero crossproduct with this average; but nothing about the biological setting guarantees that the first important dimension of variation around an average needs to have a pattern descriptor that is orthogonal to that average. *Biological and statistical decompositions of measurements on complex organized systems such as organisms have no necessary relation to one another; any ostensibly "simplifying" computation must be checked against the corresponding biological explanations.* See Figure 4.3.

Summary of Section 4.1

- The covariance between two variables x and y can be written as the expression $r_{xy}\sigma_x\sigma_y$. On a bivariate Gaussian hypothesis (a bell surface), the sampling variances and covariances of these three components can be computed all at once according to formulas Karl Pearson published in 1898.

- The error variance of the correlation r is $(1 - r^2)^2/n$, the correlation of the errors in the two σ's is r^2, and the correlation between the estimates of σ and r is $r/\sqrt{2}$.

- These computations are based on one of the two main uses of matrix algebra in morphometrics: the *matrix inverse* that refers arbitrarily correlated measurements or parameters to new linear combinations correlating only with one of the original measures or parameters. For this to be useful, the original measures or parameters have to have separable individual meanings. Pearson's invention, the information matrix of second derivatives of the loglikelihood of the data at the estimated parameter values, falls under this heading of matrix inversion when we compute its negative inverse to get the error variances of the parameters as listed in the preceding bullet point.

- The other main application of matrix algebra in morphometrics is *eigenanalysis*, which produces linear combinations of the measurements that are consistent with their own covariance-based pattern analyses. In contrast to matrix inversion, eigenanalysis presumes that the measured variables are not important by themselves but only as redundant samples from an indefinitely broad underlying space of possible measurements.

- Either technique requires that the samples over which the covariance structure was computed be homogeneous. Hidden or unacknowledged heterogeneity destroys the interpretability of all the SVD-based analyses to be introduced in the next section.

4.2 The Singular-Value Decomposition and Its Applications in Morphometrics

Almost never in geometric morphometric studies does one specific landmark or one specific distance have a scientific meaning all by itself. Instead, distances acquire meaning by virtue of their covariances with every other measured distance, and landmarks acquire meaning by their relationships to all the other landmarks, both their near neighbors and their distant counterparts. This is the case no matter how many landmarks (and semilandmarks, Section 5.5) there are. There is one substantial exception to this generalization, the study of biomechanical *indices* or *ratios* that will be discussed in Section 5.6.6. But in most other investigative styles the eigenanalysis approach to geometric morphometrics has proved the more powerful – the more likely to generate fruitful biological hypotheses for further investigation.

This section offers brief overviews and examples of the four main variants of this crucial core technique. First I introduce the singular-value decomposition (SVD), which embodies the fundamental theorem that drives this whole domain. It offers a least-squares interpretation of the partial descriptions that arise by cutting off the list of eigenvectors in various ways, and, via a different reinterpretation (principal component scores, Section 4.2.2), a way back to properties of the original specimens that seemed to have been obliterated once they contributed their crossproducts to the covariance matrix undergoing analysis. From this reconsideration of the eigenanalysis of a square covariance matrix $X'X/n$ we turn in Section 4.2.3 to the more general case of a covariance structure $X'Y/n$, the covariance of any list X of centered variables by any other conceptually distinct list Y. (This notation presumes that data matrices like X or Y have already been "centered," shifted so that every column has mean 0.) Via a quite different application of the same SVD, we arrive at an approach to the decomposition of the mutual predictive power of one block of measures for another block, a combination of regression and eigenanalysis usually called Partial Least Squares (PLS). Section 4.2.4 explains a fourth specific tool, yet another version of eigenanalysis where now the matrix under examination has one row and column for every *specimen,* not every variable: the matrix D^2 with (i,j) entry $d_{ij}^2 = \sum_k (x_{ik} - x_{jk})^2$ of *sums of squares of differences* between the values of the variables of every pair i,j of cases. This is the technique of *principal coordinates,* the explicit analysis of matrices of "squared distance" as a metaphor for *dissimilarity* among individual specimens. Following all of these applications, Section 4.3 will sketch the underlying probability theory allowing us to assess the variability of all these descriptions. The *Wishart distribution* allows one to represent the implications of bell-curve disorder for this higher algebra just as the Pearson–Filon formulation of Section 4.1 did for the a priori descriptors (standard deviations and correlations) that were our subject there.

4.2.1 The SVD Theorem and Its Component Parts

The singular-value decomposition (SVD) is the adaptation for biometrical purposes of a very old approach to mathematical lists of functions that originated well before any of these applications but that was not realized to be so central until the relatively late date of the 1930s (Eckart and Young, 1936). It is surprisingly abstract and general for a tool whose applications in organismal biology are so ubiquitous and fertile. The theorem can be put in the form of one single equation along with some corollaries, as follows.

Let X be any matrix of numbers, square or rectangular. Let the dimensions of X be $m \times n$, and write p for the smaller of m and n. Then there is an essentially unique decomposition, the *singular-value decomposition*, of X as the matrix product

$$X = UDV' \tag{4.9}$$

where U, $m \times m$, is a rotation of the space of rows of X; V, $n \times n$, is a rotation of the space of columns of X; and D, $m \times n$, is a scaling matrix with a descending list of numbers d_{ii} down the diagonal (the entries in the kth row and kth column, $k = 1, 2, \ldots, p$) and 0 everywhere else. Since D is known to be diagonal, we usually drop the duplicate subscript, writing, for instance, d_1 instead of d_{11}, etc. The entries of D are called the *singular values* of X, and the columns of U and V are its *left and right singular vectors*. Another way of saying that U and V are rotations is that either matrix is the transpose of its own inverse – we must have $U'U = I_m$, the identity matrix of order m, and likewise $V'V = I_n$. Rotations are the transformations that leave the zero vector (the place we set all the averages) unmoved and that do not change squared interspecimen distances $\sum_{k=1}^{m}(x_{ik} - x_{jk})^2$ – this is the formulation for the row space; for the column space the invariants are $\sum_{k=1}^{n}(x_{ki} - x_{kj})^2$.

Furthermore, still continuing with the theorem: If you break off this decomposition at any stage k, by setting all of the d's after the kth one to zero, then the *partial sum*

$$\sum_{i=1}^{k} U_i d_i V_i' \tag{4.10}$$

falls closest to the original X in the least-squares sense. That is, it has the minimum sum of squared mismatches $\sum_{i=1}^{m} \sum_{j=1}^{n}(X_{ij} - (\sum_{i=1}^{k} U_i d_i V_i')_{ij})^2$ of any expression like (4.10) formed out of any choice of U's, V's, and d's.

The mathematician calls k the *rank* of an approximation like this, and so this part of the SVD theorem states that the partial SVD of X of any rank k provides the least-squares approximation to X over all matrices of that rank.

What this means in a more ordinary notation, writing out the matrices involved, is that the data matrix X, $m \times n$, can be reconstructed as the sum of a set of at most $p = \min(m, n)$ rectangular structures each of the form

$$\begin{pmatrix} da_1b_1 & da_1b_2 & \ldots & da_1b_n \\ da_2b_1 & da_2b_2 & \ldots & da_2b_n \\ & & \ldots & \\ da_mb_1 & da_mb_2 & \ldots & da_mb_n \end{pmatrix} \tag{4.10a}$$

where each vector of a's is of squared length (sum of squared elements) 1.0, likewise each vector of b's, and each of the separate a-vectors is perpendicular to every other a-vector, likewise each of the b-vectors: we have $\sum_k a_{ik}a_{jk} = 0$, $i \neq j$, and likewise for the b's. That least-squares property means that the best-fitting approximation to X of a matrix of the form (4.10a) – this is equation (4.10) for $k = 1$ – is the expression where $a = U_1$, the first column of U; $b = V_1$, the first column of V; and $d = d_{11}$, the first diagonal element of D. An even better fit to X is the sum of two copies of this same expression (4.10a) where the first copy is the matrix just specified and the second is the copy with $a = U_2$, the second column of U; $b = V_2$, the second column of V; and $d = d_2$, the second diagonal element of D. And so on until, at step p (if not before), the matrix X is reconstructed exactly. Figure 4.4 shows an example with $m = 5, n = 3$.

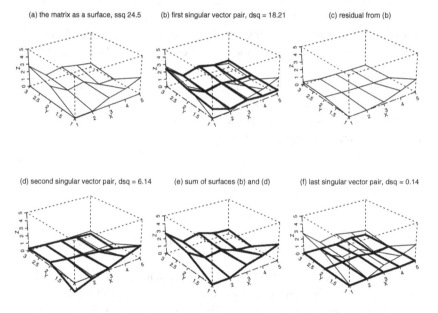

Figure 4.4 Schematic of a singular-value decomposition. (a) A 5×3 matrix to be decomposed, viewed as a facetted surface. (b) Its first singular-vector pair, drawn as the surface that is the best rank-1 approximation to the surface in (a). (You can tell it is rank-1 because every cut parallel to the x-axis is a multiple of the same pattern, and likewise every cut parallel to the y-axis.) (c) Residual from the surface in (b). (d) The second singular-vector pair, which is the best rank 1 approximation to the surface in (c). (e) The sum of (b) and (d) is the best rank-2 approximation to the original matrix. (f) The third and last singular-vector pair accounts for all the rest of the matrix in (a) by one final rank-1 term.

One useful additional property is that

$$\sum d_i^2 \equiv \sum d_{ii}^2 = \sum X_{ij}^2. \tag{4.11}$$

That is, the sum of the squared singular values equals the sum of squares of all the entries of the original matrix. (This is because orthogonal changes of basis do not change this sum of squares.[8])

Other useful properties arise when we shift our attention to the matrix $X'X$, the matrix X times its own transpose, and again require that X has the meaning of a *centered data matrix*, every row a specimen and every column a single measurement that has been "centered," meaning, taken relative to its own average. We change the letters for the size of X to correspond to the usual statistical convention: X is now n rows (specimens) by p columns (measurements). Then $X'X$ is square with counts of rows and columns both equal to p, the number of measurements. And the diagonal elements of $X'X$ are the sums of squares of each column of X – each term $(X'X)_{ii}$ is n times the variance of the ith column – whereas the off-diagonal elements are sums of products of *two* centered columns. Dividing by n, these are just the covariances of the columns in pairs. From the decomposition $X = UDV'$ we deduce $\sum d_i^2 = \operatorname{tr}(D^2) = \operatorname{tr}(D^2 UU') = \operatorname{tr}(UD^2 U') = \operatorname{tr}(UDV'VDU') = \operatorname{tr}(X'X)$, but that is just the sum of all the squares of all the centered data values. Divide these d_i^2 by n and you get a decomposition of the total variance of all the columns of X – all of the measurements going into X. In symbols, if $X = UDV'$ is any data matrix, centered or not, we have

$$\Sigma d_i^2 = \Sigma \Sigma X_{ij}^2. \tag{4.12}$$

Likewise, it follows from $X = UDV'$ that

$$X'X = (UDV')'(UDV') = VDU'UDV' = VD^2V', \tag{4.13}$$

which is itself a singular-value decomposition and hence must be the unique SVD for $X'X$. For a symmetric matrix like $X'X$, the columns of V, its singular vectors, are called its *eigenvectors*, and its singular values d_i^2 are called its *eigenvalues* and often, as in equation (4.16), are written using the different letter λ_i. So the eigenvalues of $X'X$ are the squares of the singular values of X, and thus the eigenvalues of $X'X/n$ decompose the same sum of squares as the squared eigenvalues of X do, which is to say, the total of the variances of the

---

[8] And *this* is because for square matrices A, B, $\operatorname{tr}(AB) = \operatorname{tr}(BA) = \sum_{i,j} a_{ij} b_{ji}$, and so $\operatorname{tr}(UAU') = \operatorname{tr}(AU'U) = \operatorname{tr}(A)$ whenever $U'U$ is the identity matrix, as it is in this case (a rotation times its inverse).

X-variables, the trace of the matrix $X'X/n$. (Remember that we have assumed that the mean of every column of X is zero.) To anticipate the next section just a little, this means that the *principal components* of a covariance matrix $X'X/n$ that we encounter there decompose the total variance of a set of correlated variables into a series of variances of uncorrelated variables.

There is a closely similar rule for determinants: the determinant of any square matrix A is the product of its singular values d_i.

From the basic algebraic definitions one confirms that the determinant $|AB|$ of a matrix product AB is the product $|A||B|$ of the determinants of the two matrices multiplied, and that the determinant of any square matrix equals the determinant of its transpose. The determinant of the identity matrix is just 1 – the product of the 1's down its diagonal – and so the determinant of an orthogonal matrix must also be 1 (because its square is the determinant of $UU' = I$, i.e., 1).[9] Then the determinant of any matrix A is the determinant of the matrix D in its SVD; but this is just the product of the diagonal elements of D, that is, of the d_i. It is also true that the determinant of *any* covariance matrix is equal to the following product: the variance σ_1^2 of the first variable, times the variance $\sigma_{2.1}^2$ of the residual of the second variable after regression on the first, times the variance $\sigma_{3.12}^2$ of the residual of the third variable after regression on the second together with the first, ..., times the variance $\sigma_{p.12...(p-1)}^2$ of the last variable after regression on all the others. This turns out to be a crucial step in one explication of the Wishart distribution, Section 4.3.

There will be a worked 2×2 example of this technique in Section 4.2.3 for the matrix $\begin{pmatrix} 1.0 & 0.5 \\ 0.2 & 1.4 \end{pmatrix}$ that will be imagined to be a covariance matrix there. The same matrix, subjected to the same analysis, will appear in the guise of a uniform deformation in Section 5.3, in which context the meanings of U, D, and V will all change considerably.

4.2.2 Principal Component Scores and the Biplot

Ordinarily, when a technique this common and powerful is first mentioned in a textbook, there is at least a brief sketch of its history. But, surprisingly, there seems to be no such history of the role of principal components in biology; nor is there any constructive review of its fundamental assumptions and their scientific justification. I have tried to supply a prototype of such a sketch in a recent essay (Bookstein 2017b) that is actually aimed at the supersession of principal components by a different technique, a highly modified factor

---

[9] The text tacitly assumes we are talking about *proper* orthogonal matrices, those that do not change the sign of volumes.

analysis, for GMM applications. (The suggestion is demonstrated at the very end of Section 5.6.9.) Thus while this section does indeed introduce the usual formulas and theorems, its examples are not much like everybody else's. From the several good introductions to principal components analysis as practiced in today's biometrics I would recommend one in particular, Reyment and Jöreskog (1993), that is itself conducive to the turn to factor analysis for the most sophisticated applications.

The most common application of the SVD theorem in GMM is *principal component analysis* (PCA). Anticipating the underlying change of focus involved here, from data matrices X to covariance structures like $X'X/n$, we renotate equation (4.9) in the form

$$X/\sqrt{n} = UDV' \qquad (4.9')$$

where n is the sample size that is automatically divided out in the course of computing the variance. When a column-centered data matrix X is represented this way by its singular-value decomposition as in equation (4.9'), then the columns of V (the entries of which are alled *loadings*) are the eigenvectors of Σ that we spoke of in Section 4.1.3, and the diagonal elements of D are the square roots of the associated variances (the λ's). The columns of U, each one multiplied by the corresponding diagonal element of D, are the specimen-by-specimen values of the *scores* that represent the contribution of each specimen in turn to the distribution of the eigenvector(s) under consideration.

When the SVD is applied not to the covariance matrix but instead to the original data matrix in this way, then from $X/\sqrt{n} = UDV'$ it follows that $X'X/n = VD^2V'$ – the decomposition of the data matrix engenders the decomposition of the covariance structure we had been talking about in Section 4.2.1.[10] But also we have an expression for the covariances of the columns of U themselves. From the basic identity (4.9) we have

$$UD = UDV'V = (X/\sqrt{n})V \qquad (4.14)$$

and

$$(UD)'(UD) = D'U'UD = D'D = \mathrm{diag}(d^2), \qquad (4.15)$$

---

[10] This is the easiest way to confirm the claim in connection with Figure 4.2 that the inverse Σ^{-1} of a $p \times p$ covariance matrix Σ has the same eigenvectors as Σ and eigenvalues that are the reciprocals of the eigenvalues of Σ. Writing D^{-2} for the diagonal matrix with nonzero entries $\left(\frac{1}{d_1^2}, \frac{1}{d_2^2}, \ldots, \frac{1}{d_p^2}\right)$ – the reciprocals of the diagonal entries of D^2 – it follows from $X'X/n = VD^2V'$ that $(X'X/n)(VD^{-2}V') = VD^2V'VD^{-2}V' = VD^2D^{-2}V' = VV' = I_p$, so $VD^{-2}V'$ is the inverse of VD^2V', as I already drew at the right in the figure.

meaning that the derived variables are uncorrelated and each has variance equal to the square of the corresponding singular value of $X/\sqrt{n}$ — these are the numbers we had previously called the eigenvalues of $X'X/n$. These quantities $UD = XV$, linear combinations of the original measurements, are the *principal component scores*. In the context of GMM, they are the equivalent of the *principal coordinate scores* from Procrustes distance that we will derive in Section 4.2.4, and will be interpreted there. These analyses are often presented in the form of their biplots (see below), which combine a scatterplot of pairs of columns of U with the scatterplot of the same pair of columns of V.

Because the matrix $X'X$ is derived from a sample, it must have a sampling distribution – the *Wishart distribution* that we will explore at some length in Section 4.3. At this point in the exposition, it is enough to turn to a simpler problem, the distribution of the descriptors we have just extracted: the eigenvalues and eigenvectors arising from the SVD of the matrix $X'X/n$ of variances and covariances. Derivations of the following formulas are difficult (see, for instance, T. W. Anderson, 1984), but the formulas themselves often come in useful. If the distribution being modeled really has all eigenvalues different, then the variance of the ith eigenvalue is, "in the limit of very large samples," Gaussian around the true value λ_i with error variance $2\lambda_i^2/n$, independent of the other eigenvalues of the sample. (Thus the formula is the same as for the variance of any single measured variable.) The ith loading vector of the sample, the eigenvector V_i, is distributed around the true value α_i with covariance structure

$$\frac{\lambda_i}{n} \sum_{h=1, h \neq i}^{p} \frac{\lambda_h}{(\lambda_h - \lambda_i)^2} \alpha_h \alpha_h', \tag{4.16}$$

where n is the sample size and p the count of variables whose covariance structure is being analyzed. The formula means that the sampling error of the direction of the ith eigenvector lies within the line ($p = 2$), plane ($p = 3$), or hyperplane ($p > 3$) spanned by all the *other* eigenvectors, where it is described by an interval, ellipse, or ellipsoid with squared axis lengths in every direction h other than the direction of concern being proportional to $\frac{\lambda_h}{(\lambda_h - \lambda_i)^2}$. (See figure 6.6 in Bookstein, 2014.) Finally, the sample eigenvalue λ_i and its corresponding eigenvector α_i are independent.

A simulated example. A simple example, the PCA of a set of two variables drawn as a sample of 100 from a population distributed as a bivariate

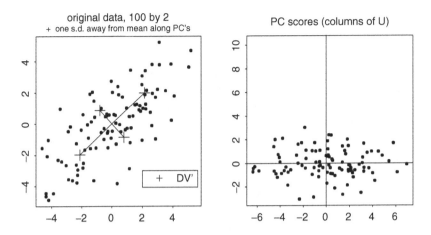

Figure 4.5 Biplot for a principal component analysis for the simplest case, two variables only. The analysis is geometrically equivalent to a rotation of the scattterplot at left to an orientation along the axes of its covariance ellipse.

normal with covariance matrix $\begin{pmatrix} 5 & 3 \\ 3 & 5 \end{pmatrix}$, illustrates the general nature of these distributions. Figure 4.5 shows the basic setup, an analysis of 100 two-vectors (paired observations). At left is the original data scatter, together with the enhancement that is generated from the SVD $X = UDV'$ of the data matrix: the axes DV' (demarcated by pairs of $+$ signs) that represent the decomposition in the geometry of this particular scatter. The first principal component $d_1 V_1$ runs along the long axis of the scatter, from southwest to northeast here, and its semilength is the first singular value d_1 (square root of the first eigenvalue of the covariance matrix $X'X/n$), which is 2.91. Orthogonal to it is the other eigenvector, of length 1.17. When we rotate this scatterplot to these new axes, as in the right-hand panel, we recover the scores U_1 and U_2 of the same SVD. Paired plots like these, which are sometimes presented in one panel rather than two, are called *biplots* (Gower and Hand, 1995).

If that is the data analysis, then the study of sampling errors of the derived vector D of singular values and the derived orthogonal matrix V of singular vectors is as in Figure 4.6. At upper left is an ensemble of 100 separate simulations of the same structure (100 observations of pairs of variables). All subsamples are drawn from the same parent Gaussian distribution with covariance structure $\begin{pmatrix} 5 & 3 \\ 3 & 5 \end{pmatrix}$, which has true eigenvalues 8 and 2, or, equivalently, represents two variables both having variance 5 and

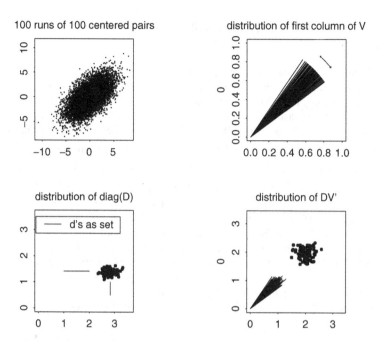

Figure 4.6 Simulation of 100 examples like the one in Figure 4.5. (upper left) 100×100 pairs from the Gaussian distribution indicated in the text. (lower left) Sampling distribution of the singular values of the hundred 100×2 subsamples. (upper right) Sampling distribution of the 100 computed unit vectors V_1. (lower right) Sampling distribution of $d_1 V_1$, the joint uncertainty of direction and length of this principal axis.

correlating 0.6. Also, just for convenience, each sample is centered at the same location $(0, 0)$. According to that designed covariance matrix, the true population eigenvectors of $X'X/n$ are the vectors $(1, \pm 1)/\sqrt{2}$ with eigenvalues (variances of the corresponding linear combinations) 8 and 2. Hence $\sqrt{d_1}V_1 = (2, 2)$ and $\sqrt{d_2}V_2 = (1, -1)$; both are close to the sample-specific evaluates shown in Figure 4.5. The distribution of the eigen*values* for the set of 100 100-case subsamples, lower left, is then Gaussian around these true values with horizontal standard deviation $\sqrt{2/100} \cdot \sqrt{8} = 0.4$ and vertical standard deviation half that. With only two measured dimensions, the distribution of the observed first eigen*vector*, upper right panel, is along the direction of the second, with variance $\frac{\lambda_1}{n} \frac{\lambda_2}{(\lambda_2 - \lambda_1)^2} = 0.02$. Both of these inferred sampling distributions match what is visible in the plotted values from the simulation. Finally, at the lower right is the joint distribution of the first eigenvalue along with the first eigenvector, in other words, the scatterplot of the now *un*normalized vector $d_1 V_1$. The distribution turns out to be circular in this plane.

> We should test the statistics of the distribution in Figure 4.5 to see if it is compatible with the model written down there. The orientation of the principal axes is evidently just what was expected — the directions at $\pm 45°$ to the original Cartesian axes. As for eigenvalues, we get those by squaring the singular values. The larger is $2.91^2 = 8.48$, versus an expected value of 8 with a standard deviation of $8\sqrt{\frac{2}{100}} \sim 1.13$; this value is clearly appropriate. For the smaller eigenvalue, $1.17^2 = 1.37$ is to be compared to an expected value of 2 with standard deviation $2\sqrt{\frac{2}{100}} \sim 0.28$. The simulation fell about 2.2 standard deviations below the expected value. A little digging indicates the reason for this: the correlation between the two variables here, which was modeled as 0.6, is actually 0.712. Transformed by Fisher's z, the comparison is of 0.69 (the model) with 0.89 (the data in Figure 4.5), for a difference of 0.20, which is just double its standard error of $1/\sqrt{97}$ for samples of size 100. In the left panel of Figure 4.5 we do indeed spy a shortage of points in the southeast quadrant. Far from being alarming, then, this particular example teaches us something quite useful about the actual variability of realizations of seemingly well-specified models.

A data example: principal components of the transects of the Vilmann rodent neurocranial octagons. As an example of this technique, still not properly set in the context of geometric morphometrics that will concern us in the next chapter, consider the SVD analysis for all 28 of the interlandmark distances of the Vilmann octagon (Figure 2.41).[11] While their average lengths vary unsystematically, their specific growth rates are relatively homogeneous. For situations of this sort, like the analysis of the Berkeley Guidance Study (Figures 2.37–2.40), an analysis goes better if the variables are replaced by their logarithms. After that modification, Figure 4.7 shows biplots for the first singular vectors left and right against each of the next three.

Inspection of these biplots shows that only the analysis of the first two dimensions of this decomposition is likely to convey a biological interpretation. By the third of these dimensions (lower middle panel) the principal component is expressing the effect of just one of the original distances (for PC3, it is IPP-Lam; for PC4, lower right panel, it is IPP-Opi), and in the corresponding plots of animal-by-animal scores in the top row these

---

[11] This is too many variables. Because there are only $k = 8$ landmarks, the full set of 28 distances involves a total of only $2k - 3 = 13$ geometric degrees of freedom. We ignore this problem until Section 5.4, where, with the aid of the shape coordinates, we construct a representation that has the correct count of parameters.

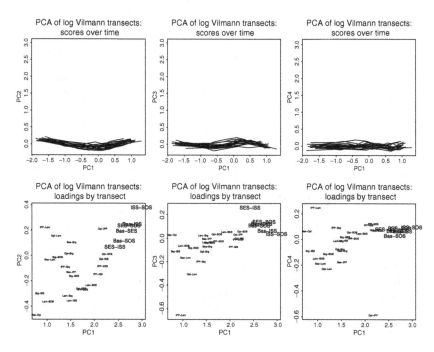

Figure 4.7 Biplots (plots of dimensions of U against each other along with the same dimensions of V against each other) for the Vilmann rodent octagon transect data after log transformation. (left) First and second singular vectors. (center) First and third. (right) First and fourth. Only the PC1–PC2 pair (left column and next figure) is likely to prove biometrically interpretable, owing to the occurrence of singletons (polar principal components) for PC3 and PC4 in the plots of the lower row. Plotted points in the lower row here and at right in Figure 4.8 have crossproduct zero not with reference to the center of the plotting region but with respect to the origin of coordinates, which is out of the frame beyond the left edge.

dimensions simply show sporadic noise at intermediate time points, suggesting a difficulty in locating the landmark IPP they share. For a principal component to deal seemingly with just one of the original variables is a *dis*qualification: the SVD analysis is not intended to individuate specific measurements in this way.

To hint at the analysis at which we will eventually arrive in Figure 5.84–5.85, Figure 4.8 presents the biplot of the first two PC's only, enlarged. The six distances that lie along the cranial base, the nearly straight line from Basion forward to SES, are printed in larger font. These six cluster together at the high end of PC1, indicating that they have high specific growth rates relative to all the other distances. The lowest loading on PC1 is for Bas-Opi,

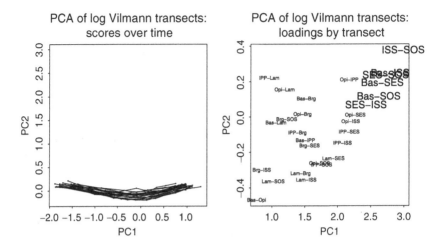

Figure 4.8 Enlargements of the two panels at left in the preceding figure. At the right, distances along the cranial base are printed in a larger font. The second principal component indicates timing of the growth spurt, from earlier (e.g., Bas-Opi) to later (the cranial base measures, also IPP-Lam and -Opi), as can be verified in an earlier plot of these dimensions as time series, Figure 2.43.

the transect across the opening of the foramen magnum. The corresponding scatter of scores over time, left panel, indicates reasonable commonality across all 18 of these growth trajectories. The nonlinearity here identifies PC2 as a component for the *timing* of these change trajectories: negative for those maturing relatively early, like Bas-Opi (compare Figure 2.43); positive for those like IPP-Lam or the measures along the cranial base that continue growing right up to the end of these series. That the corresponding charts show no trends of growth rate for PC3 (Figure 4.7, upper middle panel) or PC4 (upper right panel) cements their interpretation as high-amplitude dimensions of noise not likely to represent any interpretable integrated signal.

This example is meant here as a demonstration of PCA, not as a spatially coherent analysis of this rat growth pattern. We will return to this data set after the tools of GMM analysis per se have been introduced.

PCA versus discriminant function analysis. Section 3.5 introduced Hermon Bumpus's data for sparrows shivering through a selection event in an 1898 snowstorm in Providence, Rhode Island. Bumpus's question of 1898 concerned the apparent fitness (survival versus nonsurvival) of his sample of adult males in terms of the nine lengths he measured on these birds. An interpretable linear discriminant formula was put forward as the regression of survival on

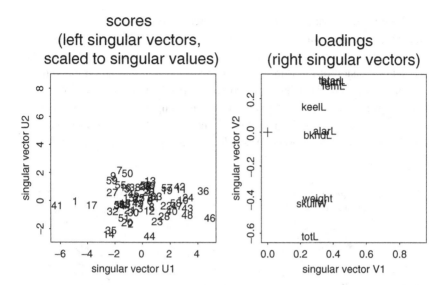

Figure 4.9 SVD of the Bumpus adult male sparrow data set, Section 3.5. (left) Scores U_1, U_2 for the first two left singular vectors. Numbers are case numbers in the original data set. (right) The corresponding loadings V_1, V_2. The cluster of three at the top of the plot are humerus length (uppermost), then toe-to-tarsus length, then femur length. The origin $(0,0)$ of the right-hand panel is marked by the + sign.

two measurements selected out of the nine: total length and femur length. The prediction took the form of a linear contrast of z-scores, or, equivalently, a proportion between the two measures.

We now return to this data set to see if the method of principal components can add any confidence or insight to this regression approach. Figure 4.9 is the usual biplot from the correlation structure of the nine measures whose cumulative distributions were shown in Figure 3.36. At left is the scatter of the first two scores after a rotation to the pair of axes whose loadings are given in the panel at the right. As is typical in analyses of multiple measured lengths, the first singular vector V_1 has all positive loadings, ranging from 0.26 to 0.40 only. The loadings of the second singular vector vary in sign, as they must, with a range from 0.31 (for humerus length and tibia-tarsus length) and 0.28 (femur length) to -0.62 (for total length). Noticing that the extremes of second singular vector loading are neatly aligned with the pair of variables we ended up with in Figure 3.39, let us inspect the association of the singular vectors themselves with survival, the dependent variable in that earlier analysis.

The first three principal component scores of the set of all nine variance-standardized lengths taken together correlate 0.05, 0.63, 0.01 with Bumpus's survival observation. So survival really does have something to do with the second dimension of the Bumpus SVD, the dimension plotted on the *vertical* axis in Figure 4.9. That direction correlates 0.847 with the gradient of the isolines in Figure 3.39, the direction that was computed by explicit attention to the survival data – of course, the second PC of the present analysis was not. We have paid a surprisingly small cost (see Figure 4.10): a correlation

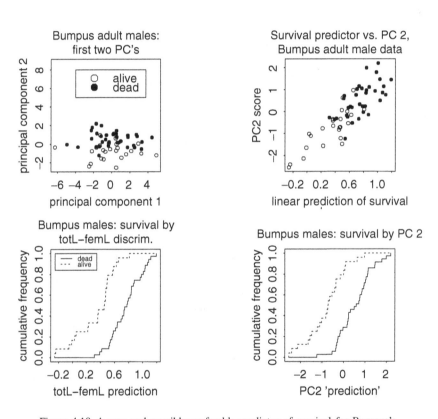

Figure 4.10 A new and possibly preferable predictor of survival for Bumpus's sparrows. (upper left) The same scatter as in Figure 4.9, enhanced now by a code for survival. Survival is correlated not at all with PC1 but substantially with PC2. Thus PC2 serves as a linear combination encoding survival well in advance of the meteorological event in question. (upper right) Comparison of the two morphometric descriptors, one computed without reference to survival per se. (lower row) Cumulative distributions of the survival groups on the linear discriminant function of Figure 3.39 (left) and the second principal component of the correlations among all the lengths (right).

of 0.653 with survival for the predictor in Figure 3.39, versus one of 0.631 for the survival-oblivious computation in Figure 4.9. In exchange, we may have demonstrated that what Bumpus called "fitness" could have been an intrinsic characteristic of these birds, not an accidental pattern of correlations as observed on one cold day in 1898. In that case, the interpretation of fitness (versus selection, on that snowy day) is explicitly encoded in the vertical dimension of Figure 4.9, the range of coefficients within the contrast. Total length, weight, and skull width all detract from survival in this sample, while the lengths of the humerus and femur and the tibiotarsal distance all correlate positively with survival. As for Darwin's finches, then (Weiner, 1995), we might tentatively speculate that this dimension of selection is present in these populations *in order to* accommodate extreme weather. Heavy wet snowstorms are not unknown in that region of the United States; perhaps this species had encountered them many times before.

4.2.3 Partial Least Squares: Least-Squares Analysis of Covariance Patterns

Partial Least Squares (PLS) is a related context for an SVD that can be explained in two different ways. In one version, PLS generalizes the connection between the SVD of a data matrix X and the SVD of the corresponding scatter matrix $X'X$ that was already introduced in Section 4.2.2. For $X/\sqrt{n} = UDV'$, we saw that $(XV)'(XV)/n = D^2$, meaning that the covariance structure of the derived scores, the right-hand panel of the biplot in Figure 4.5, is diagonal with variances in descending order. This construction neatly extends to the SVD of a matrix $X'Y/n$ conveying the averages of crossproducts of an *asymmetrical* construction, one data matrix against another that is arbitrary except for having the same count of rows. (By analogy with the formula $\Sigma(x - \bar{x})(y - \bar{y})/n$ defining a single covariance coefficient and the naming of the matrix $X'X/n$ as a "covariance structure," the matrix $X'Y/n$ where the $(i,j)^{\text{th}}$ entry is $\Sigma(x_i - \bar{x}_i)(y_j - \bar{y}_j)/n$ is called a *crosscovariance structure*.) Then if $X'Y/n = UDV'$ we have

$$(XU)'(YV)/n = U'(UDV')V = D. \tag{4.17a}$$

The covariance structure of the derived scores XU and YV is likewise diagonal, in descending order of covariance (assuming unit length for the now paired coefficient vectors involved). In fact,

$$\Sigma\Sigma(X'Y/n)_{ij}^2 = \text{tr}\left((X'Y)(Y'X)\right)/n^2 = \text{tr}(UDV'VDU') = \text{tr}(D^2) = \Sigma d_i^2, \tag{4.17b}$$

meaning that the squared singular values add up to the total of the squared original crosscovariances. (That is why one common figure of merit for reporting a PLS analysis is the ratio $d_1^2 / \Sigma d_i^2$, the "fraction of summed squared covariances explained by the first singular vector pair.") Also,

$$UD = UDV'V = (X'Y/n)V = X'(YV)/n. \qquad (4.18)$$

That is, each of the vectors U is proportional to the profile of covariances of the original X-variables with the newly derived scores YV. Conversely, each column of V is proportional to $(XU)'Y$, the profile of covariances of the new scores XU with the original measures Y. (In this setting the assumption persists that the variables included in the blocks X and Y have previously been set to mean zero. But there is no such restriction on the matrix $X'Y/n$ actually undergoing the singular-value decomposition.)

A second fruitful context for PLS runs by way of a different property of the SVD, its role in reconstructing the pattern of its argument matrix as a whole. Conceptually, this least-squares fit seems far from our earlier context for the method of least squares in the path analysis of multiple causal processes entailed in the same "dependent variable" (Section 3.1). From the normal equations we recall that that was the fit of a linear prediction formula $\sum a_i x_i$ to some predictand measurement z — the least-squares problem of minimizing $\sum(z - \sum a_i x_i)^2$ over the space of possible coefficient vectors a_i (Section 3.1). This other context for least squares would seem to be the apparently unrelated problem of fitting the sum of a whole stack of rank-1 matrices $U_i d_{ii} V_i'$ to a complete data matrix X. But, it turns out, these techniques combine in a much more fertile exegesis of the same computation we have just reviewed, the generalization of PCA to the setting of data that arise as two or more separate measurement blocks, say, the X's and the Y's.

This second approach to the method of Partial Least Squares begins with a generalization of the idea of the *arrows* in Figure 3.10 – a generalization not of measurements but of how we observe and report causation. Eventually we will be arguing via the a posteriori consistency with which the *saliences,* the coefficients of the first few columns of U and V, relate to prior knowledge of path coefficients observed in other ways.

Consider first the simplest possible setting: two blocks of two measurements each. Call them the X's, X_1 and X_2, and the Y's, Y_1 and Y_2. The X's might be length or log length measures and the Y's weight or log weight measures, or the X's might be shape measures of one organ and the Y's the same for another. Assume that all four variables have been measured on the same specimens, *that arbitrary linear combinations within each block make biological sense* (on this specific requisite, see Bookstein, 2016b), and that the covariance structure relating the X's (rows) to the Y's (columns) is

$$\begin{pmatrix} 1.0 & 0.5 \\ 0.2 & 1.4 \end{pmatrix} \tag{4.19}$$

of which the SVD is

$$\begin{pmatrix} 1.0 & 0.5 \\ 0.2 & 1.4 \end{pmatrix} = UDV'$$

with

$$U = \begin{pmatrix} .555 & -.832 \\ .832 & .555 \end{pmatrix}, \quad D = \begin{pmatrix} 1.612 & 0 \\ 0 & 0.806 \end{pmatrix}, \quad V = \begin{pmatrix} .447 & -.894 \\ .894 & .447 \end{pmatrix}. \tag{4.20}$$

The elements of the covariance matrix, squared, total 3.25. The diagonal elements of D, squared, also total 3.25, confirming that PLS is a decomposition of the sum of squared covariances, equation (4.17b). The first diagonal element d_1 of D is twice the second, and so its square accounts for $2^2/(2^2+1^2) = 80\%$ of the total; the second, for the remaining 20%. The columns of V are aligned with the directions $(1,2)$ and $(2,-1)$, which are perpendicular. The columns of U are aligned with the directions $(2,3)$ and $(3,-2)$, likewise perpendicular. We notice, for later use, that the product of the elements of D is the determinant of the original matrix, the quantity $1.0 \cdot 1.4 - 0.2 \cdot 0.5 = 1.30$, which is the factor by which the area of the starting square is increased in Figure 5.23. Recall that this is the general determinantal property of SVD's, applying as well to the principal component analysis (the SVD of a covariance structure $X'X/n$, where X is any data matrix) introduced in the previous section.

At this point the mandatory assumption about arbitrary linear combinations – that they lead to reasonable, comprehensible quantitative summaries likely to be biologically meaningful – has real bite. We need to postulate that it makes sense to imagine one linear combination $Y_1 + 2Y_2$ and another $2Y_1 - Y_2$, and two other linear combinations $2X_1 + 3X_2$ and $3X_1 - 2X_2$. Setting their coefficients to sum in square to 1, the first pair become the formulas $.447Y_1 + .894Y_2$ and $.555X_1 + .832X_2$. In the context of equation (4.20), the SVD theorem says:

- The covariance of this first pair of singular vectors is 1.612, and this is the largest possible for any pair of linear combinations, one on the X's and one on the Y's, whose coefficients each sum in square to 1;

- the rank-1 covariance matrix approximation accounted for by this pair is

$$U_1 D_{11} V_1 = \begin{pmatrix} .555 \\ .832 \end{pmatrix} (1.612)(.447, .894) = \begin{pmatrix} 0.4 & 0.8 \\ 0.6 & 1.2 \end{pmatrix}, \qquad (4.21)$$

which sum in square to $2.6 = 1.612^2$.

- the second and last singular vector pair, along $.894Y_1 - .447Y_2$ and $.832X_1 - .555X_2$, have covariance 0.806, which is the smallest possible for any such pair of constructs with coefficients that are unit vectors, and the rank-1 covariance approximation that they account for is

$$U_2 D_{22} V_2 = \begin{pmatrix} .832 \\ -.555 \end{pmatrix} (0.806)(.894, -.447) = \begin{pmatrix} 0.6 & -0.3 \\ -0.4 & 0.2 \end{pmatrix}, \qquad (4.22)$$

which sum in square to $0.65 = 0.806^2$.

- The sum of these two reconstructed rank-1 matrices is $\begin{pmatrix} 1.0 & 0.5 \\ 0.2 & 1.4 \end{pmatrix}$, the matrix with which we began.

Let us recapitulate all the assumptions that were necessary. We must presume that the sum of the squares of the coefficients of a linear combination like these is a meaningful standardization for normalizing them in regard to magnitude. This is the same as postulating a circle in the X-space of extensions that are "equivalent" in their different directions, and likewise, *but separately*, a circle in the Y-space. (Putting these together, in this 2×2 setting, gives us the topology of a torus – a bagel – as the space of joint descriptions of linear combinations in which we are operating.) This assumption does not make any obvious biological sense unless there is in fact an *actual* circle in the measurement space of the X's and the Y's, or else an equivalently symmetrical physiological measurement such as total energy. (For an example of a purported statistic that does *not* correspond to any such emergent parameter, see appendix 1 of Bookstein, 2016b.) The plausibility of meaningfulness in every direction will be the case for the shape coordinates that are the principal domain of application at which this chapter is aimed. We could equivalently have postulated that our analyses would mean the same, in biological terms, if we rotated to new axes $(X_1 \pm X_2)/\sqrt{2}$, as in the discussion of the meaning of covariance in Section 2.2. Thus the PLS assumption of rotatability of the blocks is equivalent to an assumption about the rationality of treating the rectangle on sides X_1 and X_2 as having the same area (in some biological sense, such as tissue investment) as the rectangle on sides X_2 and X_1. These assumptions can sometimes be justified when the measurements fall naturally into a Cartesian coordinate system, and may otherwise be wildly abstract and artificial, in which case the corresponding inferences risk being completely misleading or even meaningless.

We will encounter this matrix $\begin{pmatrix} 1.0 & 0.5 \\ 0.2 & 1.4 \end{pmatrix}$ again in Section 5.2 in quite a different role, the computation of a basic shape change tensor. The arithmetic of the SVD will be the same, its biometrical interpretation completely different.

Now let us generalize all this in terms of complexity, specifically, the lengths of those lists of X's and Y's. All the other symmetries I mentioned that are required for biological interpretability are unaltered.

Remember from our discussion of the quincunx (Section 2.3), how the position of a single ancestor point could explain the correlations among positions of any number of points lower down on the quincunx by manipulation of the row numbers that were supposed to express those correlations. Ignoring the row numbers themselves, we can diagram this as in the left panel of Figure 4.11: a causal factor F that accounts for the correlations r_{ij} among multiple consequences X_i as products $r_{FX_i} r_{FX_j}$ of correlations of each X with the factor F.

Suppose we have two measurement domains, one of n X-variables and the other of m Y-variables, that we believe are tied together by a single causal path after the fashion of Figure 4.11 (center). The X's and Y's separately are intended to meet the requisites for a linearly combinable, profile-able set, and furthermore are presumed *not* to meet that requirement if combined. We presume, in other words, that they are measuring two different aspects of some underlying system – for instance, they might have been generated by two different machines, one measuring form and one measuring function. The claim about the causal path is meant in the sense of "accounting for correlations." We are promulgating a vector of path coefficients $p_i, i = i, \ldots, n$

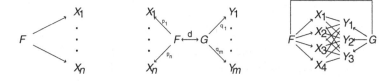

Figure 4.11 Where the least-squares aspect of a PLS analysis comes from. (left) An unmeasured factor explains multiple measured variables X_i. (center) If the X's and Y's are two different measurement blocks, we might imagine each of them to be represented by a single factor, F or G, with a covariance between F and G that links the blocks. (right) The explanatory role of F and G here is equivalent to a fit to the entire matrix of covariances between every X and every Y by a single rank-1 approximation. But that is exactly what the SVD was designed to produce.

of the X's on a factor F and a vector of path coefficients $q_j, j = 1, \ldots, m$ of the Y's on a factor G such that the covariance $\sigma_{x_i y_j}$ observed between the ith X-variable and the jth Y-variable is the product of coefficients corresponding to three of the paths in the diagram. The equation is

$$r_{x_i y_j} = d_{FG} p_i q_j. \tag{4.23}$$

We have mn equations (one for each X for each Y) but only $m+n-1$ parameters to fit (the n p's, minus one for the norming to unit length; the m q's, minus 1 for the same reason; and one path d_{FG} from F to G). So we are unlikely to be able to fit all the equations exactly. Naturally, then, we turn to the standard first cut for problems of this sort, the method of least squares. In this context, we are asking for a least-squares approximation to this rectangular matrix by an outer product of two vectors — a matrix of rank one.

But we already know how to do this. It is the same singular-value decomposition already introduced in Section 4.2.1, which yields the first pair of singular vectors (and, should we wish to proceed, a second pair, and so on).

When singular vectors are derived from correlation or covariance matrices, they can serve as coefficients of linear combinations of variables (always assuming that it makes sense to pay attention to arbitrary linear combinations of the variables in the first place). In this setting their interpretation is radically enriched. Let S, $n \times m$, now be a covariance matrix relating two sets of centered (but not necessarily z-scored) variables, a block of n measured X's and a block of m Y's on a sample of N specimens:

$$S_{ij} = N^{-1} \Sigma_k X_{ki} Y_{kj}, \quad S = X^t Y / N. \tag{4.24}$$

As before write $S = UDV^t$. Additionally, construct the matrices

$$LV_X = XU, \quad LV_Y = YV \tag{4.25}$$

(see Figure 4.12) that rotate the original centered measurements into the coordinate system of the singular vectors. Here "LV" stands for "latent variable," an ancient usage from the social sciences. These have the same formula as the numerator of the factor estimate F for the single-factor model that we have already seen in connection with Figure 4.11.

Then (in part repeating the abstract decomposition of $(XU)'(YV)$ that we have massaged already):

- Each column of U is proportional to the covariances of the block of X's with the corresponding column of the matrix LV_Y, and conversely. (By construction, $X'(YV_{.i})/N = (X'Y/N)V_{.i} = (UDV')V_{.i} = d_i U_{.i}$ and likewise $(XU_{.i})'Y/N = U'_{.i}(UDV') = d_i V'_{.i}$.) For reason of this proportionality, the

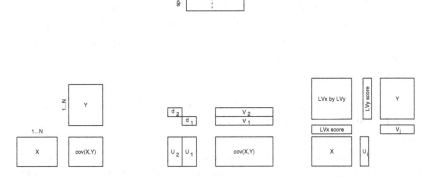

Figure 4.12 Basic structure of a two-block PLS analysis. (top) Apparent composite data matrix $(X|Y)$ assembled only to be dismantled. (lower left) From two blocks of data to their covariance matrix. (lower center) From the covariance matrix to its first one or two singular vector pairs. (lower right) From the singular vectors to paired latent variable scores and their scatterplots. Each right singular vector V_i is proportional to the covariances of the corresponding latent variable score LV_X with the variables of the Y-block, and, conversely, each left singular vector U_i is proportional to the covariances of the corresponding latent variable score LV_Y with the variables of the X-block. If the singular vectors U and V are unit vectors, the covariance of the i-th paired LV_X and LV_Y scores is d_i (center panel).

entries of singular vectors computed from correlation matrices are often called *saliences*. The subscript "$.i$" means the i-th column of the corresponding rotation matrix, U or V.

- The covariance between LV_{Xi} and LV_{Yi} is d_i. (Check: $N^{-1}(XU)^t_{.i}(YV)_{.i} = (U^tSV)_{ii} = (U^tUDV^tV)_{ii} = d_i$.) In particular, the covariance between LV_{X1} and LV_{Y1} is d_1, the maximum possible for any pair of linear combinations, one on each block, with coefficient vectors of unit length.
- An additional graphical structure becomes available beyond the U and V vectors: scatterplots of the latent variable scores. You can plot LV_X's against LV_X's and LV_Y's against LV_Y's or LV_X's against LV_Y's. Any of these can show trends, outliers, or clusters in the same way that they do for principal components scores.
- Subtle scientific signals that are not about the X's and Y's separately but rather about the relationships between the X's and the Y's often can be revealed directly when facets of the data design that are not incorporated in the matrices X or Y (for instance, subgrouping variables not explicit in the measures, or an ordering implicit but not explicit in the names of the

variables) are encoded in the icons in scatterplots of the LV scores or the biplots of the singular vectors U and V.

- Biological meaning inheres in the saliences or scores of the latent variables separately, not all together. Statistics that consider only sums of squares of covariance structures like these are unlikely to lead to any useful biological insights. This point is discussed at length in appendix 1 of Bookstein (2016b).

PLS is a much more robust multivariate technique than *canonical correlations analysis*, a cousin that produces what appear at first glance to be closely analogous scores maximizing the interblock *correlations* of the derived linear combinations rather than the covariances that PLS is maximizing. Indeed I will have occasion to mention a canonical correlation from time to time in the narratives of Chapter 5, for instance to inform the reader about the overlap in meaning of the two different analyses of mammalian evolution in Figure 5.60. But, notoriously, canonical correlations analysis requires that each of the measurement blocks being compared be of full rank – that the two separate within-block covariance structures both be invertible. As you notice from the run of formulas preceding, PLS does not refer to those within-block covariances at all. (In particular, the relation between successive columns of U or V is one of *geometric* orthogonality, not zero correlation within block.) Hence PLS is not misdirected into reporting latent variable pairs of small variance that show large correlations by chance, nor is it damaged by the presence of blocks whose explicit construction involved the removal of dimensions, such as compositional data (variables summing to 1.0) or the Procrustes shape coordinates to be introduced in the next chapter. The only effect of rank deficiency on PLS that arises is sometimes to lower the count of nonzero singular values d_i from the minimum *count* of the pair of blocks to the minimum of their *ranks*.

There are extensions of PLS to settings of more than two blocks of analysis, but we will not need to exploit them in the applications of this book. For a suggestive worked example, see Bookstein, Gunz et al. (2003). Such techniques are closely related to the more general multivariate approach to modeling of covariance structures usually called "structural equations modeling." See, for example, Bollen (1989).

There will be an example mapping one GMM domain onto an exogenous suite of measurements (in this case, neuropsychological) in Section 5.6.

From the above exegesis it should be clear that in its computational aspects the PLS method consists of treating a covariance matrix as if it were a data matrix instead, until the very end (the creation of those latent variable scores). Naturally this entails additional assumptions, specifically the linearity of all the underlying relationships. Further assumptions involve rotation in two domains of measurement, not just one. In general this complicated maneuver is likeliest to be sound when the both domains are comprised of commensurate morphometric measurements. Otherwise it is no less risky than the original PCA approach would have been. For instance, when the variables of one or the other block have no common units, it is conventional to transform nonmorphometric blocks of measurements to z-scores before computing a PLS (see, e.g., the caption to Figure 5.86), even though this maneuver makes the understanding of the saliences somewhat more difficult.

4.2.4 Principal Coordinates Analysis

Principal coordinates analysis (PCO) is an underappreciated variant of PCA that applies whenever it is most convenient to interpret the primary data in terms of "distances" (dissimilarities) among the specimens of the data set rather than, or perhaps in addition to, any representation in terms of explicit measurements specimen by specimen. The fundamental maneuvers of this topic were published by John Gower in a great paper of 1966, based on a method disseminated in another discipline by Warren Torgerson (1958). The Procrustes analysis of our GMM context appears to be its best biometric application to date.

Remember the fundamental *least-squares property* of the SVD: if the rectangular matrix S of rank r is decomposed as $S = UDV^t$, with the entries d_i of D in decreasing order, then for each rank j between 1 and $r - 1$, the approximation $M = \Sigma_{k=1}^{j} U_k d_k V_k^t$ minimizes $\Sigma_{i,j}(S_{ij} - M_{ij})^2$ over the class of matrices M of rank not greater than j. In other words, $d_1 U_1 V_1^t$ is the best-fitting rank-1 matrix to S, $d_1 U_1 V_1^t + d_2 U_2 V_2^t$, the best-fitting one of rank 2, and so on.

If the matrix S is symmetric, i.e., the same on either side of the diagonal, then its SVD must be symmetrical, too. The orthonormal matrices U and V must be the same, so that using the representation $S = UDU^t$ we are decomposing it as a sum of terms $U_i d_i U_i^t$ of outer products of a vector with itself.

Now let me pretend to change the subject for a minute. Suppose you have a set of k ordinary decimal numbers $x_1, \ldots, x_k$ that total zero. Consider the matrix of their pairwise products,:

$$S = \begin{pmatrix} x_1 x_1 & x_1 x_2 & \ldots & x_1 x_k \\ x_2 x_1 & x_2 x_2 & \ldots & x_2 x_k \\ & & \ldots & \\ x_k x_1 & x_k x_2 & \ldots & x_k x_k \end{pmatrix} \qquad (4.26)$$

where the diagonal is just the squares of the original x's. This matrix certainly has rank 1: it matches the criterion in equation (4.10a) if we take the same list of x's for both vectors, the a's and the b's, and set $d = 1$. Let us fiddle with this matrix a bit in ways that will make sense shortly. Record the diagonal, the vector $(x_1^2, x_2^2, \ldots, x_k^2)$. Multiply the original matrix S by -2. To every row of $-2S$ add the original diagonal of S, the vector we just pulled out, and also add it to every column. You end up with a matrix D^2 of which the $(i, j)^{\text{th}}$ entry is just $(x_i - x_j)^2$, the squared difference of the corresponding pair of entries in the vector of x's.

It is more interesting to run this maneuver in reverse: not from coordinates to squared distances but from squared distances back down to coordinates. Suppose you have a set of points anywhere in a plane or in space. You don't have their coordinates, but you have the squared distances $(x_i - x_j)^2$ among them in pairs, and you know that they lie on a straight line. How can you most easily put them back on that line in the right places? Well, start with the matrix D^2 of their squared interpoint Euclidean distances. D^2 has zeroes down the diagonal, but otherwise its entries are all positive, so every row has a positive average. Construct a vector whose entries are these averages. Subtract this vector from every row of D^2, and also from every column of D^2, and then, to every entry of the matrix that results, add back in the grand average of D^2 (which is the same as the average of those row averages). Finally, multiply the result by $-\frac{1}{2}$.

What you get turns out to be the matrix S we started with: a rank-one matrix whose only nontrivial singular vector is the set of point coordinates along a line with which we began. There is a relatively accessible algebraic demonstration of this assertion in Bookstein (2014:382).

In a matrix notation that is no help to the intuition but that is at least typographically concise, if D^2 is the matrix of squared distances we started with, then the rank-one matrix at which we arrive (for data that originally arose as coordinates of points on a single line) is

$$-HD^2H/2, \text{ with } H = \begin{pmatrix} 1 - \frac{1}{k} & -\frac{1}{k} & \cdots & -\frac{1}{k} \\ -\frac{1}{k} & 1 - \frac{1}{k} & \cdots & -\frac{1}{k} \\ & & \cdots & \\ -\frac{1}{k} & -\frac{1}{k} & \cdots & 1 - \frac{1}{k} \end{pmatrix} \tag{4.27}$$

H, $k \times k$, is called the *centering matrix* with diagonals all equal to $(1 - 1/k)$ and all other entries $-1/k$.

In this notation, which is Gower's, **the method of principal coordinates is the SVD of the matrix $-HD^2H/2$ where D^2 is any legitimate squared distance measure.** (A legitimate distance measure D_{ij} is a square matrix where all diagonal entries D_{ii}, the distances of the forms from themselves, are zero and where all sets of three satisfy the *triangle inequality* $D_{ij} + D_{jk} \geq D_{ik}$.) Remember that the SVD, in this application to symmetric matrices, is guaranteed to fit it by a stack of components $V_i d_i V_i^t$ where V_i is the ith column of the orthonormal matrix $U=V$ of the SVD theorem. If the matrix we were decomposing was a covariance matrix, we would say that the columns of U were "orthogonal," making an angle of $90°$ in the space of linear combinations. But in this application, the interpretation is quite a bit easier. We have singular vectors U_i that have one entry for each case of the original data set (remember the matrix D^2 is $k \times k$), and all rows and columns have mean zero (an effect of the pre-post multiplication by H), so that the word we use for orthogonality in this application is **noncorrelation.** The principal coordinates that the SVD of the matrix $-HD^2H/2$ produces are correlated zero.

But we are already aware of some quantities that correlate zero among themselves: the principal components of the original data considered as a covariance structure. If the distances you started with arose as the sums of squared differences on two variables $(x_1, \ldots, x_k)$ and $(y_1, \ldots, y_k)$, such that the x's and the y's average zero and are uncorrelated as variables, then the principal coordinates of the composite Euclidean squared distance matrix, computed as eigenvectors of $-HD^2H/2$, will just be the vectors $(x_1, \ldots, x_k)$ and $(y_1, \ldots, y_k)$ with which you began. (In the algebra we just finished, the ij^{th} entry of the matrix $-HD^2H/2$ ends up equal to $d_1 x_i x_j + d_2 y_i y_j$, which is clearly a matrix of rank two with singular vectors $(x_1 \ldots x_k)$ and $(y_1 \ldots y_k)$ on both sides of D^2.)

Principal components, because they are simply a rotation of your original data vectors, leave interspecimen distances unchanged. Then the principal component scores of any data set **are** the principal coordinates of the corresponding distance matrix. In other words: **the principal coordinates of a squared intersample Euclidean distance matrix serve at the same time as the principal component scores of the covariance matrix among the variables contributing to the Euclidean distance formula.** However many dimensions are required to explain or approximate the covariance structure or the distance structure, we can still start with a matrix of squared Euclidean distances between the cases instead of a matrix of covariances among the original coordinates, and arrive at the same ordination from the SVD of the doubly centered distance matrix $-HD^2H/2$, singular vector by singular vector, that we get from the covariance matrix of the original coordinates now treated as variables one by one.

Unless the original data really were two uncorrelated variables, $x_1 \ldots x_k$ and $y_1 \ldots y_k$ centered and with $\Sigma x_i y_i = 0$, of course we don't get back these actual x's and y's from either technique. We get a set of scores that are centered at

$(0,0)$ and rotated to put the principal coordinates (or principal components) along the Cartesian axes. Otherwise both PCA and PCO remove information about centering from the raw data, and PCO further loses the information about rotation, because that was not coded in the distances D^2.

The basic Procrustes data flow of Chapter 5 relies on PCO for the multivariate reconstruction of the Procrustes shape or form distances on which it is based. Our examples are therefore reserved for that context, beginning at Section 5.3.

Summary of Section 4.2

- Most of the matrix manipulations used in geometric morphometrics are versions of one core algorithm, the *singular-value decomposition,* which expresses any matrix X of numbers in the form $X = UDV'$ where D is diagonal and U and V are rotations.
- If X is a centered data matrix, then $X'X/n$ is the corresponding covariance structure. If $X = UDV'$, then the SVD of $X'X$ is VD^2V'. One often learns a great deal about the covariance structure $X'X/n$ by inspection of V, D, and the scores XU. This is the method of *principal components analysis.* The entries of U and V can be plotted together in combinations variously scaled by the entries of D; such diagrams are called *biplots.*
- If X and Y are two centered data matrices, their *crosscovariance matrix* $X'Y/n$ has its own SVD, again written UDV'. The relation between the X's and the Y's often can be interpreted in terms of the biology of the *saliences* U and V, the *latent variable scores* XU and YV, and the entries of D, which are the covariances of $XU_{.i}$ with $YV_{.i}$.
- If D is any *distance matrix* among k specimens (a square matrix, $k \times k$, with diagonals zero and satisfying the triangle inequality), the SVD of the product $-HD^2H/2$, where H is the centering matrix, often yields a useful matrix of scores V, the *principal coordinates* of the original distances. Our exposition of the Procrustes method in Chapter 5 will rest mainly on this computation.

4.3 The Wishart Distribution: Its Formula and a Sketch of Its Justification

For grounding their biological interpretations, the preceding tools all depend in one way or another on the underlying covariance structure of the measured data. It is unwise to proceed as if this revealed structure was inerrant, without sampling variability or its consequences for the reliability of the reported patterns. Rather, the covariance structure itself is susceptible to the same influences of noise and sampling error as are means (Section 2.1) or correlations (Section 3.4). To apply these methods of pattern analysis competently in our biometrical context, we need protocols for assessing the likely influence on our findings of the same sampling variability that underlies the interpretation of the specific arithmetic formulas applying to one or two variables at a time, the concerns of Chapters 2 and 3.

There is an analogue of the bell curve – a representation of "maximal disorder" in the same spirit – that relates specifically to patterns encountered in covariance structures. It is mathematically formidable in its details, and so is rarely taught except to professional statisticians. But its basic principles are so directly related to today's best applied practices in morphometrics that it is appropriate to communicate its principles in an intuitively accessible way: hence this section.

The informal mathematical analyses in this section are aimed at making you, the reader, comfortable (or at least much less uncomfortable than you otherwise would be) with three fundamental approaches to the interpretation of covariance matrices that are parallel to the three great themes of analysis of averages and bivariate correlations:

- a fairly simple formula (4.37) for assessing the likelihood of any a posteriori claim of a covariance pattern of any content whatsoever against a comparison hypothesis of no pattern at all;
- a fundamental formula (4.38) for the probability density (i.e., the "typicality") of encountering *any* covariance matrix in a sample from a population having a known true structure; and
- an approximate version (4.47) of the logarithm of the same formula, now intended to represent the contrast between any two covariance structures as a "distance" capable of being mapped on paper or computer screen by a variant of the principal coordinates analysis alraady introduced in Section 4.2.4.

Let's start simply, with the first property, as its explication involves only simple algebra applied to familiar Gaussian likelihood formulas like (4.2b).

4.3.1 A Handy Mathematical Fact about Gaussian Likelihoods

The method of maximum likelihood that we have adopted in this book is quite familiar to the community of practicing mathematical biologists. One of its most helpful properties is its ability to automatically discern directionality of covariance structures should that directionality exist. Suppose that we have a data set centered on some mean μ and characterized by some Gaussian distribution law $N(\mu, S)$ where S has some useful directional information in it, such as information about allometry (if at least one measured variable was a size variable) or information about the concentration of within-group variation along one or more valid biological factors. There are standard textbook results for "testing" for such information in S, but we don't need the tests, only the assurance that the maximum-likelihood method automatically identifies the "correct" description of any such directionalities of variance. The general argument requires some notation (see, for example, Mardia et al., 1979), but an intuitive appreciation can be founded well enough on the simplest case, an elliptical Gaussian distribution of just two variables around a mean of $(0, 0)$. This is the situation sketched in Figure 4.13. Without loss of generality we can take the principal components of these bivariate data as lying horizontally and

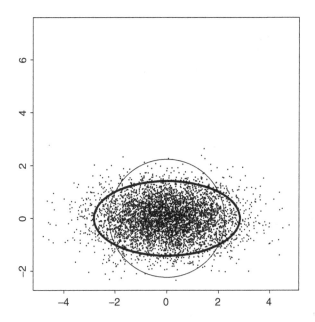

Figure 4.13 Schema for the argument that fitting an ellipse to a noncircular Gaussian distribution always has higher likelihood than fitting a circle. Dots, a 5000-point sample from a Gaussian $(N(0, 8), N(0, 2))$ of variance 8 horizontally and 2 vertically. Heavy line, isoprobability curve for 2 standard deviations in any direction. Light line, the analogous two-standard-deviation line for the optimal fit of an isotropic Gaussian (a circle) to the same data. You can see that the circle is covered too densely at left and right and too sparsely at top and bottom to serve as a plausible line of constant probability. The argument in the text derives the loglikelihood of the former model with respect to the latter.

vertically in our plane. Then the distribution can be written in the notation of Cartesian pairs (x, y) as

$$(x, y) \sim \left(N(0, s_1^2), N(0, s_2^2) \right) \tag{4.28}$$

where the two Gaussian distributions indicated are uncorrelated. We are interested in comparing two maximum-likelihood fits to this one distribution: the fit that corresponds to the true distribution model, versus the fit that uses the same standard deviation in both directions. That would be the model

$$(x, y) \sim \left(N(0, s^2), N(0, s^2) \right) \tag{4.29}$$

In the especially simple and symmetric case here, both of these models can be estimated from the data at hand. We rely on the equation of this particular bivariate Gaussian in the form

$$N(0, S) \sim K \frac{1}{s_1 s_2} e^{-\frac{x^2}{2s_1^2} - \frac{y^2}{2s_2^2}} \tag{4.30}$$

where $K = \frac{1}{2\pi}$ and $s_1 s_2$ is the square root of the determinant of the covariance matrix $S = \begin{pmatrix} s_1^2 & 0 \\ 0 & s_2^2 \end{pmatrix}$ specified in the model depicted.

We work with the *loglikelihoods* of equations (4.28) and (4.29), the expressions

$$LL_2(s_1, s_2) = \log K - \log s_1 - \log s_2 - \frac{1}{2} \left(\frac{x^2}{s_1^2} + \frac{y^2}{s_2^2} \right) \tag{4.31}$$

or the equivalent for the simpler model (4.29), which is

$$LL_1(s) = \log K - 2 \log s - \frac{1}{2} \left(\frac{x^2}{s^2} + \frac{y^2}{s^2} \right) \tag{4.32}$$

Consider first the fit of model (4.29), the circular model, to a sample of n forms from the simpler distribution. The log of the likelihood of the data on this model, according to (4.32), must be

$$LL_1(s) = n \log K - 2n \log s - \frac{1}{2} \Sigma (x^2 + y^2)/s^2, \tag{4.33}$$

where the summation indicated is over all n cases of the data set. To maximize this as a function of s (which is what Laplace's Principle, Section 2.1, says we must do), we set its derivative $\frac{dLL_1(s)}{ds}$ to zero:

$$- 2n/s + \Sigma (x^2 + y^2)/s^3 = 0 \tag{4.34}$$

or

$$s^2 = \Sigma (x^2 + y^2)/2n, \tag{4.35}$$

meaning that the squared radius of the circle in Figure 4.13 is the *arithmetic mean a* of the squared semiaxes $\Sigma x^2/n$, $\Sigma y^2/n$ of the ellipse there. For this value of s, the final term in equation (4.32) for LL_1 reduces simply to the constant 1, while the term preceding it, $-2n \log s$, reduces to $-n \log a$ where a is the arithmetic mean of the eigenvalues of S. The first term $n \log K$ does not reduce but will cancel when we subtract logs of the likelihoods below.

For the more complicated model (4.28, 4.31) our calculation is actually simpler, as the likelihood factors into a term for each Cartesian coordinate. The optimum s_1^2 must be the variance in the x-direction and the optimum s_2^2 must be the variance in the y-direction. At the optimum, the final term in (4.31), like the final term in (4.32), reduces to the constant 1, and apart from this constant and the same term $n \log K$, the remaining expression is $-n$ times the log of the *geometric mean* $g = \sqrt{s_1^2 s_2^2}$ of the variances along the eigendirections of the ellipse.

Hence the loglikelihood $LL_2 - LL_1$ according to which we compare the more complicated model of the ellipse to the simpler model of the circle is

$$- n(\log g - \log a) = n \log(a/g) \qquad (4.36)$$

where a, g are the arithmetic and geometric means of the variances along the axes of the ellipse (equivalently, the eigenvalues of the covariance matrix S in this 2×2 scenario).

With this demonstration in mind, you should be willing to accept the more general assertion (Mardia, Kent, and Bibby, 1979:134) that the loglikelihood of the correct model $N(\mu, V \operatorname{diag}(\sigma_1^2, \sigma_2^2, \ldots, \sigma_p^2) V')$ on the p-dimensional Gaussian distribution of equation (4.2c), with respect to the simpler model $N(\mu, \sigma^2 I_p)$ of the same dimensionality, is still

$$\frac{np}{2} \log(a/g). \qquad (4.37)$$

Here n is the sample size, p is the count of measurements we are examining the covariances of, V is the rotation to the basis of principal components, a is the arithmetic mean $(\sigma_1^2 + \cdots + \sigma_p^2)/p$ of the σ^2's, and g is their geometric mean $\sqrt[p]{\sigma_1^2 \times \cdots \times \sigma_p^2}$. It is an ancient mathematical fact that this logarithm cannot be negative – that the fraction a/g cannot be less than 1. For George Pólya's elegant elementary proof of this fact, the *arithmetic-geometric mean inequality*, see, for instance, Bookstein, 2014, Mathematical Note 5.2.

There is a summary formula for the net amplitude of the claim that a given covariance structure is directional (this quantity $\log a/g$). Mardia, Kent, and Bibby (1979:134) note that np times this logarithm (a product that is equal to twice the loglikelihood) is, in the limit of large samples, distributed as a chisquare (a sum of the squares of independent standard Gaussian variates) on $\frac{1}{2}(p-1)(p+2)$ degrees of freedom (the number of those squared standard Gaussians you need to summate). Here p is the count of variables and n is the count of specimens. The count $\frac{1}{2}(p-1)(p+2)$ combines the $p(p-1)/2$ degrees of freedom of rotation of the orthonormal basis λ with the $p-1$ contrasts among the no-longer-constrained set of eigenvalues s_i.

As usual, I prefer not to convert this to any sort of significance test, but rather to refer different analyses to a common standard as ratios to the expected value $\frac{1}{2}(p-1)(p+2)$ of this chisquare in order to choose among them. A generalization to any range of consecutive eigenvalues, not just the full collection, is dealt with in the difficult paper by T. W. Anderson (1963). But one particular application is straightforward: to the case of the comparison of any two consecutive eigenvalues. From the longer discussion in Bookstein (2014) I extract the useful summary chart in Figure 4.14. In this approach, no

eigenvalue ratio required for any claim to interpretability

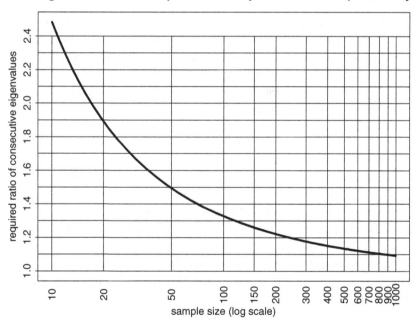

Figure 4.14 Minimum ratio of successive eigenvalues for their meaningfulness separately to be more likely than not. The corresponding threshold for a relative eigenvalue (see Section 4.3.6) is roughly $\sqrt{2}$ times the curve here. From Bookstein, 2014, Figure 5.12.

eigenvector is entitled to interpretation if its eigenvalue differs from the eigenvalue of its successor by a ratio less than that for which $2n \log (a/g)$ equals that expected value. For samples of size 100, this ratio is about 1.32. When in doubt, go with the possibility that the eigenvectors are spinning, and thus uninterpretable separately.

4.3.2 The Wishart Distribution Is Comprehensible

What follows might be called "FishWish" pedagogy. I've combined some of the more congenial elements of Ronald Fisher's great paper of 1915, the one that derived the exact distribution of the correlation coefficient on geometric principles, with aspects of John Wishart's (1928) original derivation of the eponymous distribution, a derivation likewise mainly geometric. The result does not much resemble the current textbook presentations, such as Rao (1973:597–598), which align with the mostly algebraic preferences of today's mathematical statisticians, but rather focuses on the intuitive understanding of what might be going on in actual applied contexts, such as the biometric concerns lying behind the examples on which this book is centered.

Our approach to the general study of biometric covariance structures relies on one classic model, the *Wishart distribution* of empirical covariance matrices from a sample of vectors, each element a Gaussian on its own, that collectively are controlled by a theoretically specified "true value" of that same covariance matrix. For many of our applications, that population covariance structure will be taken as the identity matrix (i.e., total noncorrelation). In practice we can always reduce a model to that case by rotating to the basis of principal components, then standardizing all their variances to 1.0.

Begin with the definition. In this context, the *Wishart distribution* $W_p(\Sigma, n)$ is the distribution of the raw sum-of-crossproducts matrix (that is, totals that were *not* divided by n) of a sample of n p-vectors from the Gaussian distribution $N(0, \Sigma)$. When Σ is the identity, as it will be here, $W_p(\Sigma, n)$ is also the distribution of $n/(n-1)$ times the centered sum-of-crossproducts matrix of n uncorrelated p-vectors of Gaussians of unit variance.

Then for this scenario of a sample of size n from the distribution $N(0, I_p)$ of p uncorrelated normals, the Wishart distribution giving the probability density at any specific empirical covariance matrix S is the comprehensible but not at all obvious formula

$$C|S|^{(n-p-2)/2}e^{-\frac{1}{2}\operatorname{tr}(nS)}. \tag{4.38}$$

Here, as before, $|\cdot|$ is the determinant function and tr is the trace operator (the sum of the diagonal elements). The probability density is taken with respect to the measure dS that is a little $\frac{p(p+1)}{2}$ –dimensional cube with one edge direction for every independent entry s_{ij} of the covariance matrix, $i \geq j$, and C is a complicated constant guaranteeing that the probability distribution integrates to 1.

> The way this equation is notated has changed over the nearly 90 years since its original publication. In most modern treatments (for instance, Mardia et al., 1979, equation 3.8.1), the exponent in the equation corresponding to (4.38) is $\frac{n-p-1}{2}$, which represents a "real sample size" of $n + 1$ specimens instead of n. The extra -1 in the presentation here corresponds to Fisher's (1915) decision to analyze correlations around a sample average value instead of around a true mean. (Graphically, this means the curve around point M in Figure 4.15 is a sphere in $n - 1$ dimensions, not in n.) This is also the interpretation of n that Wishart himself relied on in his original 1928 publication of the general formula. The corresponding degrees of freedom are thereby always reduced by 1 for every variable in the analysis. When I show just below that the $p = 1$ case of equation (4.38) corresponds to the standard formula for a chisquare, it will similarly be notated as if pertinent to a sample size smaller by 1 than the standard textbook chisquare.

My task in this short subsection is to suggest that equation (4.38) is worth trusting by demonstrating it for the explicit case $p = 2$, a pair of variables.

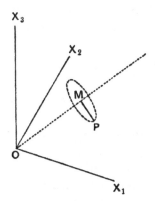

Figure 4.15 From Fisher, 1915. The situation on the x-side of the equation, for a data set of three specimens. M is the point at position $\bar{x}$ along the line of all x's equal. The observed x-vector $P = (x_1, x_2, x_3)$ lies on the circle around M of radius s_x.

To understand the general formula is not particularly difficult once the essence has been mastered via the special case $p = 2$, and in fact there is a derivation of the general formula along these lines that works essentially by mathematical induction, the passage from 2 variables to 3, 3 to 4, ..., $p - 1$ variables to p (Ghosh and Sinha, 2002).

Even simpler than this setting with $p = 2$ variables is the consideration of just one single variable. It is reassuring to see how Wishart's formula gets the right answer in that setting. Its version of the distribution formula for the sum of squares of n independent standard Gaussian variables (mean 0, variance 1) is identical to what we already know about the χ^2 (chisquare) distribution that is usually covered in a second undergraduate statistics course.

The derivation is instructive. Our concern is for the distribution of the statistic that is the sum of squares of n standard z-scores. Write Q for this quantity $\sum_1^n z_i^2$. By the independence assumption, the probability $P(z_1^2, \ldots, z_n^2)$ of any particular sequence of n squared z's is proportional to the product of their probabilities separately: this is just $e^{-z_1^2/2} \times e^{-z_2^2/2} \times \ldots \times e^{-z_n^2/2} = e^{-\Sigma z_i^2/2}$, and so the probability we seek is just a function of that sum of squares itself. We can rewrite this as $P(Q) = e^{-Q/2}$ for the Q defined above, and then further rewrite it as a function of the radius $R = \sqrt{Q}$ of the ball (in n dimensions) that spans all the sums of squares of z's that have the same total. $P(Q)$ is the n-dimensional "area" of the surface of that ball. This probability then must go as $e^{-Q/2}$ times the area of a sphere in k dimensions of radius R — this area goes as a constant times $R^{k-1} = Q^{\frac{k-1}{2}}$ – times the thickness of such a spherical shell, which is $dR = dQ/2\sqrt{Q}$. So, up to a constant factor,

$$P(Q)dQ \sim e^{-Q/2} Q^{\frac{k-1}{2} - \frac{1}{2}} dQ$$

and once you simplify that exponent to $\frac{k-2}{2}$, this is indeed the standard textbook expression for the distribution they write as χ_k^2.

But note also that this expression is identical in form to Wishart's equation (4.38) for a count of variables of $p = 1$, the lowest possible value, once we remember the correction for the missing -1 in the exponent – the correction that Fisher's derivation required for subtracting the products of sample averages. The formula for larger p at which we will shortly arrive is made up of a product of terms like $e^{-Q/2}$, the exponentiation of n times the variance of each variable in turn, times a cofactor that is modified in two ways: first, by dropping its exponent by $\frac{1}{2}$ for each additional variable under consideration; second, by replacing the product of these powered diagonals $Q^{\frac{k-p-1}{2}}$ by an expression in the determinant of the full crossproduct matrix of all the variables, a matrix that has terms like the Q's down its diagonal but also terms $\Sigma x_i y_j$ in every off-diagonal slot.

Back in the bivariate setting, my goal here is to demonstrate using only undergraduate college mathematics that for data arising as samples of two measurements x, y having a population distribution $N\left(\begin{pmatrix} 0 \\ 0 \end{pmatrix}, \begin{pmatrix} 1 & 0 \\ 0 & 1 \end{pmatrix}\right)$ (meaning: each variable has mean zero and variance, and they are uncorrelated), the probability of a covariance matrix within a small region around $\begin{pmatrix} a & h \\ h & b \end{pmatrix}$ in a sample of n 2-vectors is proportional to $(ab - h^2)^{(n-4)/2} e^{-\frac{n}{2}(a+b)} \, da \, db \, dh$. In this crucial formula, the component $e^{-\frac{n}{2}(a+b)}$ is the likelihood e^{LL_2} from which equation (4.31) was derived. The factor $|S|^{(n-p-2)/2}$ in front of it is closely related to the factor $\frac{1}{(s_1 s_2)^n}$ that appears in the denominator of equation (4.30) when it is written out separately for each case, then multiplied together; here, this adjustment takes into account the variances and covariances you find in your actual sample. (In the model, this factor is exactly 1. It becomes larger as the variances grow but smaller as the correlation grows.)

This is demonstrated in the manner of the founding generation of mathematical statisticians who thrived 90 to 100 years ago, following principles of pedagogy that remain of great value for applications to seemingly less mathematical fields like biometrics.

We will need some additional notation. Define s_x and s_y as the sample standard deviations of the x's and the y's, respectively, in the obvious way as the corresponding averages of sums of squares. Also, define r as the empirical correlation by the usual formula $n r s_x s_y = \sum (x - \bar{x})(y - \bar{y})$. We will also be making use of an angle θ having sine equal to r (note this is not the usual associated angle, the one from the formula $r = \cos \theta$, but its complement in $90°$).

The first step in the derivation is to renotate the volume of sample x-vectors $(x_1, \ldots, x_n)$ in terms of $\bar{x}$ and s_x. Fisher's (1915) illustration of this situation is in Figure 4.15. P is the observed vector of p measured x's. The point M is the sample average $\bar{x}$ of the x's times a vector of all 1's, and so the segment MP is the vector of deviations $(x_1 - \bar{x}, \ldots, x_n - \bar{x})$. The length of this segment is evidently $s_x \sqrt{n}$. Given $\bar{x}$ and s_x, P must lie on a hypersphere of radius $s_x \sqrt{n}$ around $\bar{x}$ in $n - 1$ dimensions in the hyperplane at $90°$ to the line OM through M. By the usual rule for derivatives of powers, the volume element of this hypersphere (ignoring powers of n) must be proportional to

$$s_x^{n-2} \, ds_x \, d\bar{x}.$$

We will combine this with a term for the y's, rearrange the combination rather drastically to look like the power of a determinant, then multiply by the underlying Gaussian probabilities to arrive at a probability for the covariance matrix we are aiming at. It helps to remember that on the Gaussian assumption the summary measures $\bar{x}$ and s are independent.

Now for the second step in this two-dimensional derivation: taking into account the role of the other measurement vector, the y's. We have some additional information, that correlation coefficient $r = \sin\,\theta$. In light of the restriction to correlations equal to r, which is to say, angles between the x- and y-vectors equal to $90° - \theta$, the variation of the vector of y's is restricted to a sphere of radius not $s_y\sqrt{n}$ but instead $s_y\sqrt{n}\cos\,\theta$, and centered not at the point $(\bar{y}, \bar{y}, \ldots)$, the point like M, but instead at the point $(\bar{y} + r(x_1 - \bar{x}), \ldots)$ of predicted values from that regression of the y's on the x's. (In other words, the center of this sphere is the regression prediction of the y-vector given the x-vector, and its radius is the root sum of squares of the regression residuals, not the standard deviation of the original y's.) The element of volume of this sphere is thus reduced from the analogous s_y^{n-2} by a factor (ignoring powers of n again) of $\cos^{n-2}\theta$. But the spacing ds_y of the shells for successive values of s_y must be expanded by a factor $\cos\,\theta$ to remain on the sphere we are considering. We thereby lose one of those powers of $\cos\,\theta$, leaving $n - 3$ of them. Hence the volume element over in the y-space by which we must cross the element s_x^{n-2} just computed in the x-space (Figure 4.15), is proportional to

$$s_y^{n-2} \cos^{n-3}\theta\; d\bar{y}\, ds_y\, d\theta.$$

Because on the Gaussian assumption sample means are uncorrelated with their covariance structures, by altering that prefactor C we can proceed as if the x's and y's both averaged zero. The net probability of finding a sample with parameters s_x, s_y, and θ is then proportional to

$$s_x^{n-2} s_y^{n-2} \cos^{n-3}\theta\; ds_x\, ds_y\, d\theta. \tag{4.39}$$

We want to change variables from the quantities s_x, s_y, θ from equation (4.39) to new parameters a, b, h that are just the entries of the observed covariance matrix of our sample of x's and y's. In other words, we want new variables $a = s_x^2$, $b = s_y^2$, and $h = s_x s_y \sin\,\theta$. Recall from second-year calculus that the way this is managed is to re-express the element of probability in terms of the new variables and then divide by the *Jacobian* of the transformation.

The source papers for this maneuver write that Jacobian maximally tersely as $\frac{\partial(a,b,h)}{\partial(s_x,s_y,\theta)}$ and then simply *assert* that it is proportional to $s_x^2 s_y^2 \cos\,\theta$. But it is pedagogically more effective to work out this algebra in explicit detail. For any change of variables from a list of f's to a list of g's that are a smooth and invertible function of them, the infinitesimal density $P(f_1,\ldots,f_k)\,df_1\,df_2\ldots df_k$ turns into the equivalent symbol string

$$P(g_1,\ldots,g_k)\;\frac{1}{J(g_1\ldots,g_k;\,f_1,\ldots,f_k)}\;dg_1\,dg_2\ldots dg_k$$

where, written out in full, J is the *Jacobian determinant*

$$\begin{vmatrix} \frac{\partial g_1}{\partial f_1} & \cdots & \frac{\partial g_k}{\partial f_1} \\ \cdots & \cdots & \cdots \\ \frac{\partial g_1}{\partial f_k} & \cdots & \frac{\partial g_k}{\partial f_k} \end{vmatrix}.$$

(Recall from Section 2.1 that ∂, read "del," is the standard symbol for taking a partial derivative.) In the Wishart context the f's are the list s_x, s_y, θ and the g's are the actual entries in our 2×2 covariance matrix, the functions $s_x^2, s_y^2, s_x s_y \sin\theta$. Then we have

$$J = \begin{vmatrix} \frac{\partial(s_x^2)}{\partial s_x} & \frac{\partial(s_y^2)}{\partial s_x} & \frac{\partial(s_x s_y \sin\theta)}{\partial s_x} \\ \frac{\partial(s_x^2)}{\partial s_y} & \frac{\partial(s_y^2)}{\partial s_y} & \frac{\partial(s_x s_y \sin\theta)}{\partial s_y} \\ \frac{\partial(s_x^2)}{\partial \theta} & \frac{\partial(s_y^2)}{\partial \theta} & \frac{\partial(s_x s_y \sin\theta)}{\partial \theta} \end{vmatrix} = \begin{vmatrix} 2s_x & 0 & s_y\sin\theta \\ 0 & 2s_y & s_x\sin\theta \\ 0 & 0 & s_x s_y\cos\theta \end{vmatrix} = 4s_x^2 s_y^2\cos\theta.$$

Dividing the previous volume element (4.39) of probability by this new Jacobian, we arrive at the formulation

$$\left(s_x^{n-2}s_y^{n-2}\cos^{n-3}\theta \,\Big/\, s_x^2 s_y^2\cos\theta\right)\,da\,db\,dh$$
$$= s_x^{n-4}s_y^{n-4}\cos^{n-4}\theta\,da\,db\,dh. \tag{4.40}$$

Because $\cos^{n-4}\theta = \left((\cos^2\theta)\right)^{(n-4)/2} = \left((1-\sin^2\theta)\right)^{(n-4)/2}$, we can rewrite this as

$$\left(s_x^2 s_y^2(1-\sin^2\theta)\right)^{(n-4)/2}\,da\,db\,dh. \tag{4.41}$$

But

$$s_x^2 s_y^2(1-\sin^2\theta) = ab\left(1-(h^2/ab)\right) = ab - h^2 = \left|\begin{pmatrix} a & h \\ h & b \end{pmatrix}\right|,$$

the determinant of that empirical covariance matrix. In terms of this new basis – the elements of the covariance matrix itself – the volume element is just

$$\left|\begin{pmatrix} a & h \\ h & b \end{pmatrix}\right|^{(n-4)/2}\,da\,db\,dh. \tag{4.42}$$

Wishart calls this result "very neat."[12] So in this special case of $p = 2$, two variables only, the first of the two factors in the Wishart formula, the $\frac{n-4}{2}$ power of the determinant of the empirical covariance matrix, originates in the change of variables from s_x, s_y, $\sin^{-1} r$ to $\mathrm{var}(x)$, $\mathrm{var}(y)$, $\mathrm{cov}(x, y)$. This transformation is entirely geometric in origin, making no reference to any probabilities at all. The remaining factor in the Wishart formula is the term $e^{-\frac{n}{2}(s_x^2 + s_y^2)}$, the isotropic bivariate Gaussian distribution of the observed (x, y) pairs around their own mean, as postulated.

Multiplying the probability distribution in its original coordinates by the change of variables, the probability distribution of 2×2 covariance matrices that we seek is thus proportional to

$$\left| \begin{pmatrix} a & h \\ h & b \end{pmatrix} \right|^{(n-4)/2} e^{-\frac{n}{2}(s_x^2 + s_y^2)} \, da \, db \, dh. \tag{4.43}$$

And this is the same as Wishart's actual formula (4.38) as written out for the situation of two variables only, $p = 2$.

So you see you are capable of understanding the crux of the Wishart distribution as a derivation from first principles. You needn't retreat to the far less powerful computations associated with randomization tests, permutations, matrix correlations, and the like. Instead you can actually understand the idea of the sampling distribution of a covariance matrix, and hence the distributions of its derived features (its principal components, its distance from the identity matrix), as geometric aspects of this new version of biometrical disorder, namely the implications of an extended sample of correlated bell curves that are each totally disordered separately.

This was the case of two variables. In the presentation by Ghosh and Sinha, the general case then follows almost intuitively as an induction, where going from p variables to $p + 1$ adds another term $-\frac{n}{2} s_z^2$ to the exponent in the Gaussian term and replaces the determinant of the covariance matrix on the first p variables by the determinant on all $p + 1$. But this is the same kind of maneuver that got us from a to the volume element $\det \begin{pmatrix} a & h \\ h & b \end{pmatrix}$ above. To

---

[12] It is this expression that generalizes straightforwardly to any number of dimensions, as argued with particularly appropriate diagrams by Fog (1948), among others. This is an example of the so-called *geometric approach* to the Wishart distribution. For the last half-century it has mostly been superseded by the "algebraic approach" that seems favored by the current pedagogy (e.g., Ghosh and Sinha, 2002). But I find the earlier, geometric approach by far the more congenial for explanations to a readership not necessarily fluent in the language of multivariate probability computations, a readership that includes the target audience for this book.

get from $|a|$ to $\left| \begin{pmatrix} a & h \\ h & b \end{pmatrix} \right|$ we multiplied by $s_{y \cdot x}^2 = s_y^2 (1 - r^2)$, the variance of the residual of y after regression on x. To get from the $p = 2$ case to $p = 3$, we would multiply by the variance $s_{z \cdot xy}^2$ of the new variable z after regression on x and y; and so on. Geometrically (Fog, 1948), this is just the formula for stepwise computation of the volume of a hyperparallelopiped, base area times slant height.

4.3.3 A Useful Approximation

In the form (4.38) the Wishart formula for the probability distribution of an extended covariance matrix looks formidably complicated. But it has an approximation that links it very closely to the most familiar technique in the quantitative organismal biologist's toolkit: the PCA of that same covariance structure. You will see that a simple approximate loglikelihood of any particular covariance matrix S arising from a distribution that is truly uncorrelated is almost proportional to the sum of squared logarithms of the eigenvalues of S, times $-n$.

This approximation is not too difficult to establish. The Wishart density W around the identity matrix (all zeroes except for a diagonal of 1's – the [hopelessly nonbiological] pattern of completely uncorrelated variables all of the same variance) is a function of two descriptors of a covariance matrix, the determinant and the trace. From the derivation I just sketched, the distribution of this particular W takes the asymptotic form

$$C |X|^{(n-p-2)/2} \exp \left(-\frac{1}{2} \mathrm{tr}(X) \right), \tag{4.44}$$

where X is the observed sample crossproducts matrix $nS = \Sigma x_i x_j$ and C is a constant of integration whose value, although complicated, is known exactly. (It differs from the C in equation (4.38) by a factor of n^p.)

To approximate this expression by simpler quantities it proves useful to (1) square the density, in order to remove those two divisions by 2 in the exponent; (2) take the logarithm of the resulting squared density; and (3) ignore the term $-(p + 2)$ in the exponent of $|X|$, as we will eventually divide by n under the assumption $n >> p$. We will undo the first two of these changes after we are done; the assumption $n >> p$ will remain in force.

After the term $p + 2$ has been dropped, the log of the square of the density we seek becomes, to this degree of approximation, an explicit function of constants plus a term

$$n \log |X| - \mathrm{tr}(X). \tag{4.45}$$

Now convert from X to the sample covariance structure S by dividing $|X|$ by n^p and each summand of $\text{tr}(X)$ by n. At this point, recall one of the properties of the SVD of a covariance matrix that was mentioned in Section 4.3: if the $\lambda_i, i = 1, \ldots, p$ are its p eigenvalues, then their sum is $\text{tr}(S)$, the *trace* (sum of the diagonal elements) of S, and their product is $|S|$. Using these identities, both of the terms in (4.45) can be approximated as functions of either the λ_i or their logarithms (take your pick).

Define $v_i = \lambda_i - 1$, where the λ's are still the eigenvalues of S. The v's are presumed small. If $|S| = \prod \lambda_i$, $\text{tr } S = \sum \lambda_i$, and (for λ's near 1) $\log \lambda_i \approx v_i$, then, again up to constants, the probability distribution of X/n goes as some function of

$$n \log |S| - n \, \text{tr}(S)$$
$$= n \sum \log \lambda_i - n \sum \lambda_i$$
$$\approx n \sum \left(v_i - v_i^2/2 \right) - n \sum (1 + v_i)$$
$$= -n - n \sum v_i^2/2$$
$$\approx -n - \tfrac{n}{2} \sum \log^2 \lambda_i, \qquad (4.46)$$

where the first approximation relies on the Taylor series of the log function through second order and the second approximation reverts to first order in that same Taylor series once the original first-order term has been cancelled. (The symbol $\prod$ is the analogue of $\sum$ for multiplication: it instructs us to take the product of whatever comes after.)

Hence double the logarithm of the density function of S (maneuvers 1 and 2 above) is approximately

$$-n \sum \log^2 \lambda_i \qquad (4.47)$$

up to some additive and multiplicative constants. Undoing the log and taking the square root, on the Wishart assumption with identical, uncorrelated bell curves the probability distribution of our empirical covariance matrix S around the identity I_p is approximately of the form

$$c \, \exp\left(-\frac{n}{2} \sum \log^2 \lambda_i\right), \qquad (4.48)$$

where the λ's are the eigenvalues of S. The isosurfaces of this probability are thus very nearly the isosurfaces of that sum of squared logarithms, which is also identical to what will be our version of the covariance distance from the identity (see Section 4.3.5). That is the proposition that was to be proved. It is a simplification of the exact formula from the advanced textbooks (see, e.g., formula (11) in section 13.3 of Anderson, 1984).

Relying on this approximation, we can at last put scales on the three axes of Figure 4.1 along which a 2 × 2 covariance matrix can vary around the identity (the population model of a pair of uncorrelated standard Gaussians). On either the horizontal or the vertical axis, a change of standard deviation by 1% generates a 2.01% change in its square, hence the same ratio of change in the eigenvalue in that direction, while on the assumption of a correlation remaining at 0 the other eigenvalue remains invariant at 1.0. The corresponding covariance distance (which, keep in mind, is proportional with a negative slope to the logarithm of Wishart probability) would then be $\log^2(1.0201) = 0.000396$. A change by $r\%$ along the third axis, in or out of the paper, replaces two eigenvalues of 1.0 by the pair $1 \pm r$, with logarithms approximately $\pm r$, so the sum of their squared logarithms is approximately $2r^2$. This corresponds to the same covariance distance and hence the same improbability when $r = 0.01407 \sim 0.01\sqrt{2}$. Had the left panel of Figure 4.1 been drawn exactly metrically with axes at these spacings, the surfaces of equal Wishart probability would be spheres centered on the identity matrix. The right-hand panel demonstrates this symmetry for the section of those surfaces along the horizontal plane of this coordinate system.

4.3.4 Example: Fitting a Single-Factor Model

The usefulness of this particular formulation of disorder can be tested by a simulation that systematically deviates from the model in one specific dimension. Over 1000 runs of $n = 200$ cases I simulated a set of $p = 25$ Gaussian variables that were uncorrelated with variances all 1.0 except for one direction along which the variance was set to 2.0. There are two possible biometric interpretations here, one of sphericity (directionlessness) for all 25 of the derived dimensions and one of sphericity for only the 2nd through 25th. The $np \log a/g$ statistic for the first explanation should be distributed as a chisquare on $24 \cdot 27/2 = 324$ degrees of freedom, thus with expected value 324 and variance 648.[13] For the second explanation, the distribution should be that of a chisquare on $23 \cdot 26/2 = 299$ degrees of freedom, thus should average 299 with variance 598.

The actual results of the simulation are graphed in Figure 4.16. In the upper panel of the figure is the value of the formula $np \log a/g$ for the complete set of all 25 eigenvalues. A total of 14 of the 1000 runs (1.4%) fall to the left of the Wishart-expected value of 324. At the bottom, the value of the same formula

---

[13] The mean value of a chisquare is equal to its degrees of freedom; its variance is two times this mean.

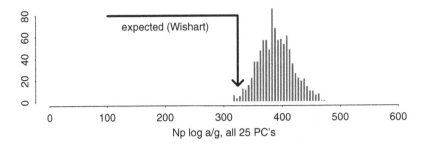

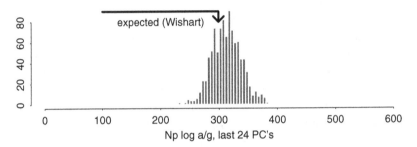

Figure 4.16 Histograms over 1000 runs of a simulation, assessing the fit of two different models for a covariance matrix on 25 uncorrelated variables in 200 cases. Twenty-four of the variables have a variance of 1.0, and the 25th, 2.0. (above) Histogram of the formula $np \log a/g$ for the set of all 25 eigenvalues of the resulting covariance matrix, together with its expected value of 324 on a spherical Wishart hypothesis of only sampling noise. Only 14 of the 1000 simulations fall below this inappropriately "expected" value. (below) The same for the last 24 eigenvalues only, corresponding to the covariance distance of the simulated structure from the actual model. The expected value of this chisquare is 299, which is close to the median of 312 over all the simulation runs. Our sample is thus quite typical under this alternative formulation (which was the situation actually simulated).

applied to the last 24 eigenvalues only, the set that should be spherical on the actual model driving the simulations. This distribution looks exactly like the chisquare it is supposed to resemble. We have thereby empirically confirmed that the Wishart model of a totally disordered covariance structure behaves in practice the way the theorems say it should. The lower panel's chisquare in Figure 4.16 is the appropriate summary of the variability of the rightmost 24 eigenvalues here. In every single one of these simulations the second principal component is meaningless (a selection from the full sphere of 24 dimensions of variation around the first component). Section 5.6.8 will show how much more useful the technique of principal components analysis becomes when components can be identified with factors such as growth gradients, which is to say, biological causes that are known, at least qualitatively, in advance.

Instead of summarizing all 25 of the eigenvalues in the $\log a/g$ formula, we might examine them one by one instead, as in the upper left panel of Figure 4.17. The first eigenvalue ought to be seen to vary around the value of 2.0 indicated by the short heavy line. In fact it is instead biased slightly upward, at a mean of 2.26. (This bias is well known – see, for instance, Jackson, 1991, formula 4.2.5.) The other 24 eigenvalues, which should all be 1.0, show a

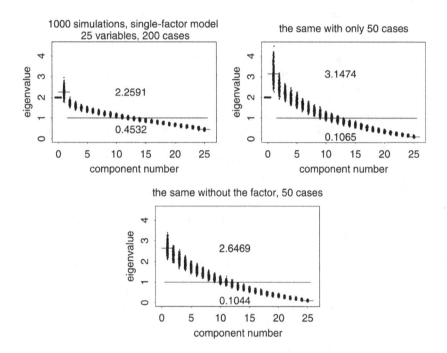

Figure 4.17 Some distributions of eigenvalues of covariance structures in Gaussian models with 25 variables. Top left, eigenvalues from 1000 simulations of 200 cases modeled by a single factor of variance double that of all the other dimensions (the same setup as in Figure 4.16). Top right, the same for a second set of 1000 simulations involving the same single factor but now only 50 cases. Bottom right, the same for a third set of 1000 simulations on 50 cases of 25 variables that now lack any shared factor. In all distributions, the horizontal coordinate of each of the 25 eigenvalues is "jittered" in order to permit visual assessment of the corresponding distributions. Averages of the largest and smallest eigenvalues are printed at their levels, which correspond to the thin little line-segments drawn through their distributions. For the simulations in the upper row, the true variance (2.0) of the single factor modeled is indicated by the thick horizontal bar to the left of the distribution of the corresponding first eigenvalue.

gradation of fully 1.25 from the average maximum (1.705 for the second) to
the average minimum (0.453 for the 25th). It is very inconvenient that this drop
is so much larger than the drop from the typical first (true) eigenvalue to the
second. This is the case even though these last 24 eigenvalues average, overall,
almost exactly what they should: 0.986 versus the theoretical setpoint of 1.0
(the height of the long horizontal rule in the figure).

All of this undesirable variation is for simulated samples of $n = 200$; most
morphometric samples are smaller. A remarkable trio of formulas concerns the
dependence on sample size of the extremes of the eigenvalues in Figure 4.17
that were all supposed to be 1. To acquaint you with this somewhat
counterintuitive phenomenon I have varied the simulation at upper left in the
figure in two ways. For the upper right panel, I reduced the count of cases from
200 to 50, which still seems "comfortably" greater than the count of 25
variables, but continued to incorporate the presence of a single factor loading
equally on all 25 variables and of double the residual variance. In the lower
right panel, the count of cases was kept at 50, but the single factor was omitted.
The crucial parameter for explaining the corresponding pathology of PCA is the
ratio γ of the variable count to the case count. For the simulations at upper left,
$\gamma = 24/200 = 0.12$; at upper right, $\gamma = 24/50 = 0.48$; at lower right,
$\gamma = 25/50 = 0.5$. (This is because there were 24 spherical variables for the two
scenarios in the top row, but 25 for the completely spherical simulations at
lower right.)

Examining the results in the right-hand column, we see that while
diminishing the count of cases from eight times the count of variables to just
double the count of variables (or, equivalently, quadrupling the count of
variables) injects an upward bias of about 40% into that first eigenvalue, it has
its main effect on the *smallest* eigenvalues, dropping their average by a factor of
more than three-quarters. It is disturbing that typically three or four of these
eigenvalues are greater than the value of 2.0 actually assigned to just the first of
them by the underlying model. (The chance that even the fourth eigenvalue is
greater than 2.0 is 41%.) Even more disturbing is the situation in the lower right
panel, for the simulations where that true factor is no longer present. Here the
dominant eigenvalue is still above 2.0 *in every simulation*, even as the smallest
is, on average, unchanged. In other words, even for a count of cases fully double
the count of variables, the inspection of eigenvalues (and, by extension,
eigenvectors) is pretty much useless as a guide to the actual factor structure of
an explanatory model supposedly accounting for the covariances.

There is a theorem relevant to this misbehavior: the *Marchenko–Pastur
Theorem* governing the limiting behavior of those extreme eigenvalues as the
count of variables and the count of cases both increase indefinitely while
maintaining the same ratio γ. Under these circumstances, and assuming a true
covariance structure that is the identity matrix (all variables uncorrelated
Gaussians of the same variance of 1.0), the largest of these misleading

eigenvalues tends to the quantity $(1 + \sqrt{\gamma})^2$ and the smallest tends to $(1 - \sqrt{\gamma})^2$. These formulas, which do not appear in the standard handbooks of principal component analysis as far as I am aware, are difficult to demonstrate except in textbooks very distant from biometry. The proposition is, for example, exercise 2.1.18 in G. W. Anderson et al. (2010), a treatise that is for graduate students in pure mathematics who also have "mastered probability theory at the graduate level." Although the theorem was originally published in 1967, apparently it went unnoticed by the biometric community until I called attention to it in Bookstein (2017a) as a prophylactic for this context of PCA interpretation. (I am quoting the version of the theorem that applies to the way we usually report principal components, in which eigenvalues are divided by the count of variables before they are printed.)

For the simulations at upper left in Figure 4.17, the second eigenvalue (the first one that "should have been" 1.0) averages 1.705, close to the limiting value of $(1 + \sqrt{.12})^2 = 1.813$, and the last, which also "should have been" 1.0, averages 0.453, versus the limiting value of $(1 - \sqrt{.12})^2 = 0.427$. The *condition number* of a matrix like this "spherical" residual, the maximum by which its inverse distorts ratios of variances, would be $\frac{1.705}{0.453} = 3.76$, not too far from its limiting expectation (lots and lots of cases with just 12% as many variables) of $\frac{1.813}{0.427} = 4.24$. For $\gamma = 0.5$, the situation at lower right in the figure, the maximum eigenvalue should average $(1 + \sqrt{0.5})^2 = 2.91$, the smallest should average $(1 - \sqrt{0.5})^2 = 0.086$, and their ratio, which here is 25.4, should approach 34.0 for the largest samples.

Of course all these values would jointly tend to 1.0 if the data of a really large sample of 25 variables had indeed been generated by uncorrelated noise of constant variance. But for organismal samples of any realistic size it is this problem with the list of eigenvalues and especially their ratios that interferes with most applications of biologically uninformed maximum-likelihood methods to the analyses of Procrustes shape coordinate data introduced in Chapter 5. The problem also sabotages other algorithms that involve inversion of covariance matrices, such as the technique of canonical variates analysis (see Mitteroecker and Bookstein, 2011) or the Lande matrix GP^{-1} that purportedly converts selection regimes into population mean shifts. Because the count of Procrustes shape coordinates dominates the count of landmarks by a factor of 2 (for planar data) or 3 (for spatial data), the Marchenko–Pastur problem becomes a good deal worse for realistic morphometric sample sizes. For instance, if you have 100 specimens each with 19 landmark points in 3D, the corresponding γ is $\frac{3 \times 19 - 7}{100} = 0.50$, the same ratio as in the lower panel of Figure 4.17. Then the expected condition number of a covariance matrix on the spherical hypothesis is likely to be close to its limiting value of 34.0, pretty much destroying the interpretability of whatever coefficients result from a linear least-squares optimization. For an exegesis of the caveats for some real morphometric analyses that derive from this deep theorem, see Bookstein (2017a).

Another consequence of the counterintuitive variability of these eigenvalues, the overlap in the distributions of the first and second eigenvalues, is particularly troublesome. Figure 4.18 scatters the drop from first to second against the drop from second to third. The line segment drawn segregates 41 of the simulations (4%) for which the first two eigenvalues are actually closer together than the second is to the third. Such an occurrence would certainly induce the biologist to interpret both of these first two, even though the programmer *knows* that only one projection of the plane through these first two eigenvectors can be meaningful: an unfortunate but predictable pitfall of any method that relies on an incomplete understanding of pattern analysis in high dimensions. The alternative will always be to rely on one's a priori biological knowledge of true (meaning, usually, experimentally demonstrable) factors of shape and shape change. We return to this concern, the pursuit of true factors of form, at the very end of Section 5.6.

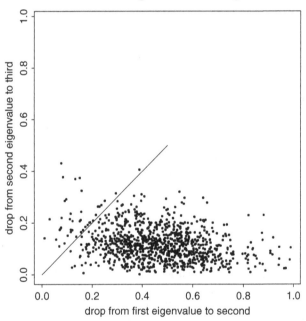

Figure 4.18 The drop from the first to the second eigenvalue in our suite of 1000 single-factor simulations varies enormously but is always less than its designed value of 1.0. That the maliciousness of chance is misdirecting us toward extraneous dimensions of no real importance across any high-dimensional sphere is systematically underappreciated by most quantitative biologists.

The confirmation of the theoretical (Wishart) result for the eigenvalues in the lower histogram of Figure 4.16 does not, of course, imply that we are capable of detecting this disorder intuitively by inspection of eigenvectors. From the formula in Anderson (1963:130), the variance of the elements of this first (and only) meaningful eigenvector around their designed value, in the limit of indefinitely large sample size n for fixed count of variables p, is $\frac{p-1}{p}\frac{2}{n}$. These are more variable than you might hope they were. Without the discipline of a specifically scripted noise model, and the corresponding $\log a/g$ statistics, the quantitative biologist is likely instead to examine the empirical principal component loadings to "see what they mean," and here the presence of multiple dimensions of noise becomes a serious problem. Figure 4.19 shows the problem more clearly by closely examining the estimated first principal component of the distribution already simulated with its true first PC having a variance of 2 along the direction $x_1 = x_2 = \ldots = x_{25}$ of "isometry" and every other dimension independent noise of variance 1. As a component, this first eigenvector should have the formula $(0.2, 0.2, \ldots, 0.2)$, 25 of those 0.2's, each with variance 0.01. (This is not an unrealistic representation of the situation in GMM, where the overwhelming majority of the dimensions of a data set *are* actually noise while the number of true biological factors is severely limited.)

As we have seen, the eigenvalue of such a first component approximates its actual setpoint well after the published bias correction. But its loadings (Figure 4.19) do not. In 25% of the simulations of this structure, at least one of those 25 loadings was at least 0.4, which is twice the value at which it was actually set. And in almost two-thirds of these simulations, at least one loading falls below zero. It is not that this is "too many variables" – the variance of each of these is still just about 0.01, just where Anderson's formula puts it. It is that, just as in the case of random walk (Figure 2.46), the biometrician finds it peculiarly difficult to appreciate the extent to which one's freedom to browse such a profile in search of biological meaning takes unfair advantage of chance, in this case, the distribution of extreme values (out of the 25) instead of their reduction to the chisquare that was correctly reported in Figure 4.16.

The objective reality of any computed principal component, however biologically suggestive, must be viewed with a great deal of skepticism until it can be confirmed by consilience with investigations of other types. In a true model where no single dimension is any more informative than any other, the temptation to interpret the result of any single empirical computation as indicating the contrary, i.e., the temptation to *interpret* a principal component pattern, will be very powerful, notwithstanding that that interpretive model

distribution of simulated PC1

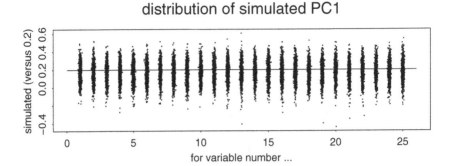

for variable number ...

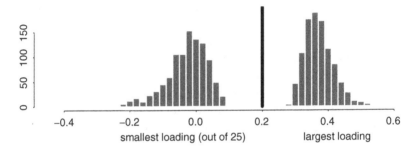

smallest loading (out of 25)   largest loading

Figure 4.19 Pitfalls of the interpretation of a strong first principal component. The simulation here is of one component with variance twice the variance of the 24 others over 1000 replicate 25-dimensional analysis for 200 cases. (top) Actual distribution of the eigenvector shows 25 nearly independent and identically distributed loadings averaging 0.2 with variance 0.01, exactly in keeping with the formulas of Anderson (1963). (bottom) Distributions of the largest and smallest elements of the first eigenvector, theoretically 0.2. Nearly two-thirds of these runs appear (misleadingly) to indicate some sort of contrast in place of the expected isometry.

was not stated at the outset of the research, and thus cannot be considered as having been "tested." Absent strong prior knowledge of true factor structure, principal components cannot be relied on to be biologically interpretable even a posteriori. For a deeper discussion of this pitfall, see the historical review in Bookstein (2015c).

4.3.5 A Special Case: Allometry

Section 2.4.4 slyly approached our present topic, the principal component of a single-factor data set, by constructing the "biorthogonal" directions for a bivariate data set with discrepant variances. This technique generalizes straightforwardly to the context of many variables whenever one of them has a variance considerably larger than the first principal component of all the others. The situation is one justification for the extension of geometric morphometrics to form space that we will study in much more detail in Section 5.3.4. In typical morphometric applications, the additional variable (the logarithm of Centroid Size, which is, in effect, the sum of all the squared distances between all pairs of landmark points) has considerably more variance than any single shape coordinate and indeed more than their first principal component. In that circumstance, the construction in Figure 2.32 extends to each of these constrained variables in turn, and, finally, to their sum. As announced in the original publication (Mitteroecker et al., 2004), the first principal component of the augmented data set then takes the form of a large multiple of this auxiliary variable accompanied by the list of all of its own regressions on the remaining variables (rather like a mother duck followed by her ducklings).

We can use the Vilmann rodent data set already introduced to illustrate this situation. The shape coordinates to be shown in Figure 5.47 have central moments (sum of x- and y-variances) with square-roots ranging from 0.011 to 0.033, as plotted in Figure 4.20. By comparison, the standard deviation of log Centroid Size is 0.1566. This dominance is adequate for the modeling to follow.

In situations like this, the formula for the first principal component is *very* close to a conceptually much simpler profile, the profile of the covariances of all of the variables with the dominant variable (i.e., 16 covariances and one variance, for the Vilmann data); this vector is then divided by the square root of its sum of squares in order to convert it to a unit vector. As you can see in Figure 4.21, the predictions of shape by RW1 or log Centroid Size are indistinguishable from one another and are very close to the actual average shapes encountered at the extremes of our range (ages 7 vs. 150 days). Nevertheless, we are not simply "predicting the average." The scatterplot of the first two components of this data set (Figure 4.22, right) is nearly a shear of the scatterplot of log Centroid Size (horizontal) by its own summary predictor in the shape space (the result of a Partial Least Squares analysis that is 16 by 1). This figure verifies the presence of allometry and also its embodiment on the first principal component. (We didn't actually need that second PC – we could have proceeded just as well using (1) log Centroid Size and (2) its predictions of shape, or the residuals from those predictions.)

This approach is not foolproof. A data set distributed with Weber and Bookstein (2011), for instance, includes 25 landmarks on a sample of human

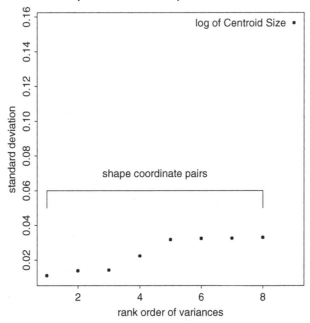

Figure 4.20 Square roots of central moments of the eight Vilmann rodent skull landmarks in the shape coordinate representation (see Figure 5.47) together with the standard deviation of log Centroid Size of these forms. Points are plotted in ascending order.

skulls. According to Figure 4.23, two of the shape coordinates for this sample are wildly more variable than the other 73 – these are the anteroposterior coordinates of the two Euryons, which is not actually an anatomical landmark at all. The variance of just one of these coordinates is indeed nearly as large as the variance of log Centroid Size itself. Under these circumstances, the matrix sent for principal components analysis is close to a matrix of the form $\begin{pmatrix} 1 & r \\ r & 1 \end{pmatrix}$, where r, the correlation between the two dimensions of greatest variance, might have any value near 0. The corresponding first principal component will have a direction like $(1, \pm 1)$ in terms of these two variables, the plus sign if $r > 0$ and the minus sign if $r < 0$, regardless of the actual regression of the offending coordinate on size (a regression that could be as weak as you like).

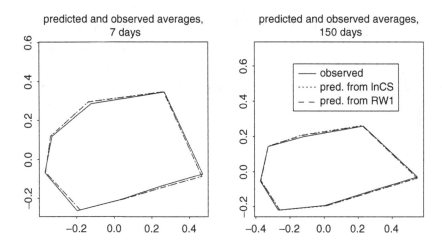

Figure 4.21 Adequacy of the allometric model for the Vilmann data: observed mean forms and average forms as predicted by size only, ages 7 and 150 days.

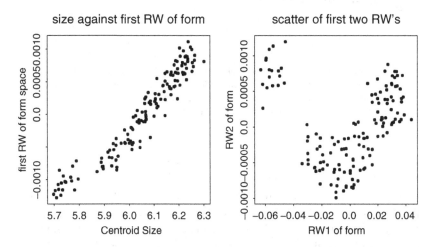

Figure 4.22 Two scatterplots, equivalently informative at the largest scale, for the representation of size allometry when size vastly dominates the diagonal of the variance matrix. (left) Log of Centroid Size plotted against the rest of the ordinary first principal component: size against allometric shape (examine the vertical scale and then compare to Figure 2.32). (right) Under these circumstances the plot of the first two principal components is a sheared version of the plot on the left to the extent that allometric shape is the first principal component of shape (a requirement that is substantially met for these data).

the problem with the allometry example

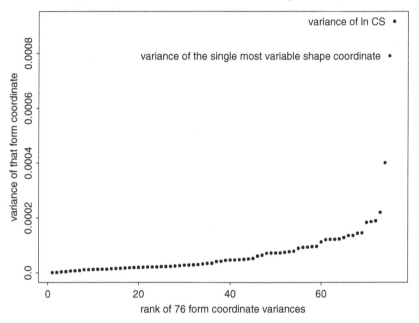

Figure 4.23 In a data set of 25 landmarks on 20 skulls distributed with Weber and Bookstein (2011), the variance of one single shape coordinate is nearly as large as the variance of log Centroid Size. This renders the conversion of the principal components analysis into a description of allometry nearly impossible.

In this situation, the implications of the previous discussion completely fail to obtain: the loading of log Centroid Size will be close to $\sqrt{.5} \cong 0.7071$ instead of to 1, the rest of the formula of the first eigenvector will not be proportional to the allometric regression (the regression of shape on size), and indeed the largest loading for log size might be on some other component than the first. We see all this from Figure 4.24, which samples from the permutation distribution of the loading of log Centroid Size on either the first or the second relative warp, whichever has the larger of those loadings, in a simulation where the actual Centroid Size of the skulls in question was randomized over their shapes (so that whatever allometry was there has been obliterated). You see that the loadings for log CS rise into the 0.90's anyway, but are enormously variable over the permutations; the loading actually encountered, about 0.81, is obviously without meaning.

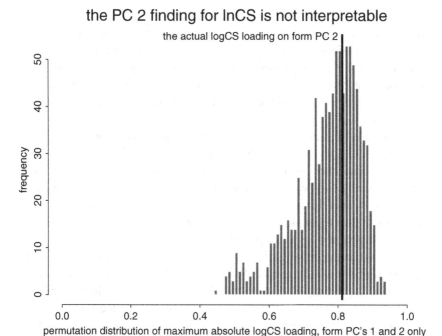

Figure 4.24 Breakdown of the preceding approach to allometry when it is not
the case that one variable has far more variance than all the others. This is a
permutation distribution, the summary from thousands of simulations that leave
the data distributions for size and shape of these specimens unchanged separately
but randomly permute the match between them (i.e., the pairing of a particular
size with a particular shape). The largest loading for log Centroid Size (here, for
the second principal component) is larger than 0.81 but nevertheless, according to
the permutation analysis here, tells us nothing whatsoever about allometry (which
actually is not present in this data set).

4.3.6 Interpreting the Sum in Equation (4.47) as a Distance

The expression $\sum \log^2 \lambda_i$ at which we arrived at the end of Section 4.3.3 plays
an additional role in GMM beyond its function here as the scaling (up to a
factor of sample size) of the improbability of a covariance matrix. Perhaps
you have already imagined thinking of it as a sort of "probability distance"
from the identity matrix (independent identically distributed Gaussians) that
we used to compute the distribution, the way the logarithm of the ordinary
bell-curve formula has a term proportional to the negative of x^2 where x is just
the distance of the underlying scalar from the population mean. In fact, the

same proves true of this term in the Wishart formula. The quantity $\sum \log^2 \lambda_i$ does indeed serve as a useful measure of the squared *distance between two covariance matrices* for any two candidates that use the same list of variables and for which the comparison makes biological sense (for instance, two subtaxa of some taxon, or males versus females, or, as in Figures 5.55 and 5.56, covariances within homogeneous age categories of growing animals studied longitudinally).

The detailed argument is a bit more nuanced than I have room for here (see Bookstein, 2014, section 6.5.3), but the gist has already been conveyed by a remark in connection with Figure 3.34, where I noted that for a likelihood ratio comparing two probability models over the same linear space, we can change the basis of that space any way we like without changing the ratio of the likelihoods. That figure was discussing the probability of an observation, but the same insight applies to the probability of a covariance matrix as a whole, which is just an integral over the appropriate regions of the linear space of all the data vectors chained together. We can diagonalize the covariance model we are using to explore the Wishart without changing the ratios of the probabilities it affords us, and then sphericize that diagonalization; hence the "shape" of this distribution is the same for any population covariance structure Σ, whether the identity I_p or not. Therefore the density with which empirical covariance matrices Σ' are distributed around their population model Σ will be the same if we transform everything to the basis in which $\Sigma = I_p$.

The λ's at which we arrive there have a name in terms of the original Σ and Σ' – they are called the *relative eigenvalues* of either with respect to the other. Bookstein (2014) argues, following the original presentation in Mitteroecker and Gunz (2009), that these λ's behave just the way you would want a distance function to work if multiples of the same single-factor model are to lie on straight lines and if models with two factors are to satisfy the Pythagorean Theorem for distances due to the two factors separately. (In fact, this formula $\sum \log^2 \lambda_i$ is the *only* squared distance function that works this way.) Principal coordinates of these distances serve as dimensions of a decomposition of the corresponding space of covariance matrices into separate processes, just like principal components of ordinary vector variables were supposed to do in Section 4.2.2. In other words, if the factor structure of a data set changes substantially, in the plot of the principal coordinates of the covariances you will see a sharp turn.

The detailed argument guaranteeing the existence and uniqueness of the λ's has a good visualization for two-dimensional data; Figure 4.25 explores a convenient example. At upper left is the general case, two arbitrary covariance matrices on the same two variables. Once they have been drawn concentrically,

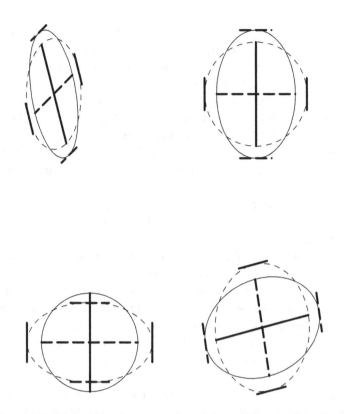

Figure 4.25 Diagram for the construction of the covariance matrix distance function $\sqrt{\sum \log^2 \lambda_i}$ in two dimensions. The covariance distance of the example here is 0.3444. All panels of this display are shears of one another, and when either ellipse is sheared into a perfect circle, as in the panels at upper right and lower left, the squared covariance distance is the sum of squared logarithms of the ratios of the axes of the transformed image of the other ellipse.

it is easy to show (by the same sort of diagonalization argument as in Section 4.2) that there exists a unique pair of directions, the thick solid and thick dashed lines, such that in *both* ellipses either line is parallel to the tangents to the ellipse at the points where the other line intersects it. Recall that these directions are called *conjugate directions*. (In higher dimensions, the uniqueness is the same but the tangent lines become tangent planes or hyperplanes.) The proof is based on the simple observation that shears leave tangency unchanged, and so we can transform the figure so that ellipse 1, say, becomes a circle, as in the upper right panel. But now the proposition is obvious: the directions we seek are just the axes of the ellipse into which ellipse 2 is sheared as ellipse 1 is circularized. You must get the same answer if you choose to circularize ellipse 2 instead (lower left). The squared distance we compute in this example, $\log^2(1.3) + \log^2(0.8) = 0.3444^2$, must be the same for *every* shear of any of these frames; at the lower right is the same comparison for another arbirarily selected basis.

In the extension to higher-dimensional covariance structures, the geometry is the same except that ellipses are replaced by ellipsoids or hyperellipsoids. The sole requisite is that these ellipsoids not be "flat": that neither Σ nor Σ' have any eigenvalues equal to zero (which does not have a logarithm). I will show the workaround for this in the GMM context where this formula is applied: see Section 5.4.5.

Because single-factor families of covariance structures lie on straight lines in this geometry, the ordination by principle coordinates that Section 4.3.4 already introduced for data can be used for covariance matrices as well. Such an analysis could tell us, for example, if a collection of these matrices for different subsets of a sample seem to scatter without pattern or instead lie on a possibly meaningful curve. We return to this construction near the end of the next chapter when we consider ordination of covariance structures on longitudinal data, an important new methodology for studies of canalization and growth regulation. These and other examples are the topic of the more thorough review of this maneuver in a variety of contexts, not all morphometric, in Bookstein and Mitteroecker (2014).

Here ends our survey of the multivariate tactics on which we will rely to analyze and make sense of GMM data. We have inspected the basic algebra of the singular-value decomposition and three distinct applications to the biological setting in which multiple analogous variables have been measured on a sample of organisms, and we have explored the Wishart distribution of covariance matrices, which describes how these structures vary around their true values, how that variation may be approximated as a sum of squares, and what this situation implies for the biological interpretation of principal components. The final chapter of this book is devoted to the foundations of the corresponding biometric inferences – the data formats, the hypotheses, and the arithmetic that generate its most elegant findings – for the special circumstances of data arising as Cartesian coordinates of corresponding points, curves, or surfaces: the data type we call *geometric morphometrics*.

Summary of Section 4.3

- Just as the multivariate Gaussian distribution generalizes the bell curve, which embodies maximum disorder for a single measurement, so the

Wishart distribution generalizes the Pearson formulas for uncertainties of variances and correlations to the setting of arbitrarily many arbitrarily correlated Gaussian measures.

• We motivate this discussion by examining the formula according to which one assesses a single covariance structure for sphericity.

• The formula for the *complete* distribution of a 2×2 covariance matrix (the Wishart distribution with $p = 2$) can be derived in a couple of pages using only elementary college mathematics. The general case is harder to notate, but conceptually it is mainly an iteration of these geometric arguments dimension by dimension.

• There is a good approximation to the Wishart density formula near the uncorrelated standardized model of equation (4.2b) that involves only the logarithms of the eigenvalues of the sample covariance matrix, squared and summed.

• These basic facts about high-dimensional covariance structures are easily confirmed in simulations of models with a single factor, such as allometric growth. Both the eigenvalues and the eigenvectors of the corresponding principal components analysis are substantially more variable than the organismal biologist would prefer, particularly if one underlying variable has much more variance than all the others do. In general, principal components should be considered reliable only when they correspond to developmental, functional, or selective factors known a priori.

• That Wishart approximation (the sum of squared logarithms of eigenvalues) serves as a robust and natural squared *covariance distance* for comparison of multiple covariance structures on the same variables (for instance, over different ages of a growth series, or between related species).

5

Geometric Morphometrics:
Its Geometry and Its Pattern Analysis

> Geometric morphometrics carefully weaves information from geom-
> etry together with information from biology in order to more clearly
> highlight a type of pattern that the viewing eye (even the trained
> organismal biologist's eye) can see only dimly: the endlessly infor-
> mative spatial patterning of biological shape and shape change.

Keep in mind the main purpose of the basic tools this book talks about: to
pass from arithmetic based in images of organisms to biological understanding
of the forms of those organisms. Two themes are equally pertinent to these
quantifications. One arises from the semiotics of diagrams in science and art,
the other from algebra. The link between the two involves both geometry
and biology, or, better, the geometry *of* biology. Here the "biology" can
be evolution, biomechanics, morphogenesis, medicine, or plain old human
variability, studied either as basic science or as applied science, while the
word "geometry," ignoring the "geo-" part, is meant in today's mathematical
meaning of the word, the locations of features with respect to one another or
in reference to the walls of a laboratory or the edges of a map. Our task in this
chapter is to outline the elements of this combination. As *aides-mémoires* I
offer the following pair of images. The first is your basic **biostereometric baby**
(Figure 5.1), and the other is the notion of an icon for explicit comparisons.
Anticipating the schema of the *transformation grid* in Section 5.5, Figure 5.2
shows one of these together with the pair of specimen images it bridges.

Figure 5.1 shows an example of a "biostereometric baby": a three-
dimensional geometric representation (here by contours of distance from
the camera into the page) of the forward-facing surface of a squirming solid
organism that every reader instantly recognizes. Our topic in this chapter is
the reduction of highly prolix and redundant representations like this one to
quantifications of much lower complexity that can benefit from the multivariate
biometric analyses introduced in previous chapters – structured lists of

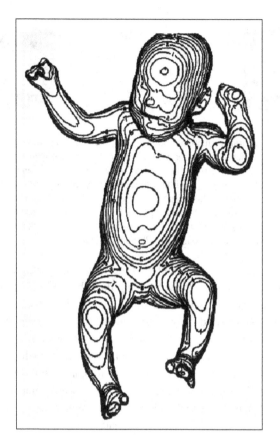

Figure 5.1 A "biostereometric baby." Image copyright Dan McCoy/ DoctorStock.com, photo 15027.

quantifications that can be averaged, correlated with other such measures or with any other type of assessment, or passed through a singular-value decomposition in the search for patterns of integrated covariation. No matter what kind of scheme there might be for standardizing the position of a baby being imaged (cf. Figure 3.46), this baby is in no such standardized position; coping with the squirming is a major component of the morphometrician's task.

The icon in the center of Figure 5.2 is an explicit descriptor applying to a novel conceptual notion, the *change of form*, that is different from all the quantifications that have preceded it in this book. Those were quantifications that applied to *measurements of extent of the individual form* – length, weight, volume, circumference, and the like. After a bit of practice, the tools introduced in this final chapter will enable you to find this middle figure legible (i.e., to "read" it), to discern the several components of the biological message(s) it

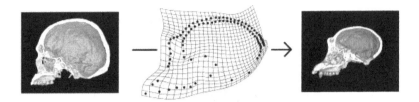

Figure 5.2 The transformation grid, our fundamental icon for explicit comparisons of geometric shape representations, is always a bridge between two forms. Here the left and right images render carefully prepared and positioned scientific objects; their job is to illustrate forms, not necessarily to expedite their comparison. The notion this chapter explores for biometric applications is the newer scientific icon in the middle panel. As an explicit representation of a comparison, it is a function of two original forms, not just one. Yet it is not any kind of subtraction. Image courtesy of Philipp Mitteroecker.

encodes, and to report it competently as the culminating diagram of a basic or applied research project. It even exemplifies the lowered dimensionality referred to in connection with Figure 5.1, in that it is based on only the information from the solid dots in the middle diagram (and their starting positions on the grid when it was square), not any other information from either figure. The icon is often called a "deformation," for which the graphic in Figure 5.3 plays the role of the *deformable template*. But as we will see in Sections 5.5 and 5.6, the deformation in question is wholly unreal, a matter of graphical statistics, not an actual biological phenomenon such as tissue strain.

First, though, the new methodology demands a detour back into the history of our subject. A theme needs to be made explicit that was left implicit through the preceding three chapters. To this point we have been exploring fundamental techniques of numerical inference that apply across most of biology. Averages, path coefficients, bell curves and correlations all help us report explanations in terms of measured extents (lengths, areas, weights) in this domain, and the information matrix and the Wishart distribution (and its approximations) supplement these classic techniques wherever they systematize the contemporary pattern analyses (and their uncertainties) invented for the organized numerical tableaux we call covariance matrices. But when the numbers involved in an analysis instead quantify *the locations of multiple organismal features in an image or in space*, these techniques all specialize further. In serving this domain, the tools introduced in Chapters 2, 3, and 4 have made their deepest penetration to date into biology. This nexus is the workbench of **geometric morphometrics** (GMM), the central concern of this final chapter.

The argument proceeds in six sections plus a coda. I begin (Section 5.1) with a discussion of the nature of the raw data of geometric morphometrics –

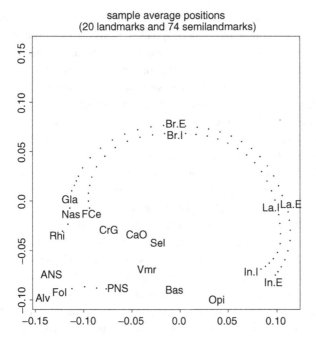

Figure 5.3 Typical example of a *template*, guide for interpreting a GMM analysis. The data driving Figures 5.51 and 5.52 (Procrustes shape coordinates and their dominant principal component for 22 specimens of *Homo sapiens*) are indicated here as they might trace a typical form of the sample (in the original study, these were synthetic midsagittal images derived from CT scans). Landmark names and operational definitions: Alv, alveolare, inferior tip of the bony septum between the two maxillary central incisors; ANS, anterior nasal spine, top of the spina nasalis anterior; Bas, basion, midsagittal point on the anterior margin of the foramen magnum; BrE, BrI, external and internal bregma, outermost and innermost intersections of sagittal and lambdoidal sutures; CaO, canalis opticus intersection, intersection point of a chord connecting the two canalis opticus landmarks with the midsagittal plane; CrG, crista galli, point at the posterior base of the crista galli; FCe, foramen caecum, anterior margin of foramen caecum in the midsagittal plane; FoI, fossa incisiva, midsagittal point on the posterior margin of the fossa incisiva; Gla, glabella, most anterior point of the frontal in the midsagittal; InE, InI, external and internal inion, most prominent projections of the occipital bone in the midsagittal; LaE, LaI, external and internal lambda, outermost and innermost intersections of sagittal and lambdoidal sutures; Nas, nasion, highest point on the nasal bones in the midsagittal plane; Opi, opisthion, midsagittal point on the posterior margin of the foramen magnum; PNS, posterior nasal spine, most posterior point of the spina nasalis; Rhi, rhinion, lowest point of the internasal suture in the midsagittal plane; Sel, sella turcica, top of dorsum sellae; Vmr, vomer, sphenobasilar suture in the midsagittal plane. Dotted lines sketch the curving of this form between the landmarks. Once standardized, these 74 unnamed dots turn into *semilandmarks* in a later version of this same data set explained in Section 5.5.4. Diagrams like this are often

not measured extents, as in earlier chapters, but *landmark locations* encoding an understanding of how points correspond from specimen to specimen. Here "correspondence" is not to be construed wholly in the biologist's sense, a matter of embryological, biomechanical, or functional arguments, but involves some aspects of geometry as well, specifically the appropriateness of a *deformable model* assembling manifold measures of extents into an seamlessly smooth, differentiable whole. These characteristic points and extents have a history far older than any other part of contemporary biological science – as old as the paleolithic origins of art and visual culture. From this review we pass, in Section 5.2, to a first pair of explicitly geometrical descriptors. One, the *strain tensor*, reduces, as Section 5.2.1 shows, to a new interpretation of the SVD already exercised at length in Chapter 4. But the desired comparison can also be computed entirely geometrically, in a construction that leads to our first example of a suite of shape coordinates, the *two-point* or *Bookstein* coordinates, Section 5.2.2. Section 5.3 turns to a crucial formalism intended to code the biologist's a priori understanding of "dissimilarity": the *Procrustes distances* among pairs of forms. These numbers, which end up filling a square matrix, can be analyzed by another of the variants of the SVD, the *principal coordinates* already introduced in Chapter 4. Procrustes distance not only drives the principal coordinates analyses but also, via John Gower's *generalized Procrustes analysis,* supplies a second suite of shape variables, the *Procrustes shape coordinates,* for which these principal coordinates serve as the *relative warps* (principal components). This coincidence of rhetorics is the subject of Section 5.4, along with an extension that restores the component of size so carelessly suppressed when we shifted from Euclidean distance to Procrustes distance in the first place.

Section 5.5 introduces a crucial diagrammatic icon invented only 30 years ago: my *thin-plate spline transformation grid* that converts all of these computations from algebra back into the geometry of the organismal image and thence (some of the time) to biology. That was the icon exemplified in the middle of Figure 5.2. With its aid, Section 5.6 concludes the analysis of our two main running examples, Vilmann's growing rats and the Gunz human skull sample, by visualizing or revisualizing all of the pattern findings they can support, and finishes with some thoughts on a current frontier of quantification, "integration." The book concludes with an Envoi, Section 5.7, sketching some open issues and sending the reader off with every good wish.

---

referred to as *deformable templates,* but, as in Figure 5.2, the "deformations" in question are purely formal, not biophysical. For a color version also indicating the conventional subdivisions of the bones of the midsagittal skull, see figure 1 of Bookstein, Gunz et al. (2003).

5.1 The Data of Geometric Morphometrics: How We Keep Our Place in an Anatomy

Our initial topic is **anatomical variability.** Indeed this section could as well have been headed "The biomathematical rhetoric of anatomical variability," except that keywords like "biomathematical" or "rhetoric" are offputting in a running head. Even though anatomical variation has been a concern of one profession or another for thousands of years, this chapter will have new things to say about it.

Students of either human or comparative anatomy typically identify what they are looking at by names, mostly in Latin, for distinct structures. These named parts provide the "homologous entities" subject to the largest-scale developmental or evolutionary explanations. To tie these resources to biometry, a different formalism than Latin nomenclature is necessary. We will end up representing *part* of the available information by the *Cartesian coordinates* developed in the 1630s as a philosophical innovation. Because the coordinate pairs or triples that represent a single integrated organism can be arbitrarily numerous, a linking scheme is necessary so that we can keep track of them. This is the role of the *landmark,* the point formalism introduced in this section.

We have already seen one classic example of a landmark configuration: the eight neurocranial points of the Vilmann rodent octagon (Figure 2.41). Figure 5.3, a more anthropological template, underlies a data set of $N = 29$ (ultimately winnowed to 22) midsagittal skull forms that will be the testbed for many computational examples in this chapter. ("Sagittal," in craniometrics, is the dimension from left to right; the "midsagittal plane" is the plane up the middle of the solid head, the plane with respect to which we are approximately symmetric.) These data were originally published in Bookstein, Gunz et al. (2003), to which the reader may refer for the scientific context of the work.

Landmark points provide concentrated information about curves or surfaces and the relationships of the tissues they trace or delimit. They are not presumed causal in the sense of the discussion in Section 3.1 – one does not usually intervene on their positions in order to produce functional effects – but only express the developmental or evolutionary or phylogenetic processes that generated their locations, as well as the locations of the continuum of points in neighboring tissue, according to morphogenetic, selective, or ecophenetic mechanisms. Moving a landmark to a new location usually does not have the effects that we might claim to be precomputing as singular vectors in an SVD analysis. If it did, we'd be doing biomechanics, not morphometrics. For more on this contrast, see Oxnard (1984). In his interpretations, curves, via the moments of the muscles that attach to them, sometimes really *do* do things. But this reasoning does not apply to evolutionary comparisons (Bookstein, 2015c).

Displays like Figure 5.3 are based on many prior agreements between presenter and audience – many *scientific conventions,* most of which are tacit. Some are conventions of *viewing.* We might be photographing a specimen from a fixed direction, for instance, the *mediolateral view* of a symmetrical skull taken perpendicular to its plane of symmetry. A particularly well-known version of this view for primates is the *Frankfurt Horizontal,* which rotates that mediolateral image so that a line from above the ear to below the eye socket is horizontal. (A detailed criticism of this convention is set down in Bookstein, 2016a.) The view might be a guide to placement of the investigator's actual fingers or digital probe in the three dimensions of the laboratory, or instead an equivalent guide to the placement of a cursor on an image of the same structure, perhaps in two dimensions, perhaps in three; the images in Figure 5.2 are "virtual slices" in that sense. Landmarks are easiest to place when they arise as intersections of sharply delineated surfaces, like the boundary between bone and air on the dried skull. It is difficult if not impossible to operationalize their placement when an actual bounding edge or surface is not available: examples include the "margin" of the diaphragm, or the "edge" of a tendon. Even when the organism clearly draws these curves or surfaces for you, the semilandmarks of Section 5.5.4 or the edge-gradient models of Bookstein (2001) are required if the available information is to drive the icon of a deformation.

Other conventions represent conventions of *detail.* In Figures 5.4 and 5.5, we see two different representations, nearly a century apart, of the human corpus callosum, the "waist" of the brain's white matter where it crosses the cerebral midline. For the purpose of morphometric measurement, these both reduce to schemes such as that in Figure 5.6 (a three-dimensional scene in the original **ewsh** output, here reproduced in one selected projection only). The task was to extract a *symmetry curve* or *midcurve* up the centerline of this structure (Bookstein et al., 2001, 2002a). This sort of representation, in turn, generated the abstraction in Figure 3.43, from which all the individualizing texture, parcellation, etc. is gone, leaving only the underlying geometry of a finite number of points presampling this prespecified boundary formalism, from which, finally, a single pair of points was identified and reduced to a separation vector for the purpose of the quadratic discriminant analysis explained there. Thus the ultimate purpose of the morphometric exercise was to extract the information that will prove relevant in functional or biomechanical analyses of these structures as they align with the course of human development, aging, or disease.

The raw data for both panels in Figure 5.6 is the NIH's Visible Female, an 8-gigabyte color image of a single human female. She was solidly frozen

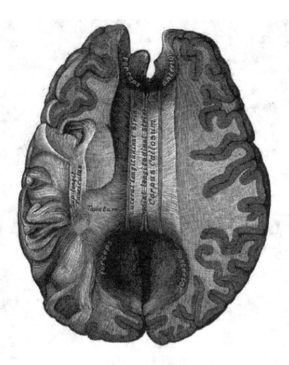

Corpus callosum from above.

Figure 5.4 A normal human corpus callosum, from *Gray's Anatomy*, 1918 edition, figure 733. (For a wry comment comparing the style of this drawing to that of representations of the same structure in contemporary atlases of human anatomy, see Bookstein, 2017c.)

after death, sliced head to toe by a huge microtome, and the cut surfaces scanned and converted to a volume of $300\mu \times 300\mu \times 300\mu$ voxels that was then reformatted for convenient exploration by dynamic tumbling trihedra using W. D. K. Green's ewsh software package (Bookstein and Green, 2002). The *morphometric* structure of interest runs roughly along the surface of this approximate central section of the *anatomical* structure of interest, which is the light-colored downward-oriented C-shaped arch of myelin (yellow in the original photographic record; red in the synthetic color version of Figure 5.5).

In the vicinity of an approximate backplane (left-hand panel), the points of the symmetry curve are traced as the intersections of the callosum's upper surface with lines normal to the surface such that the planes through them that cut the curve perpendicularly have the greatest apparent symmetry across these normals as midlines of the section. A sample of these normal planes,

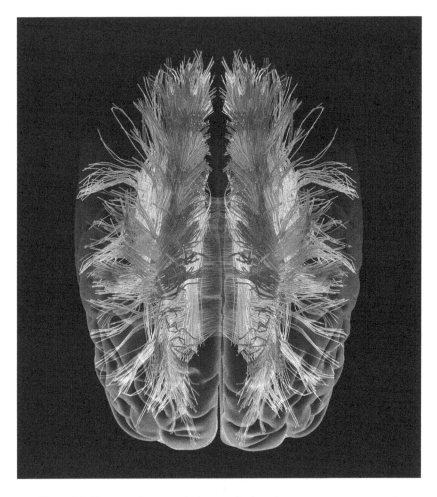

Figure 5.5 The same, from a typical recent display of a *connectome*, a structural image of the brain's actual nerve fibers. Copyright Alfred Pasieka/Science Photo Library/Getty Images.

stringently foreshortened, appears in the panel at right. In the example actually published, Bookstein et al. (2002a), which is a study of the variability of this structure in people with a fetal alcohol diagnosis, there are not seven but forty of these planes, only one of which involved an actual landmark (Rostrum, the re-entrant corner at lower left), and the source medical imagery is cranial MRI, not photography. There is enough information just in a pair of dimensions of this curve to discriminate between normal and fetal-alcohol-affected adult males in the course of forensic applications of morphometrics (Figure 3.44).

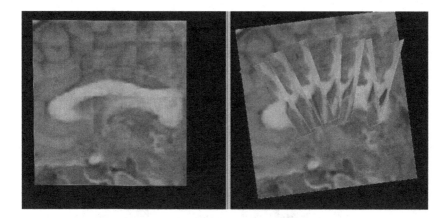

Figure 5.6 One suggested morphometric scheme for formalizing the geometric information of a single curve from Figures 5.4 and 5.5, the "callosal midcurve." See text. In the color version of this figure (online) there is a region of wholly nonbiological blue at the lower right; this is latex injected to keep the frozen specimen from deforming under the pressure of the microtome producing the series of facets exposed for photography.

Another version of the right-hand image appears on the cover of the issue of *New Anatomist* in which Bookstein et al. (2002a), was published.

The technological requirements for transforming the original anatomical understanding into Cartesian coordinates of symmetry curves like these, and then the strenuous statistical modeling required to retrace the journey back to a biomedical interpretation, are typical of what is required to bridge arithmetic to organismal understanding in applications to biomedical imaging. For one attempt at an epistemology of such transitions, emphasizing the bridge from the arithmetic of points like these to the Latin of anatomy atlases, see Section 5.6.9.2.

For a more familiar example, this one superimposed over a classic Florentine painting, consider Figure 5.7 (inspired by but not copied from the cover of Farkas, 1994). In addition to its role in clinical anthropometry, this represented an intermediate stage in the construction of a new branch of applied biometry, *face recognition,* intended as a component of "industrial biometrics" (identification of individuals by distinctive patterns of arbitrary features in very large numbers). Figure 5.8 is an example from 2014 (identification of a celebrity from an arbitrarily posed photograph) indicating the evolution of this scheme over the last twenty years. See, in general, Li and Jain (2011) or Ross et al. (2006).

And indeed today's technologies for representing information from biomedical images of living or dead surfaces or solids were anticipated hundreds or

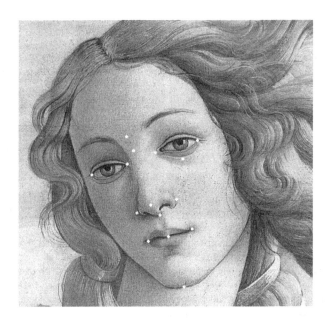

Figure 5.7 Enhancement (?) of Sandro Botticelli's *Birth of Venus* by a collection
of landmarks on the surface of the goddess's face.

even thousands of years ago by representations produced for other reasons
entirely. For instance, the thin-plate spline explained in Section 5.5 as a sturdy
graphical metaphor for shape *comparison* was present (albeit implicitly) in the
mode of artistic production known as *caricature,* and the emphasis on female
secondary sexual characteristics as clues to fecundity has been apparent ever
since the dawn of sculpture. The Venus of Willendorf (Figure 5.9) for example,
is typical of a wide range of "venuses," similarly exaggerated depictions of
female fertility or attractiveness, that arose all over Eurasia at roughly the same
time. Other famous examples include artifacts from Lespugue (France), Dolní
Věstonice (Czech Republic), and Galgenberg (Austria). One could consider
these to connote the dawn of biometrics, tens of millennia before any other
aspect of science showed any cognitive presence in the human arts or crafts.
We cannot really know the *mentalité* of the artists who sculpted the venuses,
but later examples include some individuals whose names are now in all
the textbooks (cf. da Vinci's experiments, Figure 5.10) in connection with
the then-new craft of individualized portraiture. Others were attempting to
teach principles of "human proportion" using the new technology of printed
woodcuts (Figure 5.11), and still others were simply trying to make a living
in the newly emerging mass market for images with a social sting in their tail

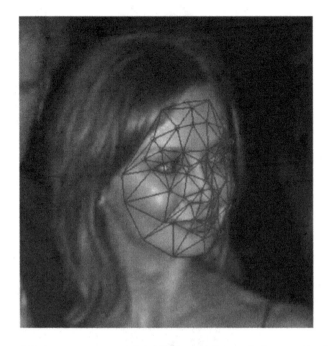

Figure 5.8 A contemporary update: a snapshot (unposed photograph) of the actress Calista Flockhart, marked up as part of a data set of four million images on four thousand individuals. Copyright 2014, IEEE. Reprinted with permission from Taigman et al. (2014).

(Figure 5.12). Examples like these could be multiplied indefinitely beginning in ancient Rome and not omitting to note Jacques Callot, George Cruikshank, and James Gillray. (Indeed, one modern technology of caricature defines it as the quantitative exaggeration of an individual's features that are already found to be the most abnormal, in order to speed recognition along with a sense of visual wit: see Brennan, 1985.) Of course examples of biometry like these arose long before there was any such notion as biological statistics.

One concise way to summarize the new morphometrics is simply to announce the conversion of the preceding intellectual-artistic tendency into a formal technoscience. We now have a reproducible digital version of what caricaturists knew how to do long before the twentieth century. A representation of the variation of human form is possible that meets all of the following central criteria:

- it is **intuitive,** exploiting a broadly human cognitive faculty while incorporating an innate but approximately valid neurocognitive segmentation process;

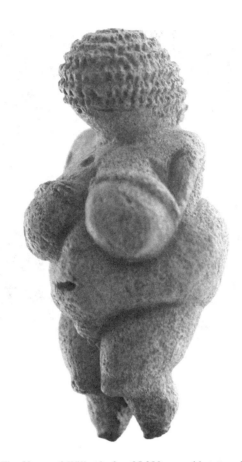

Figure 5.9 The Venus of Willendorf, a 25,000-year-old statue about 10 cm in height, representing an extrapolation of some features of the anatomy of the human female that were of particular importance in the Paleolithic. Photo by MatthiasKabel / CC BY.

- it is **quantifiable,** articulating to a formal probability theory (multivariate normality of the shape coordinates) and a formally multilinear statistical method along the lines of what we have been reviewing in Chapters 2, 3, and 4; and
- it is **consilient with explanatory biological theories,** meaning, consistent with the dominant rhetorical style of both the basic sciences of biology and their medical, ecological, and industrial applications today.

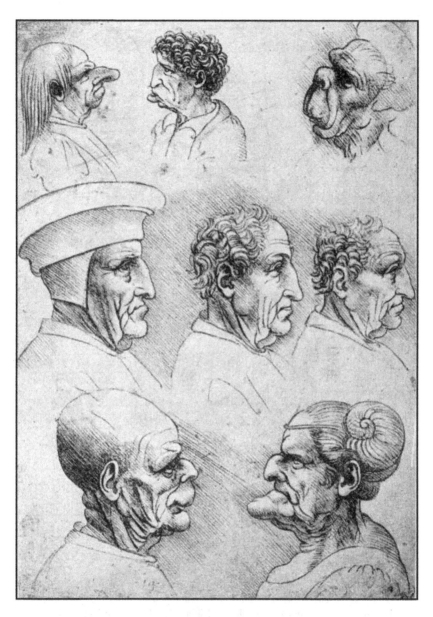

Figure 5.10 The origins of caricature: examples from the sketchbooks of Leonardo da Vinci, before 1500. Copyright Ilbusca/DigitalVision Vectors/Getty Images.

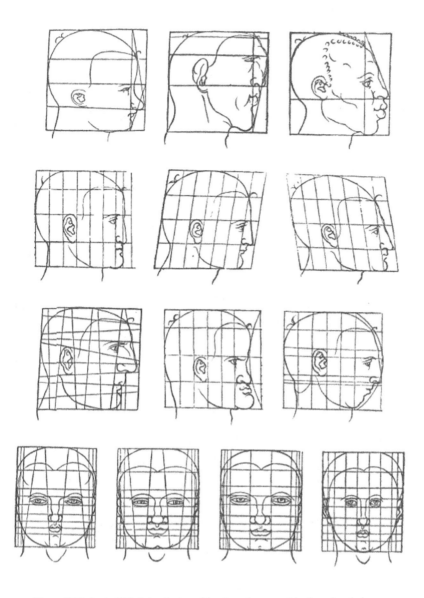

Figure 5.11 Just a little later, the transition to anthropometrics has already begun. These diagrams (compiled from Albrecht Dürer, *Vier Bücher von Menschlicher Proportion*, 1528) were intended as instruction.

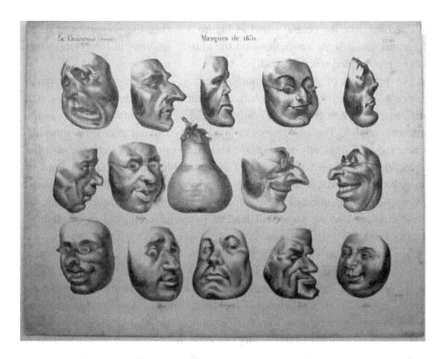

Figure 5.12 From about 300 years later than those, a bouquet of caricatures of French politicians: *Masques de 1831,* published in *La Caricature* in 1832 by Honoré Daumier. The fruit in the center is a symbol for the King of France at the time, Louis XVIII, whose face was indeed somewhat pear-shaped, but whom it was illegal to mock in this fashion. Courtesy of The Metropolitan Museum of Art, Gift of Louise Bechtel, 1958.

The preceding list of three requisites is just what GMM builds for you in a broad (but not unbounded) range of studies of organisms. GMM is a technology by which most of the questions we used to be able to ask and statistically answer about measured "extents" (lengths, areas, volumes) can now be asked and answered better by talking explicitly about shape as well.

5.1.1 Hints about the Limits of Geometric Morphometrics

Our morphometric questions are usually launched by diagrams that resemble figures from anatomy atlases. But not all of those pages are usable for our purpose. Owing to its dependence on multivariate linear statistics, the morphometrician's attention is necessarily limited to those aspects of anatomy that can be modeled by *continuous deformations* – those that do not require topological changes. If our representations are to take the schematic form of diagrams like the central panel in Figure 5.2, then the properties of those diagrams entail some restrictions on the sort of anatomical information that can be represented with their aid.

For purposes of geometric morphometrics, our instructions must be to *ignore all texture*, to *prohibit changes in the roster of visible objects*, and otherwise to *attach geometry to only those structures that have names in the anatomy atlases*. The basic observational entity driving geometric morphometrics is a biologically meaningful boundary (a curve, a surface) or a list of loci derivable from one or more of these boundaries. The manipulations of linear biometrics will be interpreted as *infinitely divisible, arbitrarily correlated changes in the location of these structures*. It is the covariance structure of these changes that we hope will lead us to useful biological or biomedical explanations.

The information encoded in boundary locations is a rather small fraction of the information content of interest to quantitative biology (cf. Cook et al., 2013). All the other formalisms of biological structure (e.g., textures, colors, energy flows, frequencies of inclusions, chemical and molecular components) are ignored unless imported separately via case labels or other data registers. You can think of the history of GMM, in general terms, as a sustained attempt to circumvent the difficulties for scientific explanation that follow from these omissions.

Then many pages of those atlases involve aspects of human variation that *cannot* be usefully treated by GMM methods.[1] Some aspects of our anatomy vary irreducibly in terms of branching order (Figure 5.13) or branching entanglement in three dimensions. Variations of the folding of the cortex of the human brain are analogous to the variations in Figure 5.13 – the subdivision by gyri and sulci beyond the first few is not stable over persons (Ono et al., 1990), and intense arguments can continue for decades about specific claims of homology (e.g., for *Homo floresiensis*). Other component organs simply vary too greatly to comport with our linear statistics (Figure 5.14), including, as every cosmetic plastic surgeon knows, the female breast. This is not just the case within species – even when homology can be granted, evolutionary variation of structures can be even greater than the variation shown for viscera in Figure 5.14. And sometimes the extension of one structure "along" or "over" another, while it can be modeled as an extent, nevertheless varies too greatly with respect to its neighbors for the composite to be usefully modeled as a

---

[1] The following discussion owes a great deal to Williams (1956), who first raised many of these issues in the larger context of biochemical variability before noting the analogy with the anatomical domain that was just beginning to be quantified via medical imaging.

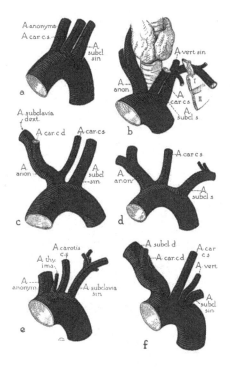

Branches of the aortic arch. Variation in the pattern of origin.

a and *b*, Common pattern; *c* and *d*, left common carotid artery from the innominate (long and short stem); *e*, separate origin of a thyreoidea ima artery; *f*, independent origin of a left vertebral.

Figure 5.13 Situations unsuited for GMM. (1) Topological variation of a branching structure. Reprinted from page 197 of *An Atlas of Human Anatomy*, by Barry J. Anson, copyright 1950, W. B. Saunders Co.

diffeomorphism (Figure 5.15). All these situations are thereby excluded from the domain of morphometrics to which this chapter is extending the methods of Chapters 2 through 4.

5.1.2 The Role of Words Today: The "Foundational Model for Anatomy"

As GMM begins with anatomical terminology, the place to begin a formal exposition is with the theory of that terminology. A clothbound book, *Terminologia Anatomica* (1998, 2011), operationalizes some 7,500 Latin terms in a format suitable for classes in medical anatomy. This resource is now online at http://www.unifr.ch/ifaa/. What proved more

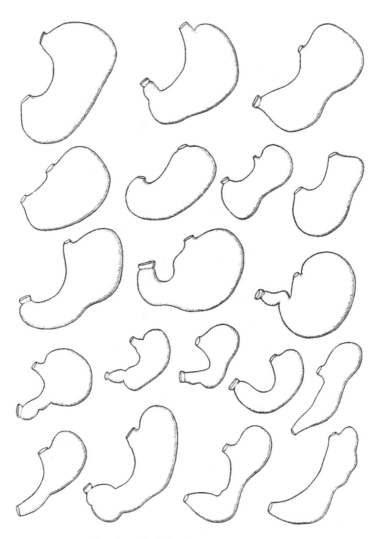

Stomach; variations in form. From laboratory specimens.

Figure 5.14 Situations unsuited for GMM. (2) Metrical variation an order of magnitude too large for the linear approximations of Chapters 2, 3, and 4: the normal range of human stomachs (left) and livers (right). Reprinted from pages 287–288 of *An Atlas of Human Anatomy*, by Barry J. Anson, copyright 1950, W. B. Saunders Co.

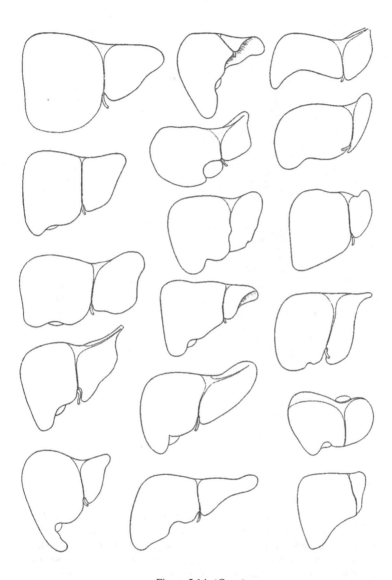

Figure 5.14 *(Cont.)*

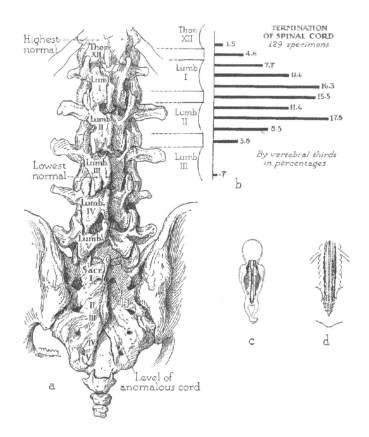

Vertebral level of termination of the spinal cord. Variation in the adult; fetal position.

a, Posterior aspect of the lumbosacral vertebral column in an adult. *b*, Graph, recording point of termination of the spinal cord in 129 specimens. *c*, Posterior aspect of the spinal cord, exposed by laminectomy, in a fetus of two and a half months. *d*, Lumbosacral area of the same specimen. The spinal cord occupies the entire length of the vertebral canal.

Figure 5.15 Situations unsuited for GMM. (3) Landmark locations on embryologically distinct structures such that their relative variations are incompatible with a smoothly deformable topology. (left) Spinal cord versus vertebral column, intrahuman variation. Reprinted from page 229 of *An Atlas of Human Anatomy*, by Barry J. Anson, copyright 1950, W. B. Saunders Co. (right) Bony skull versus superficial musculature. Arrows: effect of heterochrony, adult male gorilla to human infant, along the two shells. From Charles Oxnard and O'Higgins, "Biology Clearly Needs Morphometrics. Does Morphometrics Need Biology?" *Biological Theory*, 2009, figure 8, with permission of Springer.

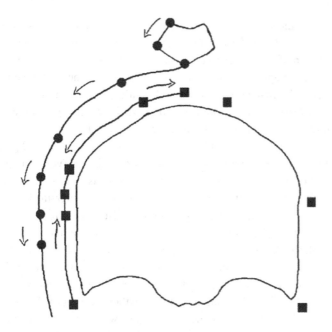

Composite diagram of all landmarks in Figure 5, columns (A)–(C), with the same conventions. Arrows indicate how the positions of the landmarks are related in the sequence from the large adult male gorilla to the human infant when the landmarks are considered as two separate shells.

Figure 5.15 *(Cont.)*

important was the so-called *foundational model of anatomy,* Cornelius Rosse's extension of *Terminologia* by incorporating the spatial relationships among these entities (in a list extended to some 75,000). See Rosse and Mejino (2001), or `http://sig.biostr.washington.edu/projects/fm/Publications.html`.

Today the main context for efforts of this sort is the construction of "ontologies" that serve the need of medical informatics more than the needs of organismal biologists. An ontology, in general, is a computer-readable directory of the uses of words across multiple disciplines that share an overlapping vocabulary. For instance, the concept of "aorta" ties together articles that deal with embryology, cardiovascular physiology, radiology, atherosclerosis, and aneurysms, and the concept of "retina" links discussions of its size and shape with aspects of its innervation, its ultrastructure, and its visual functions and dysfunctions, all as conveyed by the words used in article abstracts, figure captions, and the like. Thus a system like the one reported in Puget et al. (2012), ostensibly on the topic of spatial relations among anatomical entities, is actually about the *computerized retrieval of information about* such spatial relations, as embodied in "a semantic web service and spatial query processor." Here the notion of spatial relations is purely verbal, e.g., "anterior to," not the more quantitative approach via coordinates that will be the central concern of this chapter. (The potential transition to quantification for notions from this rhetoric was broached to theoretical biologists long ago by Jardine, 1969.) In a comment accompanying the Puget presentation, Rosse (2012) notes the direct relevance of discussions like theirs to the provenance of "a 3D graphical canonical human," but continues to subordinate the issues (which are deeper, in my view) of comparisons and explanations to the issues of navigation and identification more important to the surgeon or the lecturer in the anatomy dissection lab than to the biologist or anthropologist looking for patterns.

In other words, even today's best resources of "visible humans," however richly visualized, fail to articulate properly with the quantitative explanatory purposes that drive modern biometrics. Some additional structure needs to be attached. This overlay has a history of its own, beginning about a hundred years ago with the first European anthropology textbooks. Section 5.1.3 reviews the extension of anatomical nomenclature that was required – to the level of characterizing the individual measurement points (*Meßpunkte*) that we now call landmarks – and Section 5.1.4 reviews the consequent improvised system of shape measurement via "indices" (angles, proportions) that was not superseded by GMM until the 1990s.

5.1.3 From the Last Century, I: Standardizing Where We Point within an Image

The table of contents of Rudolf Martin's great classical treatise *Lehrbuch der Anthropologie in Systematischer Darstellung,* 1928, volume 2, "Kraniologie, Osteologie" (originally part of the one-volume edition of 1914), highlights the main localization tools exploited in the anthropometric praxis of the early twentieth century: planes and lines, standardized views (norma verticalis, norma basilaris, norma lateralis, norma frontalis, norma occipitalis, norma sagittalis), and a great diversity of points and lines in one or more of those standardized views. These loci had not arisen as parameters from anybody's theory of human evolution, growth, or variation. Instead they had accrued over the preceding several decades of applied anthropology to take advantage of chance aspects of local form in the course of specific anthropometric comparisons (ethnic groups, children versus adults, men versus women, extant versus fossil hominids). In this context, the role of the indices often turned out to be one of advocacy: to help convey the biologist's

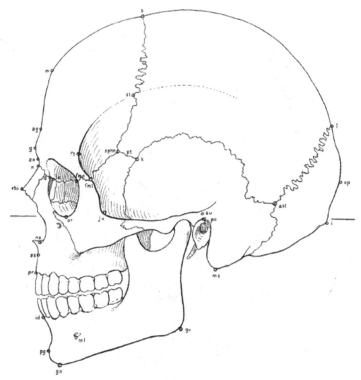

Fig. 286. Schädel in der Norma lateralis mit eingezeichneten Meßpunkten.

ast Asterion, *au* Auriculare, *b* Bregma, *d* Dakryon, *fmo* Frontomalare orbitale, *fmt* Fronto-malare temporale, *ft* Frontotemporale, *g* Glabella, *gn* Gnathion, *go* Gonion, *id* Infradentale, *i* Inion, *ju* Jugale, *k* Krotaphion, *la* Lakrimale, *l* Lambda, *ms* Mastoideale, *ml* Mentale, *m* Metopion, *n* Nasion, *ns* Nasospinale, *op* Opisthokranion, *or* Orbitale, *pg* Pogonion, *po* Porion, *pr* Prosthion, *pt* Pterion, *rhi* Rhinion, *sphn* Sphenion, *st* Stephanion, *ss* Sub-spinale, *sg* Supraglabellare, *so* Supraorbitale.

Figure 5.16 Two of Rudolf Martin's schemes for identifying potential landmark points in his six standard views. (left) Lateralis. (right) Frontalis.

pre-existing intuitions about anatomically global or regional similarity or dissimilarity of the forms on the table before him. One high point in their contemporary applications was the insights afforded for the understanding of the Neanderthals. For instance, the analyses in Gorjanović-Kramberger (1906) are based firmly in the kind of representations Martin was reviewing – see Figures 5.19–5.20.

The interested reader is urged to find a copy of Martin's treatise if only to marvel at the astonishing prescience of these figures, which were decades ahead of their time. Throughout organismal biology, in agreement with Martin's emphasis, landmarks are typically characterized in the standard views – Martin conveys 68 of these points in seven drawings. (In other fields,

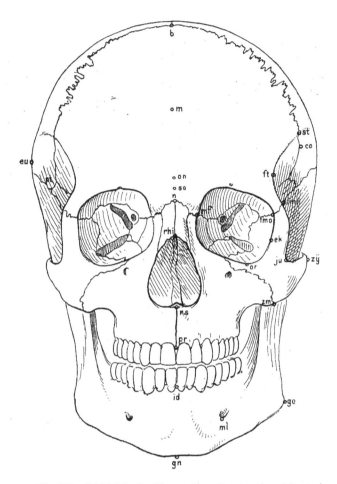

Fig. 290. Schädel in der Norma frontalis mit eingezeichneten Meßpunkten.

b Bregma, *co* Coronale, *ek* Ektokonchion, *eu* Euryon, *fmo* Frontomalare orbitale, *fmt* Frontomalare temporale, *ft* Frontotemporale, *gn* Gnathion, *mf* Maxillofrontale, *ml* Mentale, *m* Metopion, *go* Gonion, *id* Infradentale, *ju* Jugale, *n* Nasion, *ns* Nasospinale, *on* Ophryon, *or* Orbitale, *pr* Prosthion, *pt* Pterion, *rhi* Rhinion, *st* Stephanion, *so* Supraorbitale, *zy* Zygion, *zm* Zygomaxillare.

Figure 5.16 *(Cont.)*

like micropaleontology, the characterization is by overlays on photographs instead, and, in radiology, by arrows pointing to variably fuzzy features of real images.) Many of the constructions lie in the midsagittal plane (not surprisingly, in view of the role of the midcurve in landmark definitions), but surprisingly many points appear in two, three, or even four of Martin's plates.

Martin did not formalize any protocol by which points emerged from drawings of this sort. Over the ensuing century, the erection of a scheme for them required a detour from the geometry of points to the geometry of curves, as follows. (Either way, we are not yet aligned with the somewhat different purposes of the "ontology" that was the concern of Rosse in the preceding section.)

5.1.3.1 Curves

Although Martin seems never to have noticed this, it is crucial for today's routine applications that nearly all of Martin's 68 points actually arise on *curves*. Based on this observation, a few years ago (Weber and Bookstein, 2011, chapter 4) I suggested a new formalism that places the processing of curves logically prior to the processing of discrete points that may lie upon them. This affords a tighter link between the language of curves and the language of measurement than seemed needed in Martin's day, and also serves as an *aperçu* to the present, when curves themselves are extracted with equal celerity from surface representations as from the actual interior boundaries visualized in CT or MR images. Specific reference to **types of curves** (a typology that Martin does not invoke) augments the list of landmark points per se by constructions that account for curves or surfaces and for symmetry in more flexible ways than were classically available. The landmarks are the same, but we have changed the language of their statistical combination, and also incorporated information from the locations in-between the landmarks, all in a principled way.

It is convenient to sort the range of curves into three types with different origins in image geometry and different protocols for landmark point extraction: observed curves, ridge lines, and symmetry curves.

Observed curves generally arise as intersections of two actual biological surfaces or of one smooth surface with a standardized plane, or as centerlines of extended tubular structures.

> *Examples* (from the human skull). Sutures; outlines in the standard planes; center of the spinal canal, nerves.

Ridge curves, also called "crest lines" in the medical imaging literature, are curves of points at each of which the *perpendicular* curvature is a local maximum along that perpendicular direction.

> *Examples.* Brow ridge, foramen magnum, mandibular line, alveolar ridge (at a specific range of scales), auditory meatus, orbits, pyriform aperture.

Symmetry curves, introduced in Bookstein et al. (2001), are a new construction borrowed from medical imaging (specifically, from brain imaging) to handle curves on medial surfaces with greater precision than is possible using the language of "a midsagittal plane." A symmetry curve is an ordinary smooth curve together with a perpendicular direction at every point such that every plane through that direction looks (approximately) symmetric in the vicinity of the curve.

Examples. Symphysis, falx, aspects of neuroanatomy "in the midplane," postcranial medial structures, deformed midline (in the synostoses).

5.1.3.2 Six Types of Landmark Points

In one convenient typology the roster of conventional landmark points may be divided into six types intended to replace the three types set out in Bookstein (1991). The new classification corresponds to different operational origins of the points upon the curve or curves on which they lie.

Type 1: discrete juxtapositions of tissues. Good points can be defined by the intersection of three surfaces in space, a curve and a surface through which it passes, or any other combination of constraints on Cartesian coordinates that add up to the correct count. Centers of "sufficiently small" inclusions serve as valid landmarks in 2D, in 3D, and in the 2D surfaces of 3D objects.

Type 2: extremes of curvature characterizing a single structure. For data that arise directly in the form of curves, whether in 2D or in 3D, these are the points classically called "vertices" (extremes of one-dimensional curvature). For data arising as surfaces in 3D, these are usually the extrema of directional or Gaussian curvature: peaks, points, pits, or passes.

Type 3: landmark points characterized locally by information from multiple curves and by symmetry. *3a.* Intersection of a ridge curve and the midcurve on the same surface. These are points at which a structure characterized by a sharp fold of the surface, like foramen magnum, cuts the midsurface: the point at which that structure is itself symmetric with respect to its own (local) midline. *3b.* Intersection of an observed curve and the midcurve. The observed curve may be a self-contained curve in space, like the posterior border of the hard palate, or it may be itself a curve on a surface, such as any of the curves that try to follow a centerline of the dental occlusion. *3c.* Intersection of a ridge curve and an observed curve on the same surface. These typically arise where an extended anatomical boundary surface, such as a suture, crosses a ridge curve.

Type 4: Semilandmarks on curves. These points are the subject of a recent advance in Procrustes analysis (Bookstein, 1997; Bookstein et al., 1999) that we will describe at length in Section 5.5.4. Semilandmarks are matched between specimens under control of some global energy term, such as the bending energy of the thin-plate spline; typically this computation is with respect to a sample Procrustes average. The number of semilandmarks needs to be sufficient to capture the spatial nature of variation or covariation that will ultimately emerge from multivariate analysis of their shape coordinates.

Type 5: Semilandmarks on surfaces. These points have been the subject of intensive experimentation by the "Vienna–Leipzig morphometrics working group" since about 2000. Semilandmarks constrained to surfaces can slide with respect to any combination of point landmarks and curve semilandmarks.

Type 6: Constructed semilandmarks. This is a portmanteau category collecting various familiar loci that appear not to qualify for any of the preceding categories. It includes projections of one structure onto another, construction points yielding places that curves can be deemed to "start" or "finish" for digitizing purposes, places where some curve comes nearest to another, loci of greatest width of bilaterally symmetric structures, and other special circumstances.

5.1.3.3 Recent Examples

Riolo et al. (1974), present growth curves of some 200 scalar measurements derived from the scheme of 45 points in Figure 5.17. I have previously critiqued this specific measurement system in Moyers and Bookstein (1979) for its inheritance of many of the less desirable features of Martin's method, including arbitrary choices from the set of loci that could actually be defined unambiguously on histological grounds and the absence of any coherent protocol for a transformation to measurements. A new problem, not inherited from Martin, arises via the origin of these data in transmission radiographs, not surface representations: the emergence of points like #36, #40, #42, or #43 that represent features of curving surfaces that do not reduce to points at all. (Here, #42 is a double tangent and #43 a quadruply tangent line, while #36 is the intersection of one curve along the midplane with a bundle of tangents from a bilateral feature, and #40, "Orbitale," seems not really to have a 3D operational definition.) There are also "points" like #28 that lie in air, not on the skull. Point #11 likewise never had any operational definition at all, not even according to the original authors. For deeper discussion along these lines see Bookstein (2016a).

More recently, one large federally funded US research project called CAESAR (for "Civilian American and European Surface Anthropometry

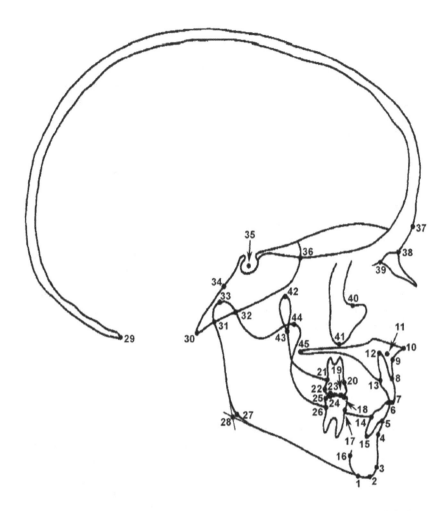

Figure 5.17 A typical modern version of Martin's suggestion: system of 45 points from a typical "lateral cephalogram tracing" of the head of an orthodontic patient. Notice that these points do not lie on any single plane; those that are not midsagittal are actually averages of bilateral pairs. Most points lie upon curved lines in the tracing, but many of those curves do not actually exist on the bony skull ostensibly being traced. See text. From Riolo, M. L., Moyers, R. E., McNamara, J. A. Jr., Hunter, W. S., *An Atlas of Cranofacial Growth,* Monograph 2, Cranofacial Growth Series, Center for Human Growth and Development, University of Michigan, 1974, with permission.

Resource" – quite a baroque acronym) has attempted to build an archive of some dozens of measured extents over a data base of many thousand body surfaces that together comprise an approximately representative sample of the contemporary US population (see Robinette, Daanen, and Paquet, 1999;

Harrison and Robinette, 2002). The extension to so huge a sample is at the cost of detail in the surface representations so averaged. As of this writing, and in spite of very suggestive experiments such as Allen et al. 2003), there do not yet seem to be such representative samples for more than a very few purposes of applied anthropology (e.g., protection of the faces or the heads of soldiers [D. E. Slice, personal communication, 2014], or standardized garment sizing).

By accepting the criteria whose violations are noted in critiques such as those in the preceding paragraph, we can learn what makes a version likelier to withstand such criticisms. A landmark configuration should be designed as a coherent whole, balanced in its coverage of spatial details but also incorporating enough global information to be used in support of a wide range of explanations, not just the group differences or growth gradients that you think are your principal topic of analysis. For a list to make sense, each landmark, individually, must be operationally defined to sufficient spatial accuracy upon any form where it appears. But it is not enough to treat the landmarks individually. The set of all those participating in any analysis, whether point landmarks, semilandmarks, or a mix, needs to make sense both as a data set of Procrustes shape coordinates (Section 5.4) and as the nodes of a thin-plate spline deformation (Section 5.5). For instance, landmarks can never "coincide" (or the spline cannot be computed beginning from that form, and the grid is necessarily folded in transformations *to* that form): points that are in different locations in any form can never have the same location in any other form that will be deformed into it. Curves must be homologous as biological structures from specimen to specimen of a data set, or from species to species. And landmarks must be distributed relatively evenly over the area and especially the circumference of the form, to escape the pathologies of centering and scaling that will be dissected at Figure 5.57.

5.1.4 From the Last Century, II: The Origin of Morphometric Quantifications

From a concern with point locations per se we move on to consider the ways that specific quantifications can emerge from those systems. In this respect the pioneers of morphometrics were on somewhat firmer ground. They generally adapted existing methods of descriptive geometry, an engineering technology for annotating blueprints that had proven its usefulness since the days of Denis Diderot's *Encyclopédie*. The quantifications that applied to those drawings included distances of points to points, distances of points to lines or curves, areas, angles, radii of curvature, and a few other primary measurements that were directly relevant to the construction of physical objects (components of machines or buildings) or the engineering assessment of their strength or suitability for an intended function.

Martin himself, although limited by the statistical technology of his time mostly to averages and standard deviations – he eschewed, among other notions, the Pearson correlation that had been common in British biometrics for some time already – showed no analogous limits in his primary quantifications. Direct measures were plotted by their operational definitions directly on his canonical views, while the formulas for many other quantities were written out explicitly as ratios among pairs of these primary measurements (see Figure 5.18). In so doing, Martin attempted to incorporate nearly every quantity that anyone had ever mentioned in the literature of the late nineteenth and early twentieth centuries as ever applying to any reasonable comparison of fossil or recent bones of children or adults. In other words, the impetus to speak directly to evolutionary explanations was present even though no grammar for such comparisons existed yet. I have excerpted a particularly interesting application, Gorjanović-Kramberger's analysis of *"Homo primigenius"* (his suggested name for the Krapina [Croatia] Neanderthals), in Figures 5.19–5.20. We see an earnest attempt to hint at group differences but no protocol for the generation of these formulas and no rules of multivariate inference. In the 1920s and 1930s, Mahalanobis and others developed much of the core of today's multivariate biometry in the course of establishing a rigorous language for *statistical* inference based in such data. A combined rhetoric fusing the statistical (variation) with the biometric (formulation of quantities in the first place) had to wait for my work toward the end of the century.

Martin offers no protocol by which these rosters of indices can be generated or, more importantly, winnowed. If there are m multiple candidates for a distance measure, such as "height above the earhole,"[2] and likewise n alternate

---

[2] Of which one commonly encountered realization is vertical distance as measured from that Frankfurt Horizontal (which Martin calls the "Ohr–Augen Ebene," the ear–eye plane). In Martin's day, the principal role of these planes was as baselines for perpendicular measurements. The alternate interpretation as rules for *registration*, meaning coordinate transformations for following the repositioning of particular landmarks or curves, did not emerge as a community theme until later, in projects such as Biegert (1957) or Delattre and Fenart (1960). Separately this orientation played a role in the emergence in 1931 of the *Broadbent–Bolton* system for three-dimensionalization of head measurements by simultaneous two-plane cephalometry, including defining precisely what was meant by a frontal projection as captured by photograph or radiograph. (This was the system generating the landmarks viewed in Figure 5.90, for example.) The illusion that registrations permit the reporting of landmark-specific changes as displacements did not survive the formalization of shape coordinates in the 1980s and 1990s, which involved, among other observations, the realization that in the absence of strong prior knowledge any such analysis inextricably entangled the "moving" and the "fixed" structures. The critique of registration rules in general is implicit in analyses such as Figures 5.57–5.58, while the remedy, the explicit construction of measurements that align with particular contrasts, is the subject of the tensor formalism for uniform transformations (Section 5.3) and then the thin-plate splines (Section 5.5). Regarding the nonexistence of the Frankfurt Horizontal plane per se, see Bookstein (2016a).

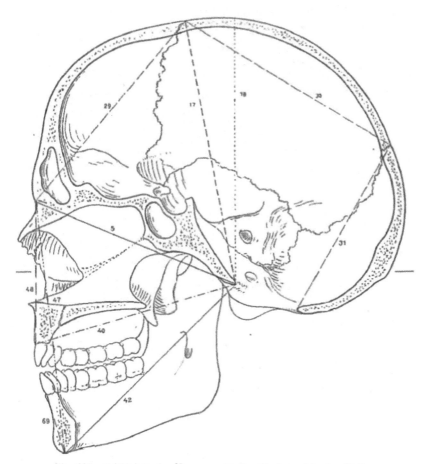

Fig. 295. Schädel in der Norma sagittalis mit eingezeichneten Maßen.

Figure 5.18 Overview of Rudolf Martin's general approach to morphometry.
(left) Each standard view (cf. Figure 5.16) sustains a collection of systems of
primary quantification – distances between points, distances of points from lines,
angles among lines. (right) From the distances arise collections of "indices" that
are computed as ratios of distances, and also categories created by arbitrary cuts
within the range of the indices or the measured angles.

candidates for a measure of skull length, then there will be mn candidates for
a "length-height ratio." In the absence of graphical evidence (cf. Figures 5.48,
5.49) conveying the extent of information transfer to some domain exogenous
to morphometrics, it is unclear how the biologist is supposed to select among
these alternatives.

Längenhöhen-Index (JAGDHOLD):

$$= \frac{\text{Gesamthöhe } [18\ (1)] \times 100}{\text{Größte Schädellänge } [1]}$$

chamaekran   x—72,9
orthokran   73,0—77,9
hypsikran   78,0—x

Breitenhöhen-Index des Schädels (Indice transverso-vertical):

$$= \frac{\text{Basion-Bregma-Höhe } [17] \times 100}{\text{Größte Schädelbreite } [8]}$$

Einteilung:

tapeinokephal (besser tapeinokran)   x—91,9
metriokephal (,,   metriokran)   92,0—97,9
akrokephal (,:   akrokran)   98,0—x

Andere Einteilungen:
eurykran   x— 95,0
mesoeurykran   95,1—100,0
stenokran   101,0—x   (v. TÖRÖK)

Ferner:

ultrabrachystenokephal   x— 89,9
hyperbrachystenokephal   90,0— 94,9
brachystenokephal   95,0— 99,9
orthostenokephal   100,0—104,9
hypsistenokephal   105,0—109.9
hyperhypsistenokephal   110,0—114,9
ultrahypsistenokephal   115,0—x   (DAVIS, WELCKER)

Gelegentlich sind auch andere Höhen als die Basion-Bregma-Höhe zur Berechnung dieses Index benützt worden.

Längen-Ohr-Bregma-Höhen-Index des Schädels (Auriculo-vertical-Index):

$$= \frac{\text{Ohr-Bregma-Höhe } [20] \times 100}{\text{Größte Schädellänge } [1]}$$

Einteilung:

chamaekephal (besser chamaekran)   x—57,9
orthokephal (,,   orthokran)   58,0—62,9
hypsikephal (,,   hypsikran)   63,0—x

G (I) = 1,0; G (I₁—I₂) = 1,4 × G (I) = 1,4.

Breiten-Ohr-Bregma-Höhen-Index:

$$= \frac{\text{Ohr-Bregma-Höhe } [20] \times 100}{\text{Größte Schädelbreite } [1]}$$

Einteilung:

tapeinokran =   x—79,9   (JAGDHOLD).
metriokran = 80,0—85,9
akrokran = 86,0—x.

Als Variante ist auch häufig verwendet worden:

$$= \frac{\text{Ganze Ohrhöhe } [21] \times 100}{\text{Gerade Schädellänge } [1a]}$$

Figure 5.18 *(Cont.)*

From these historical examples it may be useful to turn to one of the running examples of this book, the Vilmann data on rodent neurocranial growth.

As an initial guess at a quantification in imitation of Martin's style, Section 2.6 considered the net area of this form of eight landmarks for each

Ein Vergleich dieser Dimensionen, Indices und Winkel mit solchen an rezenten und bekannten fossilen (diluvialen) Menschenschädeln wird uns am besten über den Typus des Krapinaer-Schädels belehren. Ich werde zu diesem Zwecke unsere Ausmaße mit denjenigen Schwalbes über den Schädel von Neandertal und den Angaben desselben Autors über den Schädel von Spy II vergleichend vorführen:

	Rezent	Spy II.	Krapina	Neander
			Millimeter	
Glabella-Inion Länge:	—	—	197,5	199,0
Längen-Breiten-Index:	—	81,1	85,5	79,0
Kalotten-Höhe:	84,0	87,0	83,5	80.5
Kalotten-Höhe-Index:	52,3—68,9	44,3	42,2	40,4
Lambda-Kalottenhöhe-Index:	29,4—43,0	31,3	29,3	29,4
Lageindex des Bregma:	22,2—35,2	35,2	31,8	38,4
Differenz d. Glabella-Inion u. d. Glabella-Lambda-Länge:	—	7,0	17,0	14,0
Frontobiorbital-Index:	82,9—über 90	87,9	87,3	88,8
Stirnwinkel:	78—110°	67°	66°	62°
Bregmawinkel:	53°	50,5°	50°	44°
Lambdawinkel:	78—85°	—	65°	66,5°
Opisthionwinkel:	31—40°	—	57°	51,5°

Diese Tabelle belehrt uns, daß unser rekonstruierter Schädel D zweifellos der Art *Homo primigenius* angehört, und daß er zwischen den Schädeln des Neandertalers und des Spy II steht. Bemerkenswert ist jedenfalls seine große Breite, resp. dessen Längen-Breiten-Index mit 85,5. Nachdem aber auch unser C-Schädel einen hohen derartigen Wert mit 83,7 aufweist, müssen wir annehmen, daß der Homo von Krapina jedenfalls einen breiteren Schädel als der Mensch von Neandertal und Spy II besaß. Doch bilden alle diese diluvialen Schädel eine kontinuierliche Reihe allmählich breiter werdender Schädel, wovon der Neandertaler der längste, der Krapina-D-Schädel der breiteste war. Bezüglich der übrigen Verhältnisse aber schließt sich unser rekonstruierter Schädel dem Spy II an.

Figure 5.19 A typical application of Martin's style of methodology: one of Gorjanović-Kramberger's (1906:119) comparisons of his specimens of "Homo primigenius" from Krapina with other instances of Neanderthals known by that time and with "recent" *H. sapiens*. The list of measurements is presented without any justification.

of the 144 outlines of the complete data subset. By studying the extent to which interlandmark distances could predict a biotheoretically important quantity (the apparent extent of brain tissue in this view), Figure 3.32 managed to reduce this list of 28 distances to just two. Section 4.2.2, continuing with the comparative analysis of multiple candidate distances, demonstrated principal component analysis by examining the patterns of covariation of all 28 of these transects at the same time. Neither of these approaches proved

Tabellarische Übersicht

der

Ausmaasse einiger wichtigeren diluvialen Unterkiefer.

	Malar-naud	d'Arcy	La Nau-lette	Spy I.	Ochos	Krapina D	E	F	G	H	J
Höhe an der Symphyse	26,0	28,0	31,0	38,0	–	33	35,0	c. 31,0	30,4—31,5	40	42,3
Höhe beim M₂	22,0	24,0	23,0	33,0	–	c. 28	24,1	–	28,0	33 - 34,3	32,2
Dicke an der Symphyse	13,0	15,5	14,0	15,0	18,0	13,6	13,1	14,5	14,1	15,4	15,0
Dicke beim M₂	15,0	17,0	16,0	14,0	–	–	–	–	14,9	–	–
Dicke unter dem C	–	–	–	–	–	–	14,1	16,7	14,8; 15,5	16,4	–
Entfernung der Außenränder der M₂	–	–	–	–	–	–	–	–	–	70,9	77,0
„ „ „ M₁	–	–	–	66,0	–	–	–	–	–	66,5	74,0
Gerade Entfernung der mittleren Berührungsfläche der J von der distalen Fläche des M₃ . . .	–	–	–	60,0	65,0	–	–	–	–	65,5	64,0
Abstand d. Mittelpunkte d. Condyli untereinander	–	–	–	–	–	–	–	–	–	–	121,8
„ „ „ v. d. Incisiven	–	–	–	–	–	–	–	–	–	–	c. 125,0
Höhe des Proc. coronoideus über der Basis . .	–	–	–	–	–	–	–	–	–	–	73,0
Breite des Ramus in der Mitte (geringste Breite)	–	–	–	–	–	–	–	–	–	–	37,0
„ „ „ beim Condylus (größte Breite)	–	–	–	–	–	–	–	–	–	–	44,4
„ „ „ in den Winkeln	–	–	–	–	–	–	–	–	–	–	38,3—40,0
M₁ { lang	–	–	–	–	11,5; 12	11,0	12,9	–	12,3	11,3; 11,5	11,4—11,0
M₁ { breit	–	–	–	–	10,0; 11	10,6	12,1	–	11,4	10,9; 11,0	11,3—11,1
M₂ { lang	–	–	–	–	12,0; 12	10	12,8	–	12,6	12,0; 11,6	11,5—12,5
M₂ { breit	–	–	–	–	11,0; 11	–	11,5	–	11,4	11,5; 11,5	12,2—11,6
M₃ { lang	–	–	–	–	12	–	–	–	11,6	12,2; 12,0	11,6
M₃ { breit	–	–	–	–	11	–	–	–	10,0	10,8; 10,5	c. 10,3

Figure 5.20 The same for the lower jaw, with the same typical motley of measurements and specimens. From Gorjanović-Kramberger (1906:167). The word "Ausmaasse" in the table title is a misprint for "Ausmasse," meaning "extents" or "dimensions."

powerful enough to properly assess the geometric organization of this data set. (Figure 2.43, for instance, is meaningless without the template in Figure 2.41 that indicates the placement of these eight endpoints on a typical form.) So, rather than the presentation in that figure, which wastes the two-dimensionality of the paper, we explore a representation (Figure 5.21) that sets out growth ratios of every separate interlandmark segment over pairs of ages from the data set (a range of 28 choices, the same number as the choice of landmark transects, because the count of ages happens to be the same as the count of landmarks).

The hundreds of indices Rudolf Martin offered were assembled seemingly without any system. Nowadays we are not so restricted in our choices: our computers can examine thousands or millions all at once, then sort the results for salience in order to winnow the list down. Before we leave this domain of what is now called "traditional morphometrics" (see Marcus, 1990), it is instructive to touch on Martin's other theme, the selection of indices (most of which were ratios) to serve as evidence in the course of scientific arguments. Over in this domain the problem is not computation, but choice. From just eight landmarks, for instance, there are 378 possible distance-ratios among

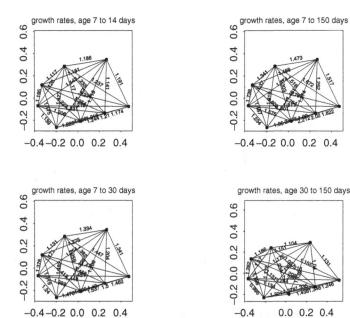

Figure 5.21 Growth ratios along all possible interlandmark distances for four different time intervals in the development of the Vilmann neurocranial octagons. Borrowing from a technique to be introduced later, each one is drawn on a graph corresponding to the Procrustes average shape for its starting age class. Analysis of the extremes among the printed ratios is the focus of the elementary technique known as EDMA, for Euclidean Distance Matrix Analysis. In general it is much less efficient than the techniques to be introduced later in this chapter (this point will be argued explicitly in Section 5.2.4).

combinations of various points (756, if you also count their reciprocals) and also 168 distinct three-point angles. From this riot of possibilities I extract just two to indicate the general nature of the problem he was facing.

Figure 5.22 demonstrates Martin's approach in a way that elucidates our problem particularly well. At left is shown the *aspect ratio* of these forms, the ratio of height to width, both directions defined by the extreme landmarks along the cranial base. The analysis at right corresponds to one version of the classic "orthocephalization ratio," length of the top of the calva in relation to the length of that same cranial base. Hence the two ratios have the same denominator.

The displays here agree in the general description of the growth trend in these aspects of "shape." They differ, however, both in the specific timing of their secular decline (fastest earlier? or later?) and in the pattern of age-by-age

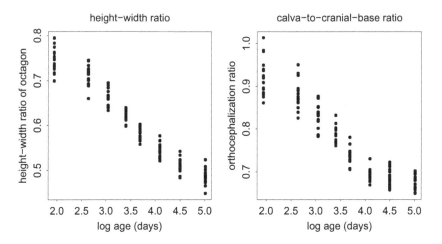

Figure 5.22 Continuing to analyze the rat growth data after the fashion of Martin: two arbitrarily selected indices. See text.

variances superimposed over those declines (the notion of *canalization,* which is proving of increasing interest for evo-devo biologists right now). We cannot tell if one of these candidate indices is more informative than the other. More crucially, we cannot yet produce formally optimal descriptors of whatever processes we have reason to believe are working to govern data resources like these. To do so we will need to exploit to a far greater extent a technology that was barely imagined (except by one eccentric expert, Karl Pearson) at the time Martin was compiling his treatise: the multivariate approach introduced in Chapter 4. To use it, however, we will need to replace Martin's discipline of multiple measured *lengths* by a modern technology that centers instead on a replacement of the whole idea of point locations as delimiters of segments. The function of a landmark point is no longer as a spot for placement of the endpoint of a dividers (or, for Figure 5.7, a flexible measuring tape); it is as a location whose explicit Cartesian coordinates are to be archived for later reference via the once-novel technology of *digitizing.*

The technology of linear statistical modeling will supersede Martin's improvised recourse to distances in great part by organizing the discussion of those distances – by offering ways to specify more generally the combinations of distances we should be most concerned with for specific explanatory contexts. For instance, we will see in Section 5.2 that there are special advantages to combining distances like these in orthogonal pairs, because, loosely speaking, if one of the distances bears the lowest ratio over some comparison of interest, then the orthogonal one will bear a ratio close to the highest, and vice versa. Even if we could expedite the generation of those extreme ratios, however, we see that they vary from segment to segment over the duration of the growth processes reviewed here. Compare the 7-to-30-day chart for growth ratios of those rodent skulls with the 30-to-150-day chart, for instance (Figure 5.21, bottom row). Extrema of growth rate are not in the same locations between these frames. Should we therefore emphasize more holistic measures, like the "net" change of cranial base length, weighted average of the three subsegmental rates along the bottom of the diagram? Likewise, for a net measure of change of "height," should we somehow try to average the transects that run more or less vertically? Questions like these will have no useful answers until we liberate ourselves from this language of "primary measurements," the interlandmark distances, and replace them by the much more flexible schemes of shape coordinates introduced in the next three sections.

In other words, even though we can highlight distances that show the greatest and least rates of change among our 28, we are still not making enough progress. The information in these distance measurements does not "speak for itself" in any biologically meaningful sense. We need a method that **combines information about the typical landmark configuration with information about its patterns of change,** a method that makes sense both analytically and graphically. Only such a method is capable of bringing a stronger order to the representation of our questions – an order that is grounded in the scenario generating our measurements, the spacing of those eight landmarks along growth trajectories of Vilmann's 18 rats.

Why is D'Arcy Thompson's notion of "Cartesian transformations" absent from this survey? The knowledgeable reader might be startled that chapter XVII, "On the theory of transformations, or the comparison of related forms," of D'Arcy Thompson's celebrated book-length essay, *On Growth and Form* (1917, 1961), goes unmentioned in the survey of techniques and iconic images just concluded. Many earlier discussions of computational anatomy, including the review I myself wrote in the course of my doctoral dissertation (Bookstein, 1978), reproduce some of Thompson's figures, often the "deformation" of the porcupinefish *Diodon* into the sunfish *Mola,* and thereafter attempt to account for much of the subsequent century of developments in morphometrics as a response to the impetus of his ideas.

I now believe that such an attribution is inappropriate. While this book is not the right place for an extended argument along these lines (see Bookstein, Khambay, et al., 2017), a brief summary might not be amiss. Thompson's thesis was that a good grid diagram will permit, as a "comparatively easy task," an assessment of "the direction and magnitude of the force capable of effecting the required transformation" (Thompson 1961;272). Assume that "the form of the entire structure under investigation should be found to vary in a more or less uniform manner, after the fashion of an approximately homogeneous and isotropic body ... and that our structure vary in its entirety, or at least that 'independent variants' should be relatively few" (ibid., 274). Then, if diverse and dissimilar fishes [or other organisms] can be referred as a whole to identical functions of very different co-ordinate systems, this fact will of itself constitute a proof that variation had proceeded on definite and orderly lines, that a comprehensive 'law of growth' has pervaded the whole structure in its integrity, and that some more or less simple and recognisable system of forces has been in control. It will not only show how real and deep-seated is the phenomenon of 'correlation,' in regard to form, but it will also demonstrate the fact that a correlation which had seemed too complex for analysis or comprehension is, in many cases, capable of very simple graphical expression. (ibid., 275–276; emphasis in the original)

Thompson's key idea, then, was to work with pairs of drawings of organisms rather than with measurements. To show the comparison, Thompson would draw a grid of vertical and horizontal lines over the picture of one organism in some orientation, then deform these verticals and horizontals over the picture of a second organism so that grid blocks that corresponded graphically would roughly correspond morphologically as well. He liked to interpret these graphical patterns via a metaphor, the explanation of form change as the result of a "system of forces."

The problem is that the method does not result in biological insights, quantitative or otherwise. As Peter Medawar (1958:231) said long ago, "The reason why D'Arcy's method has been so little used in practice (only I and one or two others have tried to develop it at all) is because it is analytically unwieldy." Thompson's examples often involve ludicrously distorted forms (e.g., the "human skull" on page 318 of the 1961 edition) or systematically misrepresent the matching of identifiable locations between the grids of a pair. But when diagrams are produced with adequate care (Sokal and Sneath, 1963:83), "not only are the grid lines deformed in several ways, but the deformation is different in different parts." In other words, when these grids are accurate, they cannot be reduced to cogent verbal or numerical reports; when they are legible, it is because they are inaccurate.

As Medawar had put it fourteen years earlier (Medawar 1944:139), "the purpose of [Thompson's] analysis is primarily and fundamentally descriptive. The need for an accurate technique of descriptive analysis is justified by the belief that a knowledge of *what happens* in any physiological process should precede an inquiry into how it comes about." (Emphasis in the original.) And "how it comes about" is a matter of endless details, not integral summaries. Any comparison of biological shapes must go forward at *multiple scales simultaneously* – but such comparisons do not conform to Thompson's thesis of variation "in a more or less uniform manner, after the fashion of an approximately homogeneous and isotropic body."

Thompson was concerned with outline drawings, but GMM deals with landmark configurations, which are a far more stylized measurement channel; Thompson attended to the shape and spacing of the coordinate curves per se, but GMM concerns the little grid cells per se as they deviate from the sizes and shapes of their neighbors; Thompson was interested in pairs of forms, whereas GMM embraces analysis of patterns across samples of arbitrarily many landmark configurations. To Thompson there is only one Cartesian transformation per biological comparison, and it *is* the explanation; whereas in GMM, you will learn by the end of this chapter, transformations are considered in groups, as sets of mutually helpful diagrams that might lead the investigator to explanations later that take the form of group comparisons, trends, growth gradients (or their complement, the focal transformations), responses to variations of the environment, or any other coherently reported cause. What our grids have in common with Thompson's is this powerful cognitive property of *suggesting* explanations. The price of preserving that cognitive power was transferring the technique out of Thompson's naïve setting, the single organism-to-organism comparison, into the rigorous context of statistical signal processing.

For all these reasons, this book does not attribute any important aspect of the foundation of geometric morphometrics to D'Arcy Thompson's *On Growth and Form*. He did not anticipate any of the technologies that drive our actual computations, nor the rhetoric by which we report our typical findings and the corresponding explanations. In light of today's understandings of the actual evolutionary and developmental mechanisms that produce organismal form, anatomical insight needs to be supplied reductionistically, not holistically; today's GMM does not draw from Thompson's practice in any meaningful way.

Summary of Section 5.1

- In addition to its algebraic, geometric, and statistical machinery, geometric morphometrics draws from the knowledge base and terminology of comparative anatomy and from the art and visual psychology of caricature.
- The anatomical structures best suited to a GMM analysis are those that vary in extent, not in presence–absence, meristics, seriation (sequence along an outline or an axis), or topology, and for which the analyst can ignore histology or its imaging equivalent except where it underlies the delineation of anatomical boundaries.
- The biology informing landmark points is the biology of the curves or surfaces upon which they have been specified.
- Originally the "G" of GMM, the geometry, was limited to the simplest measurements, distances and angles among two or three points at a time. These could show trends or group differences, but there were no protocols for generating them from drawings or for organizing them into lists.

5.2 Pattern Descriptors for Landmarks Taken Three at a Time

Historically, geometric morphometrics emerged as a bridge between the two pillars of Martin's methodology, the locations of landmarks and the statistics of "indices." It was constructed in two phases: a first version emphasizing configurations of three landmarks only (Bookstein 1984), and a second generalizing these constructions from three landmarks to "many" (Bookstein, 1986; Marcus et al., 1996). The methods for analysis of triangles are simpler than those that apply to the general case and so are better for reports and diagrams whenever they lead to satisfactory pattern analyses and explanations.

These simpler methods were developed in two parallel variants. One approach, the subject of Section 5.2.1, remained within the general domain of "indices" but turned explicitly to the specification problem, constructing optimal selections of those distances for the numerator and denominator of ratios, or, equivalently, optimal selections of angles to show either the maximum contrast or else precisely zero contrast across the poles of a comparison. The other approach to triangles, the subject of Section 5.2.2, skipped first to a thrust that was not present in Martin's archive, the construction of a biometric space of new variables from which the interesting distances or other indices could be extracted by statistical, not necessarily geometric, methods. Shapes of the same landmark triangles can be re-expressed as ordered pairs of two new variables, the *two-point* or *Bookstein shape coordinates*, that submit to direct applications of the methods of Chapters 2, 3, and 4. Bookstein (1991), the earliest monograph on this new GMM, emphasized both of these thrusts equally, as Procrustes coordinates (Section 5.4) had not yet been properly understood as the more symmetric (hence more powerful) solution to the second problem, the generation of a *shape space* that brought with it a mathematically tractable metric (a formula for distance between any two shapes). Discussion of whether the formula is also *biologically* meaningful is deferred until Section 5.6.8.

5.2.1 Tensors as Morphometric Pattern Descriptors

Return to Section 4.2 for a moment, where equations (4.19) and (4.20) presented (in full detail) the singular-value decomposition of the 2×2 matrix $S = \begin{pmatrix} 1.0 & 0.5 \\ 0.2 & 1.4 \end{pmatrix}$ interpreted as the pattern of covariances between a pair of variables X_1, X_2 and another pair Y_1, Y_2. We found that S could be expressed as UDV^t with

$$U = \begin{pmatrix} .555 & -.832 \\ .832 & .555 \end{pmatrix}, \quad D = \begin{pmatrix} 1.612 & 0 \\ 0 & 0.806 \end{pmatrix}, \quad V = \begin{pmatrix} .447 & -.894 \\ .894 & .447 \end{pmatrix}$$

$$(4.20)$$

and interpreted this as the production of two new pairs of measurements (latent variables), $(.555X_1 + .832X_2), (.832X_1 - .555X_2)$ and $(.447Y_1 + .894Y_2)$,

$(.894Y_1 - .447Y_2)$, such that (1) each pair was geometrically orthogonal and (2) the first X-score was uncorrelated with the second Y-score, and vice versa. It followed that the covariance 1.612 between the first X-score and the first Y-score, $.555X_1 + .832X_2$ and $.447Y_1 + .894Y_2$, was the largest possible for two linear combinations whose coefficients each summed in square to 1.0, and the covariance between the second X and the second Y, $.832X_1 - .555X_2$ and $.894Y_1 - .447Y_2$, was 0.806, the smallest for any similarly normalized pair of scores.

We now *radically* reinterpret this same computation as the generation of a pair of distance measurements optimally describing the shape change in Figure 5.23.

analysis of one single tensor

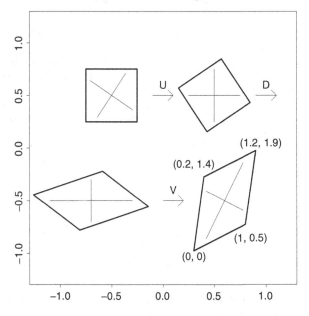

Figure 5.23 Reinterpretation of an earlier singular-value decomposition $S = UDV^t$ as the canonical description of how a square is sheared into a parallelogram. Upper left: starting square of graph paper. Upper right: the rotation U puts the biorthogonal directions (light lines) horizontal and vertical. Lower left: the diagonal stretches D extend the light lines by multiples d_1, d_2. In doing so, the transformation alters the size and shape of the starting square into those of the target parallelogram. Lower right: the second rotation V rotates the form UD into the coordinate system of the original target parallelogram S. The SVD produces the distances that begin and end at 90° while reproducing this transformation.

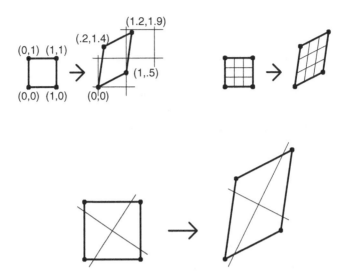

Figure 5.24 Clarification of the final scene in Figure 5.23 in showing "distances of greatest and least ratio of change across the transformation." Upper left: original data. Note that the northeast corner location $(1.2, 1.9)$ is the vector sum of the northwest and southeast corner locations $(1, 0.5)$ and $(0.2, 1.4)$. Upper right: The same in the metaphor of a "uniform shape change" linking the interior of the square to the interior of the parallelogram. Lower: interpretation of the SVD from Figure 5.23 as the pair of directions *across the interior* that show the maximum and minimum distance-ratios (and that thus, by the SVD theorem, must lie at 90° in both forms). In this realization the distances could be measured (in principle) on a real biological specimen in your laboratory. Figure 5.25 will show us an even better strategy for the same task.

In Figures 5.23 and 5.24 the singular values $d_1, d_2 = 1.612, 0.806$ that were the covariances of the latent variables $(.555X_1 + .832X_2)$ and $(.832X_1 - .555X_2)$ with their mates $.447Y_1 + .894Y_2$ and $.894Y_1 - .447Y_2$ now play an entirely different scientific role, the *lengths of lines* across the parallelogram that were of unit length across the square. Distances along the more vertical direction are multiplied by 1.612, distances along the perpendicular (which remains perpendicular) are shrunk to 0.806 of their starting length, *and these are the largest and smallest possible ratios of change, respectively.*

We are not quite finished – we still need explicit instructions for measuring the distances thus indicated on our actual samples of specimens – but we have come most of the way to our goal, which is the explicit merging of Martin's two separate biometrical concerns.

We encountered this sort of coincidence before in Section 3.1 when we found that three completely different rhetorics of explanation were associated with the same system of normal equations in the context of linear multiple regression. For instance, recall from that previous discussion of the SVD that the entries of the diagonal matrix in the SVD, squared, sum to the sum of squares of the entries of the original covariance matrix. In the present context, where the entries are not covariances but coordinates, we infer that the sum of the squares of the maximum and minimum scale factors equals the sum of squared lengths of the vectors into which any pair of adjacent sides of the starting unit square are transformed.

There is also an identity between either of these two analyses and a third, the principal components analysis of the two variables that are the x- and y-coordinates of the four corners of the parallelogram at lower right in Figure 5.23 or 5.24. For the data set

$$(0,0), (0.2, 1.4), (1.2, 1.9), (1.0, 0.5), \qquad (5.1)$$

we find eigenvalues 0.806 and 0.403 – exactly half the singular values of the PLS, since covariances are divided by the count of "cases," which is 4, and the square root of 4 is 2. The directions of the eigenvectors are (.447, .894) and (−.894, .447), the same as for the U-block of the PLS, and the scores are the four points (−1.12, 0.11), (0.22, 0.56), (1.12, −0.11), (−.22, −.56), which form a configuration identical in shape and in orientation to the lozenge at lower left in Figure 5.23 or 5.24. The PCA was aimed at maximizing and minimizing *variance*, the PLS at maximizing and minimizing *covariance*, and the tensor analysis is apparently maximizing and minimizing rate of change of length (the quantity usually called *strain rate* in bioengineering). The fact that these three tasks are numerically interchangeable ought to give thoughtful students pause, much as did the way that the least-squares analysis of Section 3.1 proved arithmetically identical to Sewall Wright's path analysis on the same data. Another way to put all this is that statisticians are very efficient in reusing the algebra of eigenanalyses just as they were in reusing the matrix inversion approach that drives the multiple interpretations of multiple regression. So it becomes the job of the biologist, not the statistician, to keep these interpretations separate and determine which, if any, apply in the case at hand.

The same type of cautionary note applies, then, that we have already encountered in Chapter 4. We will see, for instance, that if a transformation is not geometrically uniform, then the distance-ratios we are about to derive do not apply to individual patches of tissue. Analogously, if covariance structures are not consistent across the sample space, then the PLS analysis computed there likewise fails to apply to any particular pair of numerical scores – the implied regressions would no longer be linear with constant coefficients.

In this context it is instructive to verify an important property of the 2×2 eigenanalysis that we will need in the sequel: that the directions of greatest and least rate of change of length are at 90° in both the starting square and the ending parallelogram. To do this, write out the general problem as analysis of the map from a square to the form with corners at $(0, 0)$, (a_x, a_y), (b_x, b_y), and $(a_x + b_x, a_y + b_y)$. Consider a line through $(0, 0)$ in the direction of the point $(1, \alpha)$ on the square – this is a line that makes an angle with the horizontal there having tangent equal to α. The squared length of this segment is $1 + \alpha^2$. It is transformed into a line through $(0, 0)$ and $(a_x + \alpha b_x, a_y + \alpha b_y)$ on the parallelogram, a line having squared length $(a_x + \alpha b_x)^2 + (a_y + \alpha b_y)^2$. We want to maximize the ratio of these lengths: the fraction

$$\frac{(a_x + \alpha b_x)^2 + (a_y + \alpha b_y)^2}{1 + \alpha^2} \tag{5.2}$$

One finds the maximum and minimum of this ratio by setting its derivative with respect to α equal to zero. You remember from elementary calculus that the differential of a ratio u/v is $\frac{v\,du - u\,dv}{v^2}$, and so is zero where the numerator $v\,du - u\,dv$ is zero. (A similar equation emerged in the course of our study of the tangent lines to ellipses, Section 2.3.) Substituting for the u and v at hand, and taking derivatives with respect to α, this becomes

$$\begin{aligned}
(1 + \alpha^2)&d((a_x + \alpha b_x)^2 + (a_y + \alpha b_y)^2 \\
&- ((a_x + \alpha b_x)^2 + (a_y + \alpha b_y)^2)d(1 + \alpha^2) \\
&= (1 + \alpha^2)(2b_x(a_x + \alpha b_x) + 2b_y(a_y + \alpha b_y)) \\
&- ((a_x + \alpha b_x)^2 + (a_y + \alpha b_y)^2)(2\alpha).
\end{aligned} \tag{5.3}$$

The two pairs of terms in α^3 cancel. We are left with

$$\alpha^2(a_x a_y + b_x b_y) + \alpha(a_x^2 + a_y^2 - b_x^2 - b_y^2) - (a_x a_y + b_x b_y) = 0. \tag{5.4}$$

Call the coefficient of the α^2 term D – this is the dot product of the two sides of the parallelogram adjacent to $(0, 0)$. It is the same as the constant term except for a minus sign. The coefficient of α is the difference in the squared lengths $L_x^2 = a_x^2 + a_y^2$ and $L_y^2 = b_x^2 + b_y^2$ of the same two sides. In other words, the equation for the directions of extreme strain ratio is

$$D\alpha^2 + \alpha(L_x^2 - L_y^2) - D = 0. \tag{5.5}$$

As long as $D \neq 0$, this equation has two roots. Their product must be the ratio of the last coefficient to the first, $(-D)/D = -1$, meaning that the two directions we are interested in can be written $(1, \alpha)$ and $(1, -1/\alpha)$. The dot product of these two two-vectors is zero, meaning that they are perpendicular (equivalently, they lie along directions whose tangents multiply to -1, which guarantees the same perpendicularity).

Special case. If $D = 0$ – if we are starting with a square that turns into a rectangle – we can't get to equation (5.5). Instead, the strain ratios L_x in the x-direction and L_y in the y-direction are themselves the maximum and the minimum, and, generally, the strain in the direction at angle θ to the first side of the square is $\sqrt{L_x^2 \cos^2 \theta + L_y^2 \sin^2 \theta}$.

Example. (From Figure 5.23.) We have $(a_x, a_y) = (1, 0.5)$, $(b_x, b_y) = (.2, 1.4)$. This gives us $L_x^2 = 1.25$, $L_y^2 = 2.0$, and $D = .9$. The equation (5.5) is thus $.9\alpha^2 h + .75\alpha - .9 = 0$ or $6\alpha^2 + 5\alpha - 6 = 0$, with roots $\frac{2}{3}$ and $-\frac{3}{2}$. These are proportional to the directions of the columns of U in the eigenanalysis reported in Section 4.6 that corresponded to the SVD of $\begin{pmatrix} 1.0 & 0.5 \\ 0.2 & 1.4 \end{pmatrix}$.

5.2.2 The Circle Construction for Triangles

In this section the problem of the description of two triangles on the same three landmarks is reduced to the algebra of the eigenanalysis in the preceding section. In doing so, we will have carried out a **fundamental reinterpretation of the idea of a landmark configuration,** as I promised at the outset of this chapter. It is no longer the case that landmark locations are merely reference points for measurements, as they were in Martin's methodology. Now they will serve also as **instructions for measurements yet to be made** – for parameters driving the design of a measurement scheme matched to the signal being analyzed.

We continue with this theme by offering a different analysis of the same situation that was our focus in Section 5.2.1: a perfectly uniform shape change (one sending parallel lines into parallel lines, and thereby preserving all collinear proportions). Switching from parallelograms to triangles would seem like it is changing the question, but we will arrive at the same answer, this time by recourse to geometry rather than algebra. You may follow the argument in either row of Figure 5.25.

We began with a parallelogram of landmarks, Figure 5.23 or 5.24, but we never actually used the fourth landmark, only the first three. So in this presentation the relevant data really are a triangle of landmarks, not a quadrilateral. In fact, we can arrange things so that the triangles share two of their three landmarks, differing only in the location of the third. We manage this by picking up one of them (either one) and translating, rotating, and scaling an edge (any one, but the same, anatomically, in both of the triangles) so that its two landmarks exactly overlie the same two points of the other triangle.

principal axes for a pair of triangles

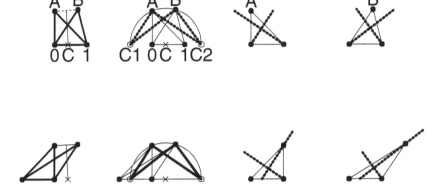

Figure 5.25 (top row) Figure for the construction of the principal axes for any pair of triangles by substituting lines and circles for the squares and parallelograms of Section 5.2.1. The heavy dotted lines are at 90° in both forms. See the text for the explanation of the steps from left to right. (bottom row) The same for the data in Figure 5.24.

At upper left in Figure 5.25, the triangles share the two landmarks marked "0" and "1" in anticipation of Figure 5.26, but one has third vertex at A and the other at B. These are drawn as the superimposed triangles of heavy lines. We construct a new point C (which will stand for "center" in a moment) that is the intersection with the line 01 of the *perpendicular bisector* of AB, the line through its midpoint perpendicular to the segment AB itself. In the lower row is the same construction for the data from Figure 5.23. It will be a bit more cluttered, as the center C falls outside the baseline of either triangle to the right.

Now enhance the diagram as in the second column. It is an ancient theorem (one from the actual geometry textbook written by Euclid himself) that the point C is at the same distance from A as it is from B. Draw a circle around C with this radius, as shown, and let it intersect the line 01 in two points C1, C2. (It will not matter much whether the C's are inside the segment 01 or outside it, and, if outside, which side they are on, or how far away.) Connect the points A and B, separately, to these new points C1 and C2 with the dotted lines shown.

The triangles C1–A–C2 and C1–B–C2 are both triangles inscribed on a diameter of the circle. Hence, by another theorem of Euclid's, each of these is a right triangle.

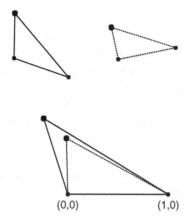

(0,0) (1,0)

Figure 5.26 Construction of the Bookstein coordinates (large dots, bottom panel) for two triangles of landmarks. In a drastic further simplification of Figure 5.25, there is no further need for either the lines or the circles; all the information about the shape of two or more triangles inheres in the two Cartesian coordinates of this single variable point.

Hence these are the directions we are looking for!

If they are perpendicular both before and after the shape change, then one is the direction of greatest ratio of change of length and the other is the direction of least such change. The actual strains in these directions are easily computed as $b(BC_1/AC_1)$ and $b(BC_2/AC_2)$, where b is the ratio of the baseline length 01 in the second form to its length in the first.

In both examples here, it is the direction through C1 that shows the greatest ratio, and the direction through C2 that shows the least. We convert them to Martin-style proportions by taking explicitly measureable parallels as shown in the two rightmost columns. Let's narrate the panels in the upper row first. The length that grows by the greatest fraction of its starting extent runs from the $(0, 0)$ corner – perhaps this was landmark 1 – to a point about 40% of the way from $(0, 1)$ to $(1, 0)$ on the square (and the corresponding point on the corresponding segment of the second geometry). The length that shrinks by the greatest fraction of its starting length is the length from corner $(1, 0)$ – maybe this was landmark 2 – to the line that divides the originally vertical edge in a ratio of about 0.7 to 0.3. It is still obvious that these are the distances we wish to measure, as they are evidently at 90° in both forms, just like the corresponding directions in Figure 5.24.

In the second row, the analysis corresponding to the actual geometry of Figures 5.23 and 5.24, the measurement instructions are little bit different.

The first measurement, the one showing the greatest ratio of increase, now runs from the *third* landmark (the "moving" one, although this is just an arbitrary decision for the purpose of drawing the figure) through a point dividing the baseline about 30% of the way along its length. Because the baseline increased in length by a ratio of $\sqrt{1.25} = 1.118$, the increases in the figure must divide the previous strain ratios of 1.612 and 0.806 by that scaling factor; thus in the second row of the figure the dimension aligned with the NW-SE diagonal increases in length by a ratio of $1.612/1.118 = 1.442$. Perpendicular to it is a segment that would be measured from the second (righthand) baseline landmark through a point about a third of the way from landmark 1 to landmark 3, and the length measurement in the figure should represent a ratio of change of $0.806/1.118 = 0.721$.

> When the segment AB is exactly vertical, the point C is "at infinity," and then the two directions we seek to compute are the directions along the baseline 01 and the perpendicular to it through the movable landmark A. This construction will be shown in panel (c) of Figure 5.28.

To link this construction to the Gaussian machinery of earlier chapters, I make use of a mathematical convenience I had no occasion to mention earlier. *Everything I have noted about the statistics of Gaussian distributions generalizes from variables that are real numbers to variables that are complex numbers,* which is to say, coordinate *pairs.*

> **A quick review.** The more mathematically adept among you first saw this notation in high school, but unless you're a geometer, an engineer, or a physicist, you may not have thought about it since then. If X is a complex number, $X = X_1 + X_2 i$ where $i = \sqrt{-1}$, we call X_1 the *real part* of X and X_2 the *imaginary part*. Then the statistics of the single quantity X are just the statistics of the ordered pair (X_1, X_2) that visualizes X on the ordinary Argand plane (the plane with X_1 plotted horizontally and X_2 vertically). Keep in mind the usual conventions for complex arithmetic. We treat real numbers like X_1 as the corresponding complex numbers $X_1 + 0i$, the same value but with a zero imaginary part. Adding and subtracting are easy – two complex numbers $X = (X_1, X_2)$ and $Y = (Y_1, Y_2)$ are added or subtracted vectorwise: $X \pm Y = (X_1 \pm Y_1, X_2 \pm Y_2)$. Where it gets interesting is multiplication and division. To describe these, it helps to refer to three auxiliary quantities associated with $X = X_1 + X_2 i$. The **conjugate** $\overline{X} = X_1 - X_2 i$ results from changing the sign of the imaginary part only. The **modulus** of X, $\mathrm{Mod}(X)$, is defined as its length in the Argand plane, $\mathrm{Mod}(X) = \sqrt{X_1^2 + X_2^2}$. And the **argument** of X is the angle made by its vector (X_1, X_2) with respect to the horizontal, $\mathrm{Arg}(X) = \tan^{-1}(X_1, X_2)$ in the usual convention for notating that angle (the Fortran function `atan2`). In this context, the **product** XY of two complex numbers $X = (X_1, X_2)$ and $Y = (Y_1, Y_2)$ is the new complex number

$(X_1Y_1 - X_2Y_2, X_1Y_2 + X_2Y_1)$. This is the same as YX, the product in the other order. Geometrically, to multiply by X is to simultaneously rescale by $\text{Mod}(X)$ and rotate *counterclockwise* by $\text{Arg}(X)$. One can check that $X\overline{X} = (X_1^2 + X_2^2) + 0i$, the real number $\text{Mod}^2(X)$. Then if Y is defined as $\overline{X}/\text{Mod}^2(X)$, we have $XY = 1 + 0i$. So, by analogy with the ordinary real numbers you already know, to divide by X is the same as multiplying by a quantity we define as $X^{-1} = \overline{X}/\text{Mod}^2(X)$. Geometrically, we are dividing by $\text{Mod}(X)$ and at the same time rotating *clockwise* by $\text{Arg}(X)$, the exact opposite of the two steps for multiplying. Check your mastery of these rules by verifying that $i^2 = -1$, justifying the identity $i = \sqrt{-1}$ with which we began. Geometrically, we are asserting that the result of two consecutive $90°$ rotations is replacement of every number X by its opposite $-X$.

Let Z_1, Z_2, Z_3 be three landmark locations $(X_1, Y_1), (X_2, Y_2), (X_3, Y_3)$ in a plane, each one consisting of two ordinary coordinates such as might be measured by some digitizing apparatus in some Cartesian coordinate system, and construct the **single new complex variable** $W = (Z_3 - Z_1)/(Z_2 - Z_1)$. We can write out the value of W in full by expanding the formulas for multiplication and division just reviewed:

$$(Z_3 - Z_1)/(Z_2 - Z_1) = (W_1, W_2) \text{ for}$$

$$W_1 = \frac{(X_3 - X_1)(X_2 - X_1) + (Y_3 - Y_1)(Y_2 - Y_1)}{(X_2 - X_1)^2 + (Y_2 - Y_1)^2},$$

$$W_2 = \frac{(X_3 - X_1)(Y_2 - Y_1) - (Y_3 - Y_1)(X_2 - X_1)}{(X_2 - X_1)^2 + (Y_2 - Y_1)^2}. \tag{5.6}$$

The resulting point $W = (W_1, W_2)$ is called the *shape coordinate pair of Z_3 to the baseline from Z_1 to Z_2*. As Figure 5.26 shows, the corresponding geometric construction is conceptually very simple. One picks up the triangle Z_1, Z_2, Z_3 and puts it down again after changing its size and its orientation, **but not its shape,** so that Z_1 now falls at the point $(0, 0)$ and Z_2 at the point $(1, 0)$. Whatever information we had about the shape of the original triangle $Z_1Z_2Z_3$ must now be coded in the only two coordinates left to vary, the coordinates W_1 and W_2.

Then it is an important fact that, for small circular variations in the locations of all of the original Z's around different mean locations in the original digitizing plane, the resulting shape coordinates (W_1, W_2) are **also** distributed with circular symmetry in their plane. And if the Z-distributions were all circular Gaussian, then so, approximately, is the distribution of the W's. The situation is as in Figure 5.27. (For a proof, see Bookstein, 1991, Section 5.1.1, or Dryden and Mardia, 2016.) The W's are called **two-point shape coordinates** or, after Stuart and Ord (1994:279), **Bookstein coordinates** of the

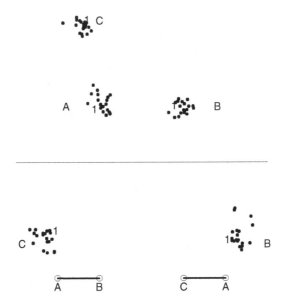

Figure 5.27 If three landmarks vary around different average locations by circular Gaussian variation of the same small standard deviation, then so do the Bookstein coordinates of their shape to any baseline. Above: three landmark locations distributed as independent circular Gaussians of the same variance, for 20 cases. Below: shape coordinates to two different baselines. These scatters correspond point for point under a transform $z_2 = z_1/(z_1 - 1)$ that is close to a similarity transform (a combination of translation, rotation and rescaling) whenever the shape scatter is sufficiently small. To ease the perception of that near-similarity transform, the first of the 20 cases has been printed with the character "1" in all three panels.

triangle $Z_1 Z_2 Z_3$ to the baseline from Z_1 to Z_2. (I was not the person to name them that; it was originally Kanti Mardia's idea.)

Just as these scatters simplify to a quasilinear version when shape variation is small, so does the exact construction in Figure 5.25 simplify. Suppose the treatment of the shape coordinates by the methods of Chapters 2 through 4 results in a direction of dominant interest – a contrast of group mean shapes, a regression on some exogenous measurement like ecology, a dependence on the information about baseline length that has been divided out of the current analysis, or a principal component of an interesting single-factor shape coordinate scatter. If we assume that the points A and B of Figure 5.25 are close enough together, we can fuse them in one single location (Figure 5.28) while still drawing the direction of interest as the short, heavy line through that location. Then, using Euclid again to skip the step that required constructing

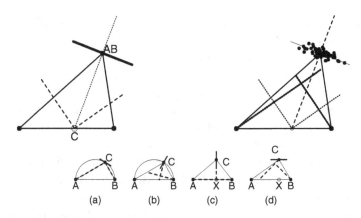

Figure 5.28 Simplifying Figure 5.25 when shape variation is small. (top row) For sufficiently small shape variation, the axes in Figure 5.25 that represent the proper distances for measuring variation along the heavy line through AB simplify to the bisectors (the dashed lines) of the angles between the perpendicular to the direction of interest of the mean form and the baseline. We have thereby solved Martin's index construction problem. (bottom row) Some special cases lead to simpler reports (see text). Heavy dashed lines indicate the result of the construction in the upper panel.

the circle, we can jump directly to the directions of interest as the bisectors of the angles made by the perpendicular to this direction of interest (dotted line) where it intersects the baseline of the construction (the point C we had before). It remains only to translate these bisectors (dashed lines through C) so that each one passes through a vertex of the triangle while properly intersecting the opposite edge.

Thus it was only one more construction step to solving the problem that Rudolf Martin implicitly proposed a century ago, the explicit construction of an index (here, a distance ratio). We simply need to move those dashed lines inside the outline of the averaged triangle. As already demonstrated in Figure 5.25, moving the dashed lines inside the outline of the averaged triangle is a straightforward matter of parallel transport until the line goes through one of the triangle's vertices along with a point properly upon the opposite edge. In the example at the top of Figure 5.28, the principal component drawn in light line through the middle of the shape coordinate scatter is represented by the ratio of distances shown in the heavy dotted lines. One of these distances connects the lower right corner to a point about two-thirds of the way up the edge opposite, and the other connects the lower left corner to a point about one-sixth of the way down the edge opposite to *it*. From the geometry of this panel of the figure we can see that, to a degree of approximation depending on the range of the shape coordinate scatter, these distances remain perpendicular throughout the range of forms in the sample. We have thereby solved Martin's index construction problem: the indicated distance ratio must correlate nearly perfectly with the principal component score along the long axis of the scatter shown. The price to be paid is that the ratio we've constructed is no longer a ratio of interlandmark distances, but of the distances between one landmark and some weighted average of the other two. In this way we have reversed the conventional temporal ordering of the stages of a biometric analysis: not "variables first, then statistics" but "statistics first, then variables." I do not know why it took so long for this possibility to become a recognized biostatistical strategy.

The upper panel in Figure 5.28 exemplifies this general construction. There are a few special cases that lead to simpler reports. From left to right in the bottom row of Figure 5.28, these go as follows. (a) If the line along which C appears to shift is tangent to the semicircle on baseline AB, then the ratio of sides CA:CB is the best measure of the change, while the angle between the sides is invariant at 90°. (b) If the line of shift at C is perpendicular to that semicircle, then the best measure of the change is the ratio of the lengths intercepted by the two angle bisectors at C (the two transects shown in dotted line); for small changes their ratio is statistically equivalent to the angle at C between the edges of the triangle ABC there. (c) If the direction of shift at C is perpendicular to the baseline, the best scalar measure of the change is the ratio of the altitude CX to the length AB of the baseline. (d) But if the direction of shift at C is parallel to the baseline AB, the best measure of the change is the ratio AX:XB, or, equivalently, the ratio of transects at 45° to the baseline, as shown by the dotted lines. See, in general, Bookstein (1991:220–223).

Exactly the same construction will apply to the comparison of any two group means, the extraction of a ratio that aligns with a regression of the Bookstein coordinates on any exogenous measurement, and so forth. Instances of all of these maneuvers will follow in the course of the examples that follow.

5.2.3 Extensions and Examples

The principal reason for being interested in these triangles and their Bookstein coordinates is that in the multivariate space of shape coordinates to be built in Section 5.4 every transformation has a component, the *uniform component,* that accords with these restrictions. (These lie in the subspace spanned by the fifth and sixth rows of the *J*-matrix in equation (5.7) of Section 5.4.4.) The explanation of this fact must await the complete explanation (Section 5.5) of the sorts of transformations that are *not* uniform (those described by the partial warps of nonzero bending), but even at this point we can explore some examples of contrasts that are "mostly uniform" in ways that lead to interesting explanations.

When transformations are uniform, analyses of any three landmark locations lead to the same tensor representation. (This fact renders more reasonable the assertion to come in Section 5.5 that there exists a sort of averaging procedure over all such representations that has, in general, a smaller standard error of estimate than would be afforded by restricting our attention to any single triangle.) It will also be the case that the uniform transformations turn out to be maximally *integrated* in the sense of Section 5.6.8. Mostly, however, they serve the useful role of linking to *possible explanations of uniformity*, which are typically biomechanical, identifying the directions of optimal distance-ratios with the principal strains of biophysical causes of the shape changes encountered.

5.2.3.1 Vilmann Analysis, Continued

We can now show aspects of the spatial organization of the skein of inter-landmark growth rates already displayed in Figure 5.21. I will be exploring two different families of two-point shape coordinates that visualize the shape aspects of this single coordinated growth regimen. In one approach, we will concentrate on representations of the outer margin of these neurocrania, as represented by the set of eight shape coordinate pairs arising from every triangle of three consecutive outline points (Figure 5.29). The other approach (Figures 5.32–5.34) relies on the baselines that show minimum or maximum ratios of growth over the age range in which we are interested.

In the first approach, using circumferential shape coordinates only, one can ask about consistency in two different senses: over specimens or over time. Figure 5.30 shows the analyses of sample average changes over the eight ages at which these rodents were imaged. (The division into two sets is simply by outline order, as explained in the caption of Figure 5.29.) This visual summary shows considerable heterogeneity. The trajectories of Bregma (upper right in the left panel) and Opisthion and SES (far left and far right in the right panel) are nearly collinear in this representation, implying consistency of tensor descriptors over the seven age intervals here. In contrast, the trajectories for Basion (left panel, lower left corner) and Lambda (right panel, upper edge) are highly curved, and the trajectories for ISS (left panel, lower right edge) and SOS (right panel, lower edge) show hardly any variation at all, implying proportionate growth without bending all along the cranial base. Figure 5.31, replicating these plots for each animal separately, confirms the linearity for Bregma and for SES, and the near-invariance along the cranial base at ISS

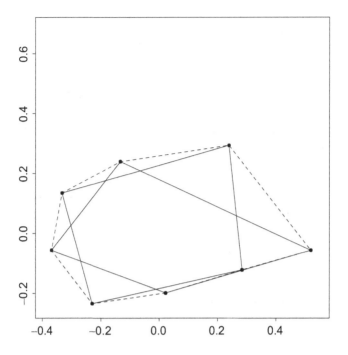

Figure 5.29 A scheme of eight Bookstein coordinate pairs jointly circumam-
bulating the Vilmann rodent neurocranial data set of Figure 2.41. (dotted lines)
Actual outline scheme. (solid lines) Baselines for representing each landmark as
it deviates from the adjacent outline chord. These chords can be divided into two
sets of four each; for clarity, these will be diagrammed separately, first for the
sample average and then for the 18 animals one by one, in the next two figures.

and SOS, but indicates that corresponding to the nonlinear trajectories in
Figure 5.30, there is also considerable animal-to-animal heterogeneity. The
pooled trajectories in this figure have roughly the same width on the plots,
suggesting that there may be a model for these data available in terms of two
longitudinal factors together with noise. We return to the consideration of these
same 18 octagon histories in Section 5.6, using the most advanced methods put
forward there, varieties of the analysis of relative warps.

From this circumferential analysis we turn to the other variant, the one
emphasizing homogeneity of this tensor representation over the whole configuration. Figure 5.32 analyzes just the initial period of growth of these octagons,
from age 7 days to 14, using as the pair of alternate baselines the directions
not on the convex hull (i.e., cutting across the interior) that show the extremes
of growth ratio according to the corresponding frame of Figure 5.21. In the
difference between the frames of the lower row we see clear confirmation of

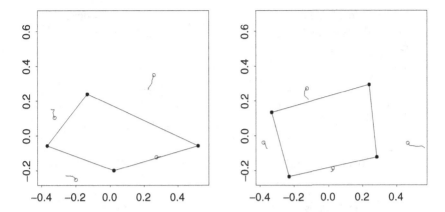

Figure 5.30 Analysis of circumferential Vilmann histories, version 1: sample mean shape coordinates at the eight ages of the measurement design. Open circles mark average locations from the age-7 data.

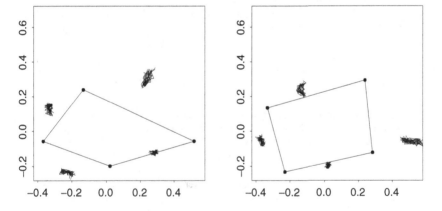

Figure 5.31 Analysis of circumferential Vilmann histories, version 2: individual shape trajectories, 18 rats, eight ages.

our baseline choices: at left, every mean coordinate pair moves away from the baseline; at right, every pair moves toward the baseline. In general, pairs are moving in parallel vectors, regardless of baseline, and by extents that seem approximately proportional to distance *from* the baseline. Hence this growth process is somewhat uniform (to be specific, 83% uniform, in the Procrustes metric; the net shape change between these two ages is as in Figure 5.69, upper left).

We can contrast this analysis with the corresponding display for the full time course of this data set, from age 7 days to 150 (Figure 5.33). The

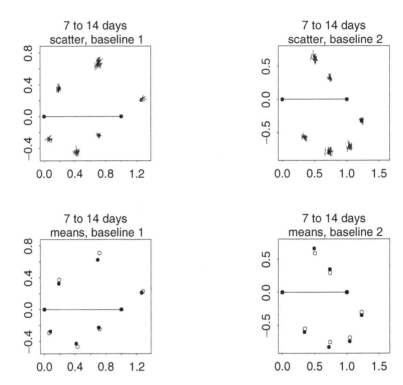

Figure 5.32 Analysis of multiple Bookstein coordinates, Vilmann data, I. Age 7 to age 14 days. (left) To the baseline from Interparietal Point to ISS, the segment with the highest specific mean growth rate (1.254) over this interval according to the upper left panel in Figure 5.21. (right) To the baseline from Bregma to SOS, having the shortest specific ratio of mean growth (1.118) over this interval. (upper row) Detailed histories animal by animal. (lower row) Averages for the two ages only.

analysis is divided into two subintervals, 7 to 30 days and 30 to 150, and the baseline I have chosen is now the distance from Lambda to ISS, the transversal showing the slowest net mean growth ratio over the full 143-day growth record according to the upper right panel of Figure 5.21. It remains the case that the individual animals' trajectories are very highly aligned (upper row), both over the earlier age interval and over the later interval, and that the group mean displacements appear to roughly fit a model of proportionate parallel vectors both above and below the baseline. But these parallel vectors, which convert to tensors or distance-ratios according to the geometry of Figure 5.28, are not the same whether compared from above to below this baseline (anterior to posterior of the neurocranium) or from the earlier time period to the later. The methods of Section 5.6 are required if we are to disentangle this curvature.

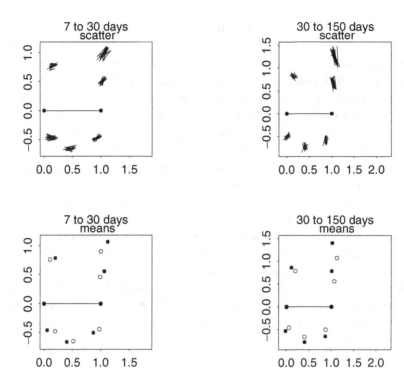

Figure 5.33 Analysis of multiple Bookstein coordinates, Vilmann data, II. The baseline is now the segment from ISS to Lambda. (upper row) Animal by animal. (lower row) Sample means only. (left column) Age 7 to age 30 days. (right column) Age 30 to age 150 days. The vertical coordinate of these shifts (which is anatomically horizontal, as the baseline is actually vertical in the laboratory frame) persists, but the horizontal coordinate reverses over this time interval, and the tensor describing the anterior component here seems inconsistent with that describing the posterior component.

5.2.3.2 Another Example: Craniofacial Growth

As a second example of these useful visualizations I present a simplified version of the analysis of allometry in the human midsagittal data set to be examined more intensively in Section 5.6.3. There I will be showing representations by transformation grids based on regressions of Procrustes shape coordinates. Here it is enough to approach the same narrative by the simpler analysis of group mean differences in Bookstein coordinates to a carefully chosen baseline.

The data for this exercise correspond to the template already shown in Figure 5.3. The data set of $N = 22$ landmark configurations involves 6 children aged 2 through 10 years along with 16 adults selected haphazardly (it would be misleading to say "randomly") from the collection of the Department of Anthropology of the University of Vienna. These data have been described in several earlier publications (e.g., Bookstein, Gunz et al., 2003; Weber and Bookstein, 2011, chapter 4) to which the reader can turn for more detailed information about the sample. For present purposes it is enough to know that it is not representative of any biological population.

From the literature, or from preliminary computations, one learns that there is a direction of lowest average change in distance ratio from children to adults, the direction from internal Bregma to internal Lambda. This chord is, however, external to the rest of the configuration (it lies on the convex hull of the landmarks instead of inside it). This eccentricity limits its relevance for functional explanations. A more useful baseline that is nevertheless quite near this one is the segment from internal Bregma to internal Inion. The first of these chords is almost parallel to the baseline from Sella to Nasion that is the mainstay of conventional cephalometric representations of this same anatomical concern. Figure 5.34 shows the shape change between the average of the three infants (specimens "2y" or "4y" in Figure 5.74) and the average of the sixteen adults as a set of changes of two-point shape coordinates according to either of these baselines.

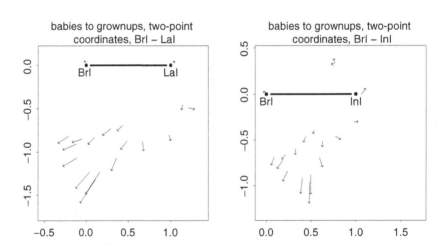

Figure 5.34 Mean changes in Bookstein coordinates, three infants versus fifteen adults, for the landmark configuration in Figure 5.3. (left) To a Bregma–Lambda baseline, transect of the minimum distance ratio between the groups. (right) To a Bregma–Inion baseline, better aligned with the conventional narrative (growth of the maxilla "directly away from" the neurocranium). Arrows at BrI stand for shifts at BrE; arrows at LaI (left panel) and InI (right panel), shifts at LaE and InE, respectively.

We know these two plots need to be visualizing exactly the same phenomenon – there is no difference in their information content – yet one is much simpler to report than the other. To the baseline on the left, from internal Bregma to internal Lambda, the points of the maxilla appear to be displaced obliquely. To the baseline on the right, now from internal Bregma to internal Inion, the displacement of those maxillary landmarks appears to be "straight down," which is the simplest special case for reporting that was already noted in Section 5.2.2. The uniform part of this shape difference is easy to summarize as the sum of the distances moved by all those landmarks away from the baseline, divided by the sum of their starting distances from the baseline and then divided again by the length of that baseline. External Inion itself does not conform to this summary according to either baseline – it remodels rather drastically in response to forces exerted by the neck muscles – and there remains nonuniform variation in the vicinity of the foramen magnum (at Opisthion and Basion) that would likewise benefit from some additional biomechanical analysis. Nevertheless, the summary at right in Figure 5.34 is a good compromise between the output of the more sophisticated analyses (Procrustes coordinates, thin-plate splines) and the additional written text needed to explain the arithmetic along with any biological argument it justifies.

5.2.4 A Further Comment on Distance Ratios

Consider an isosceles triangle changing its shape by extension of the altitude to the apex. Specifically, let us have four groups of these shapes, each one with baseline landmarks averaging locations $(0, 0)$ and $(1, 0)$ and with average third vertices at $(0, 0.6)$ (group A), $(0, 0.5)$ (group B), $(0, 0.3)$ (group C), and $(0, 0.2)$ (group D). Around each of the average forms we take 20 specimens that vary by independent circular Gaussian noise of standard deviation 0.05 in every direction at each landmark. (Thus the noise process is not aware of the bilateral symmetry of the model. For methods that handle that symmetry, see Section 5.6.7.) The net collection of 80 shapes is shown in Figure 5.35 to the obvious two-point baseline.

Suppose we are interested in an argument that the angle at the apex has changed from one sample to another (males vs. females, say). Then we can ask: Given some difference in that angle, how large a sample will be need to estimate it as a preset multiple of its own standard error, say, three times, if we proceed (a) by assessing the pair of shape coordinates representing this point to a baseline of the others, or (b) by considering only the ratios of interlandmark distances as in the method of EDMA (Figure 5.21)? The answer is that the required sample size in strategy (a) is smaller than what is required under the

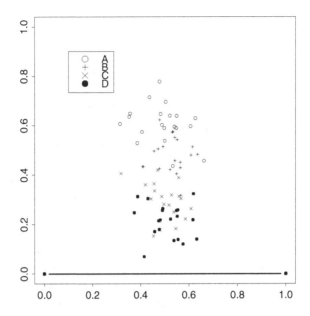

Figure 5.35 Design of a little simulation to compare two-point shape coordinates
with distance ratio methods like EDMA. There are four groups A, B, C, D, each of
20 simulated triangle of landmarks having the same independent circular Gaussian
digitizing error at every landmark. Group A will be compared to group B by two
methods, and likewise group C to group D. Squares at bottom left and bottom
right: ends of the two-point baseline shown.

inferior approach (b) by a factor that rises quickly as the height of the apex of
the triangle above its baseline decreases.

Figure 5.36 confirms this intuition. Either method offers two degrees of
freedom for comparison (for the shape coordinates, any direction in the
space; for EDMA, it is either of the two independent distance ratios). For
each comparison we select the coordinate that would do best in the limit of
very large samples. For the shape coordinates, this is the vertical coordinate
from the baseline to the apex; for EDMA, the ratio of either slant side to
the baseline. Then it is sufficient to note that observed differences are five
times their standard errors in the upper left panel, three times those errors
in the lower left and upper right panels, and less than twice their standard
errors in the lower right panel. This little analysis confirms what F. J. Rohlf
has been demonstrating now for many years in many comparative contexts
(e.g., Rohlf, 2000a, 2000b). EDMA is *never* better than the shape-coordinate
methods of this book at detecting shape changes, and in fact is inferior
whenever the landmarks and their shifts are in general position (which is

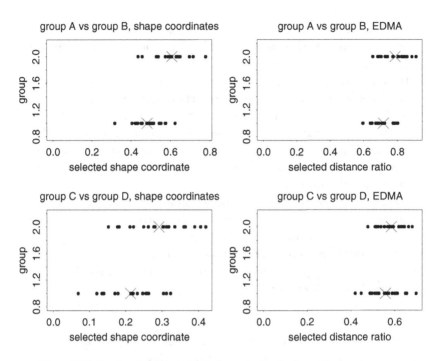

Figure 5.36 Results of a typical simulation, using method-specific descriptors as in the text. In each panel, the large X's indicates the two group averages.

usually the case) with respect to the underlying biological processes the landmarks are tracking. The simplicity of narrative style that EDMA offers comes at an unacceptable cost in efficiency of signal processing, meaning required sample size to detect a signal: a cost that furthermore is a function of the average form in quite counterintuitive ways. In short, it is long past the time when reports of interlandmark distance ratios per se should be considered appropriate in general for a morphometric communication. Also, the distance-ratio methods do not extend to representations of curving form (semilandmark data) or to biomechanical analyses of the forces that actually push the landmarks into the positions where they are observed. Enough said.

Summary of Section 5.2

- The singular-value decomposition introduced in Chapter 4 reappears in GMM as one core analysis of the *shape change tensor* describing triangles of landmarks that do not lie along or near a line. The role of the SVD is to link the landmark coordinates to the realm of *all* the potential measurements of the landmark locations, rather than having to specify any list of measurements in advance.

- These analyses go forward equivalently in algebra (a quadratic equation) or in geometry (a ruler-and-compass construction on the *two-point* or *Bookstein coordinates* of the triangle). Either way, the result is to specify particularly informative *pairs* of distances between one landmark and the weighted average of two others. The paired distances begin and end at 90° over the shape change. One distance bears the greatest ratio of change in length, the other the least.
- Particular alignments between the location of average shape coordinates and the direction in which they shift over a comparison can sometimes lead to simpler reports of the shape change observed.
- These tensor methods often are sufficient to summarize real data sets concerned with the growth of rigid skeletal complexes, such as the hominoid or the rodent skull.

5.3 Procrustes Matters: The Least-Squares Approach to Morphometrics

While this is not a book about philosophy of science, it is time to briefly sketch the distinction between theories and theorems. Informally speaking, a mathematical *theorem* is an assertion that typically refers to the necessary equivalence of two formal computations (or their empirical realizations) or the uniqueness of some numerical manipulation. In contrast, a scientific *theory* is an assertion about a biological situation or causal factor that surely could have been otherwise: growth allometry, sexual dimorphism, ecophenotypy, natural selection of hominids for brain size, and so forth.

To this point in the book I have made use of many theorems. Averages are maximum-likelihood under a Gaussian assumption; the singular vectors of a singular-value decomposition always exist, are geometrically orthogonal, and supply least-squares low-rank fits to the matrix being thus decomposed; and so on. Some theorems deal with probability theory, some with statistical procedures such as least-squares regression, and some with the conversion of landmark locations into distances that drove the previous generation of morphometrics.

This roster does not exhaust the possibilities, however. There is a group of theorems concerned with where "shape distances" come from; this will turn out to be the same question as where "shape variables" come from. While the origin of landmarks is craft knowledge, morphometrics offers an unusually sophisticated response to the generation of the corresponding distances and variables. The standard Procrustes approach guarantees the comparability of shape variables by enforcing a particular superposition, and then never refers to that superposition again in any way. The combined protocol (Procrustes shape coordinates expressing Procrustes shape distance or Procrustes form distance) lies at the core of the methodology and its claims to strengthen some scientific arguments. But it also drives a severe critique of the method as an adjunct to persuasive investigations in organismal biology, a critique based on the sheer abstraction and wholly unrealistic symmetries of the Procrustes distance formula itself.

5.3.1 The Conventional Procrustes Shape Distance

We will produce a shape distance as a monotone transformation of a quantity representing a shape (im)probability.[3] The first (and still, by far, the most popular) technique for such a probability is the *Procrustes distribution* sketched in Figure 5.37. The figure actually suggests four of these, one for each radius of the circles at the 25 suspiciously symmetric landmark locations shown by the tiny centered dots. (For larger radii the corresponding grids begin to fold over themselves, a circumstance having no biometric interpretation.)

Please turn your attention now to the chart in Figure 5.38. Shown are 100 forms that all have the connectivity of that starting 5×5 grid but with nodes assigned by random circular variation with standard deviation a series of radii like those in Figure 5.37. They have been sorted horizontally by the statistic to be introduced presently: their *Procrustes distance* from the ideal type (the arrangement of sixteen equal squares that you see isolated at the lower left corner). While it is clear that *something* is going haywire in the journey from the left column to the right, it is much less obvious what this "something" is, biologically speaking. Analytically, each column of this chart arises from a hyperspherical shell in a 46-dimensional space. Such a space is difficult to imagine, let alone the notion of a series of nested hypersurfaces within it. What a biologist should find most remarkable is that most of these little sketches, while surely representing deviations from the ideal square arrangement, nevertheless do not seem to afford "features" for the deviations – they just wouldn't make biological sense. That impression is

---

[3] This is the same strategy as the *Mahalanobis distance* for sorting cases into multiple Gaussian scatters, another name for the technique in Figure 3.52 (top right).

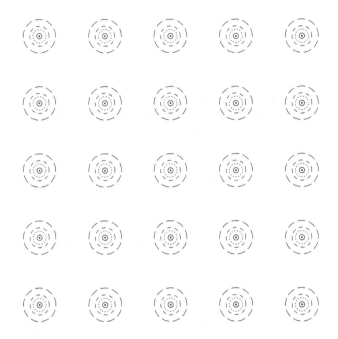

Figure 5.37 One scheme for generating samples of shapes: Procrustes models. For each of the four radii drawn here, the Procrustes scatter of that radius is the set of shapes of points distributed around the indicated 25 mean locations by independent circular Gaussians with every standard deviation equal to the radius indicated. This is called the *offset isotropic Gaussian landmark distribution*, and the shape distribution it generates is the *isotropic Mardia–Dryden* distribution.

no accident; instead, it is a specific property of the model according to which these deformations were simulated. In the model of Figure 5.37, variation is independent at every landmark individually, and at each landmark that variation is a circular Gaussian of the same variance. An explanatory biological interpretation will be found in the *deviation* of a data set from this model, specifically deviations in the form of large-scale alignments (coordinated shifts at nearby landmarks, or at all of them). That is the goal at which we are driving: a method for discerning and delineating those divergences that apply similarly across whole extended regions of the form. In short, what we seek to demonstrate in real data sets are the patterns by which data *deviate* from the axioms here.

Our first task, then, is to browse the preceding three chapters' worth of multivariate techniques to see which might be borrowed to serve this far more biological purpose – the description of the way in which a sample's shape variations are *not* disorderly in this particularly uninformative way. And indeed assorted examples of Procrustes distance

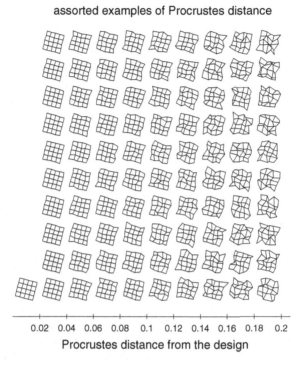

Figure 5.38 From repeated simulations as shown in Figure 5.37 we arrive at a huge variety of variations on a 5 × 5 grid that can be sorted by their actual Procrustes distance from the ideal form (compare Figure 5.41). The sorting here is correlated with the sorting by radius in the preceding figure, but it is not the same.

such a method can be retrieved from the assortment of tools in Chapter 4. It is the method of *principal coordinates analysis,* PCO, which was designed specifically for data in the form of interspecimen dissimilarities. Let us explore the ways it might be of use in this new context.

Already at this stage we can imagine modifications of Figures 5.37–5.38 that circumvent this complaint about disorganization. Figures 5.39–5.41 show one simple possibility, from Bookstein (2007). The model is hierarchical. An outer shape is modeled as a quadrangle after the fashion of Figure 5.38, but thereafter every other landmark is modeled at a scale proportionate to the geometric scale of its own little tessera. Figure 5.40 is an analogue of any single column of Figure 5.38, while Figure 5.41 replicates the whole scheme, including the gradient of increasing variance columnwise from left to right.

So how did we construct this model of "completely meaningless shape change" so as to be able to describe our samples by their contrast with it?

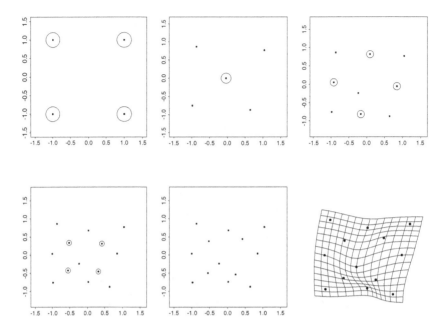

Figure 5.39 Design of an alternative probability distribution that begins with a
Procrustes change at the largest scale (the outer corners of a square) but imposes
proportionately smaller changes down the hierarchy of cells of a subdivision
(which can be extended indefinitely). Circled points are the loci of new variation
frame by frame, with perturbation proportional to radius.

It proves easiest to begin with a distance measure that has the same nonbiological meaninglessness by virtue of its explicit construction. Its mathematical underpinnings can be reviewed in Dryden and Mardia (2016) or
Kendall (1984), but for applied purposes it is sufficient to understand the
diagrammatic version in Figure 5.42.

The data for this underlying computation consist of a pair of forms having
the same landmarks, numbering k in each form; for instance, the pair in the
left column of Figure 5.42, where $k = 4$. As a preliminary, the centroid of
each form is computed, center-of-gravity of the landmarks (not of the area).
Then the two-form Procrustes fit proceeds in three steps. First, the forms
separately are rescaled so that the sum of squared distances of the landmarks
from their centroid is equal to 1 in the forms separately. Then the centroids are
superposed, and, finally, either form is rotated over the other until the sum of
squared distances between corresponding landmarks (the distances that are the
radii of the little circles at lower right) is a minimum over all such rotations.
In one formulation (they differ in exactly how they handle nonlinearities), the

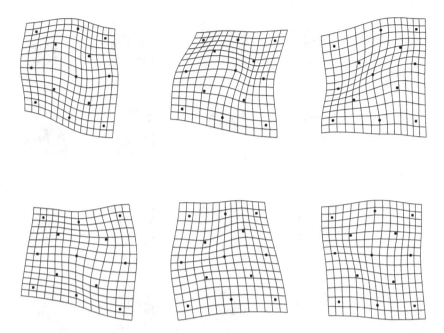

Figure 5.40 Six realizations of the simulation from the preceding figure. Notice how, in contrast to the examples in Figure 5.38, there are now hints of biologically interpretable features at a range of scales.

squared Procrustes distance between the two landmark shapes is then the sum of squares of all those little distances, landmark to homologous landmark, in this superposition; it equals the total area of the little circles drawn, divided by π. For two-dimensional data, the net outcome of all this can be closely approximated by a closed formula (Bookstein, 1991) that actually stands for the error variance of a complex regression, one set of landmark locations upon the other, and the algebra for the general case can be written out as another version of the singular-value decomposition we have already introduced in connection with pattern analysis (Rohlf and Slice, 1990). I will present an approximate formula for all this at equations (5.7) and (5.7a).

It is not only the last step, the rotation, that minimizes the summed area of those little circles. The second step, the joint centering of both forms at the same spot, must reduce that sum of areas, and, to a very good approximation, so does the first as well, the setting of the sums of squared landmark distances from their centroid to be the same for the two polygons. (It is exactly proportional, too, to the sum of *all* the squared interlandmark distances.) This quantity, which will prove very important when we come to study size and

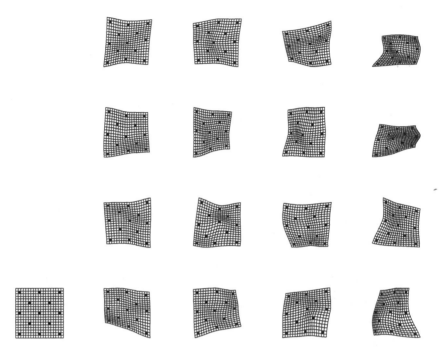

Figure 5.41 Display analogous to Figure 5.38 for the new model of discretely selfsimilar deformations around the mean configuration at lower left. These are examples of the sort of deformations that, if found to be systematic, can be detected by the method of Procrustes distance and Procrustes shape coordinates to be introduced here. Columns from left to right are produced at steadily larger multiples of the pattern of nested standard deviations schematized in Figure 5.39.

allometry, is called the squared **Centroid Size** of the polygon. In physics, it would be the *second central moment* of the set of landmarks treated as point masses. Of course we could make the areas of all of those circles as small as we wanted just by shrinking the figure. To be technically correct, then, this needs to be phrased a little more carefully: once one configuration is fixed, the minimum of summed circle areas is achieved when the second polygon has (almost exactly) the same Centroid Size as the first.

5.3.2 Principal Coordinates of Procrustes Distance

If we have a square matrix of distances between all pairs of specimens in a sample, then under reasonable assumptions the principal coordinates technique of Section 4.2.5 permits us to convert the information in that matrix to a graphical display, the *principal coordinate plot* or *metric multidimensional scaling* of the given data. Of the various interpretations afforded in Chapter 4

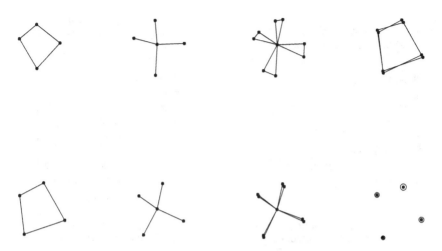

Figure 5.42 Procrustes distance between two quadrilaterals. (left column) The two quadrilaterals. (second column) Center and scale each one separately. (third column) Superimpose the centroids (upper panel), then rotate to best fit (lower panel). (right column) The resulting superposition (upper panel) has minimum summed area of the little circles shown below. The Procrustes distance we seek is the square root of this sum of areas, divided by $\sqrt{\pi}$.

about the import of the singular-value decomposition, the one most pertinent to the present context is the least-squares property set out in equation (4.10): for each count m of pairs of singular vectors, from 1 up to the rank of the matrix, the approximation using just that sublist of vectors comes closest to the original matrix of any rank-m matrix. In this application, to a symmetric matrix of reduced squared distance $-\frac{1}{2}HD^2H$, the corresponding terms of the lowered-rank sum are just the sums of squares of differences on the singular vector entries, which is to say the principal coordinate scores, themselves. In other words, the distances between points on principal coordinate scatterplots such as those in Figure 5.43 are the best possible two-dimensional fit to their squared dissimilarities as indexed by the Procrustes distances we just introduced.

The reason this is a desirable approach is that under the assumptions driving Figure 5.37 (and its analogue for any other configuration of mean landmark locations), the distribution of Procrustes distances is *spherically symmetric*, meaning that in the limit of large samples it is expected to have very nearly the same variance in *every* direction. (We have seen such a distribution already in the single-factor example that ends Chapter 4.) This is a theorem, proven in such standard reference treatises as Dryden and Mardia (2016). It can be made almost intuitive by an argument from Gaussian symmetry that will be found in Section 5.4.4 in the last bullet point after equation (5.7).

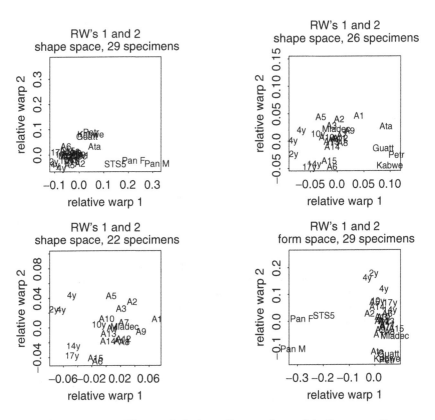

Figure 5.43 Four different principal coordinate analyses of the Procrustes distances among some skull forms. (upper left, upper right, lower left) A sequence of three principal coordinate analyses of shape on $N = 29$, 26, and 22 forms, respectively. (lower right) Analysis of a slightly different list of measurements, which augments the preceding list by one more variable, for Centroid Size (see the next section). The ordination interior to the chimpanzee subsample differs considerably, illustrating the dependence of principal component analyses on the precise list of variables involved. A, Adult *Homo sapiens*, numbered; ny, child aged n years. From Bookstein, 2014, figure 6.7.

Hence if we find a few sample principal coordinate axes that greatly dominate all the others, we have evidence of a biological structure for the sample shapes that *contradicts* the meaningless scheme in Figure 5.37 – an empirical structure that, by virtue of the apparent clusters, trend lines, elliptical elongations, or empty quarters it manifests, indicates an ordering that has constrained the range of forms that we have encountered. This interpretation immediately becomes clearer once we have access to visualizations of the principal coordinates themselves, as interesting dimensions of a linearized space of shapes. Such a visualization is the ultimate goal of the tools in Sections 5.4 and 5.5: to produce Procrustes shape coordinates as the variables whose principal coordinates are those in Figure 5.43, and then to visualize the axes of these plots as the principal components of those variables.

5.3.3 Example: The Gunz Skull Data Set, II

Let us return to the data set whose template has already been shown in Figure 5.3. The size allometry here has already been called to your attention in Figure 5.34 using groupwise averages of Bookstein coordinates. It is time to make this analysis a great deal more sophisticated.

The data here, kindly supplied by Philipp Gunz, were originally reported in the study published as Bookstein, Gunz et al. (2003). The published study dealt with 38 crania (of which we will use data from up to 29 here) bearing 20 landmark points along with 74 *semilandmarks* (see Section 5.5.4). The 2003 publication used 18 of the landmarks (all except the inions) and 66 of the semilandmarks. The data arise from a synthetic midsagittal plane extracted from solid CT scans – for a drawing in situ, please see figure 1 of the 2003 article. The example is in 2D for ease of exposition – I like being able to highlight on paper what it is that I want you to take note of. The sequence of displays recommended here is the same whether your data arises in 2D or in 3D. (In fact, they also work for data in 1D – points on a line: see Small, 1996.) The complete landmark configurations will be laid out specimen by specimen in Figure 5.74.

A sequence of analyses is displayed all at once in Figure 5.43. At upper left is the initial analysis for the starting data set of $N = 29$ specimens, including an australopithecine and two chimpanzees. The first few singular values of the analysis are 0.236, 0.0349, 0.0159, 0.0129, ..., and so it is appropriate to look at the first two dimensions (singular vectors) only.[4] The structure of this scatter is informative, but not in a way that recommends the interpretation of the principal component analysis (the SVD) per se. We see three forms quite a distance from the others. From the labels, two of these (one male, one female) are chimpanzees (genus *Pan*), and the third is the famous australopithecine specimen Sts 5 discovered at Sterkfontein in 1947, the specimen affectionately known as "Mrs. Ples" ("Ples" for "Plesianthropus," the initial scientific nomenclature, and "Mrs." because it was thought at the time to be a female [though as of this writing the issue of its gender is not yet settled]). At the left of the plot, in the direction opposite Pan M out of

---

[4] The ratio .0159/.0129 falls short of the threshold for $N = 29$ from Figure 4.14.

the grand mean at $(0, 0)$, is a mass of forms labeled either "A" followed by a number – these are all adult *Homo sapiens* specimens – or, for the six juvenile humans, by their age in years (y). Off to one side of the line between these two groups is a clear cluster of three forms all given geographical names – these three are all Neanderthals, as is a fourth form, Atapuerca (a particularly archaic Neanderthal), plotting nearby.

The information this plot conveys about the analysis by principal components is thus explicitly self-refuting. Because the sample is so obviously heterogeneous, the method of principal components should not be applied. Any findings in respect of those linear combinations are necessarily a function of the relative proportions of *H. sapiens, H. neanderthalensis,* and the other species in the sample, and these proportions are not biological phenomena. A numerical inference via PCA can make sense only if applied to a group that might be a legitimate homogeneous sample of something.

So we set aside Mrs. Ples and the chimps and repeat the data centering and the SVD, resulting in the figure in the upper right panel. The first principal component is aligned with the difference between the average Neanderthal and the average *H. sapiens* – this cannot be news, and suggests, once again, that the analysis continues to be without merit. We also delete the four Neanderthals, then, leaving only the 22 *sapiens* (21 modern forms, plus one archaic specimen, "Mladec," from the Mladeč cave in what is now the Czech Republic). In the resulting scatter of the first two columns of *U*, lower left, we see, finally, a continuum from the children on the left to the adults on the right, suggesting, at last, a biological meaning for component 1. We see no structure in RW2, but that is all right because the squared singular values of this 22-skull data set (which are proportional to its principal component variances of 0.029, 0.014, 0.011, . . . – see at Section 5.4.3.2) will suggest, according to Figure 4.14, that no dimensions after the first are interpretable anyway. (If this second dimension had been interpretable, its diagram would be that of the right-hand column in Figure 5.80.)

This example will continue in Section 5.3.4 with another set of principal coordinates, this time including size information, and again in Section 5.6 with the visualization of the axes we have produced that drive the apparent population structure of these dissimilarity scores.

5.3.4 Procrustes Form Distance

This is the most recent component of the standard Vienna syllabus we're reviewing here. Introduced in Mitteroecker et al. (2004), it was certified as part of the consensus only at the Vienna MorphoFest meeting in July 2006, where it was assigned its present name. It has two principal applications: one in studies of group differences or time trends that are confounded by allometry, and the other for studies where allometry is the principal factor of interest. Publications prior to 2006 had no practical means of access to this method, but you should switch to it anyway.

Working at the level of pairwise interspecimen distances, our concern in the present section, this involves adding a term $(\log\ CS_1 - \log\ CS_2)^2$, the square of the log of the ratio of Centroid Sizes, to the shape distances that were extracted following Figure 5.42 before proceeding with principal coordinate analysis as in Section 5.3.2. Remember that logs are to base e. Once we have the Procrustes shape coordinates that will be introduced in the next section, this same maneuver is accomplished by adding a column of log Centroid Sizes to the matrix of shape coordinates derived as in Figure 5.46, and then proceeding with the corresponding principal components analysis; the results are still dual to one another. The "presumption of maximum disorder" reviewed at Section 2.3.5 now extends to one additional clause, the absence of any prior knowledge about allometry (the dependence of shape on size).

If size could possibly be an explanatory factor for your data set, then the principal coordinates plot at upper left in Figure 5.43 needs to be augmented by a second principal coordinates plot (lower right in the same figure) in which Procrustes shape distance is replaced by Procrustes form distance. There is no effect on the shape coordinates, which have not been altered, but thin-plate spline diagrams (Section 5.5) could be modified to incorporate the correct Centroid Size relationship associated with the shape comparison vector being drawn. (The vector space carries these as logarithms, so they need to be exponentiated [to base e] before drawing, as in Figure 5.44, or simply printed as part of the legend.)

For instance, let us return to the data set of $N = 29$ anthropoid skulls (Figure 5.43) to examine what happens if we shift from shape space to the form space we have just introduced. Remember how simple the shift is: we augment the shape coordinate data set with one additional variable that represents geometric size by way of its (natural) logarithm. The result, at lower right in Figure 5.43, is quite different from that for shape space (upper left), with which we began. The singular values are .0954, .0804, .0259, ..., implying that these two dimensions bear all the interpretative weight we can get from this SVD. Now it appears that the male chimp does *not* simply represent an extrapolation of the difference of the female chimp from the humans; rather, he differs from her in a direction not too far from the direction in which the human adults differ from the three infants (the 2y specimen and the two 4y's). The subscatter of all the humans at lower right looks somewhat like a shear of

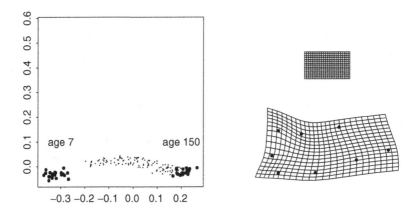

Figure 5.44 First two principal coordinates of the Vilmann rodent data set in form space. The deviation from linear allometry is still apparent toward the middle of the distribution, but now the dominant feature is far more powerful an explanation of the pattern of similarity. At right, anticipating an analysis from Section 5.5, is the grid transformation corresponding to the full length of the first (horizontal) principal coordinate. The net change of Centroid Size, a factor of about 1.89, is now encoded in the diagram. Its value compromises between a greater factor for the longitudinal increase and a lesser factor for the height above the cranial base.

the corresponding configuration at lower left, except that the archaic Mladeč specimen has shifted position in the direction of the Neanderthals. It is still the case that the chimpanzees, and then the Neanderthals, need to be ostracized. There is considerably more explanation of this specific example in chapter 4 of Weber and Bookstein (2011).

As another example of this same procedure, Figure 5.44 shows the computation of the first two form space principal coordinates (all that can be stably estimated) for the Vilmann data set whose shape space ordination will be shown in Figure 5.49. The form space ordination is far more collinear, indicating the strong presence of allometry, the model we have already discussed for these same data in Section 4.3.5. The gap between the 7-day-old and 14-day-old animals is much cleaner in this space (where they differ by about 13% in average size) than in the space of their shapes per se.

Summary of Section 5.3

• One way of launching the extension of multivariate methods to deal with shape is the notion of *Procrustes distance,* which generalizes the subtraction operation $x - y$ that applied to lengths so that it can accommodate two aspects of landmark coordinate data that usually do not carry biologically meaningful information, the location and orientation of the figure as a whole, along with a third aspect, geometrical scale, which, alas, often *is* meaningful.

- A matrix of Procrustes distances between all pairs of specimens can be analyzed by the principal coordinate methods of Section 4.2.5. The resulting dimensions are sometimes called its *relative warps*.
- An example from data about human evolution shows how the principal coordinate plots can be inspected for advice about when not to trust the corresponding biological interpretations.
- *Procrustes form distance,* a recent modification of the formula for Procrustes distance, puts back in the information about size difference that was suppressed in the original approach.

5.4 Procrustes Coordinates, a Different Set of Shape Coordinates

This section reviews the radical solution to the coordinate-system problem that was worked out among us in the geometric morphometric community, beginning with David Kendall and ending with Kanti Mardia, John Kent, and Ian Dryden, in a flurry of applied-mathematics developments over the two decades starting around 1977.

5.4.1 A Language for "Shape Coordinates," Not for "Shape"

My discussion here differs from most introductions to morphometrics by avoiding all talk about "what shape is." There is a way of talking about morphometrics in which one refers to "a shape," and even draws pictures of "shapes," but that is not how data arise from the scanners or how they get attached to biological explanations (which, as we have known since Galileo, are usually not scale-free). In the present context it seems greatly preferable, following language originally published by Mosimann (1970), to refer instead solely to shape *variables* or, for data that were originally Cartesian coordinates, to the term of art "shape coordinates," which are Cartesian coordinates of the original scanned data after being put down over the full sample average in one particular way. (In referring here to "the full sample average" we have gotten a little ahead of our story; that concept will come up at Figure 5.45.)

What differentiates shape variables from other kinds of variables (or shape coordinates from other kinds of coordinates) is their invariance under some

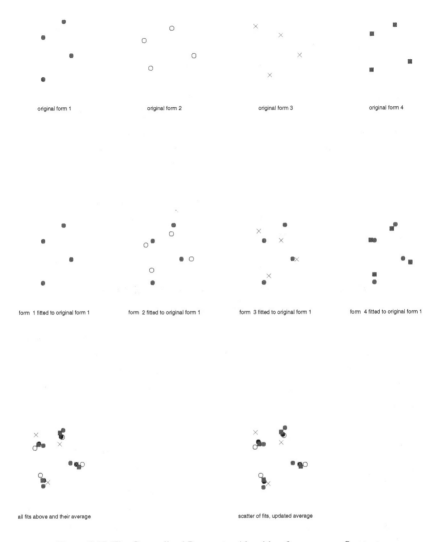

Figure 5.45 The Generalized Procrustes Algorithm for averages. See text.

kinds of transformations of the raw data. For shape variables, following Mosimann, the invariance is against scaling (changing the ruler). For shape coordinates, following Kendall (1984), the invariance is also against the everyday sorts of difficulties involved in getting an object into a scanner: where it should be put and in what direction it should be facing. We want our pattern analyses of coordinates to have both of these properties of positioning invariance, and, sometimes, the scale-free property as well.

There is an exquisite formal theory of "the geometry of shape" (cf. Small, 1996) in which shapes are objectified as "things" that are classes, namely classes of the different sets of coordinates that all have "the same shape." This is not as tautological as it sounds. Shapes in this sense have a geometry of their own, and a statistical distribution theory, but neither of those topics is germane to the discussion here. Still, that general approach has a name for what we are talking about in this chapter: it is "similarity shape," shape coordinates that do not change when the original scans are submitted to an isometric transformation (change of position and orientation, just the nuisances of scanning noted before) but likewise when they are rescaled. There are other possibilities, including "affine shape," which is independent of the way a picture is tilted before scanning, and "projective shape," which is independent of the location of a camera that is taking a 2D photograph of some 3D scene. These are important in other sciences, particularly computer vision and robotics, but we will not need them here.

5.4.2 Gower's "Generalized Procrustes Analysis"

What we *do* need to ensure is that the quantities we are calling "shape coordinates," *considered as functions of the raw Cartesian data*, are immune to the same nuisances of positioning (or scaling) to which the shape distances themselves are immune. We arrange for this by a clever trick due originally to John Kent and Fred Bookstein independently. Shape distance is *defined* as the minimum of familiar (Euclidean) distance over all possible changes of position and orientation, and then the shape coordinates are *defined* as one of the sets of Cartesian coordinates for which ordinary Euclidean distance is almost exactly identical with this minimum *for all pairs of specimens in the original sample*. Follow through the logic again, and you will see that automatically, seemingly just by wishing it, we arrive at a shape distance and a set of shape coordinates that are mutually consistent (squared distances agreeing with sums of squares of coordinate differences) and guaranteed invariant against the transformations they are supposed to ignore. For the definition to be practical there needs to be an easy algorithm. That is the task of the Generalized Procrustes Analysis (GPA) algorithm originally published by John Gower and sketched here in Figure 5.45. For an appropriately respectful discussion of all of this in full algebraic detail, see Dryden and Mardia (2016), and for Gower's own exegesis of these matters, Gower and Dijksterhuis (2004).

5.4.2.1 The Generalized Procrustes Average Shape

By leveraging a standard property of ordinary squared Euclidean distance (sums of squares of coordinate differences, like the areas of the circles in

Figure 5.42) we can get a sample average form for free at the same time we fit each form of a sample *to* that average.

This is not as paradoxical as it sounds. The Procrustes fit is defined by a least-squares criterion in sums of squares, and sample averages are already defined by such a criterion: the average of any set of n numbers x_i, which is $\Sigma_1^n x_i/n$, is the number v minimizing $\Sigma_1^n (v - x_i)^2$ over all possible v. (This is why the algorithm of Figure 5.45 begins with a superposition of the two configurations at their centroids.) This is an average in the original space of the picture or the volume in which our landmark data arose, whereas what we mean by an "average shape" would need to be some sort of shape, not some sort of point on the digitizer; but, still, the intuition is correct. The central **theorem** of all this work is the assertion that for reasonably similar landmark configurations the algorithm in Figure 5.45 converges to the shape that has the least summed squared Procrustes distances to all the configurations of any homologously labelled sample.

Step 1. Choose any specimen in your sample, for instance, the first specimen.
Step 2. Superimpose all the specimens over this specimen in the least-squares position (row 2 of the figure).
Step 3. Take the (ordinary Euclidean) average, landmark by landmark and coordinate by coordinate, of all of the superimposed specimens (row 3, left). Scale this average back up to Centroid Size 1 (it will always have turned out just a little bit less, the same way the "average" of Vienna and Paris is a point a few miles below the surface of the earth near Munich).
Step 4. Replace the first specimen by this average, and return to Step 2. That is, repeat all the fitting operations (row 3 of the figure) until the candidate average stops changing from cycle to cycle to whatever number of significant digits you set in advance.

This is **Generalized Procrustes Analysis** (GPA). For any data set that began with a competently designed landmark configuration that is not too variable, GPA converges to the selfsame average form regardless of the specimen chosen in Step 1. The reason, roughly speaking, is that each step reduces the same sum of squares, the sum of the areas of all the circles we could draw in every frame of the figure, and this minimization has to converge to a unique smallest possible value somewhere above 0.

5.4.2.2 Procrustes Shape Coordinates

Think again about the situation in the final panel of Figure 5.45, imagined as it looks when the iterations have finished. Figure 5.46 enlarges this image

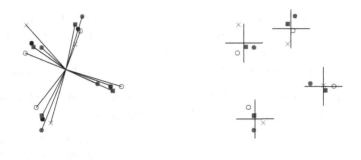

optimal Procrustes positions

the four sets of
Procrustes shape coordinates

Figure 5.46 GPA gives you shape coordinates for free. The units of plots like this are cm/cm, which is to say, dimensionless units of Procrustes shape. (left) The four superimposed shapes. (right) Their shape coordinates.

and enhances it a bit. There is a set of point locations for the average, the big black dots, and for each specimen of the sample a set of point locations around that black dot, plotted with a different symbol for each specimen, such that not only (1) is the average of the four dots for the four specimens for each landmark equal to the big black dot standing for the average shape, but also (2) for each specimen, the squared Procrustes distance from the average is the sum of squares of the coordinatewise differences over all four landmarks of the configuration. It turns out that this equality approximately obtains not only for distances from the average but for the distance between any pair of specimens. (This property is no longer guaranteed when shape variation is too large. See Figure 5.58 and the accompanying text.)

The Procrustes shape coordinates have the following very fine algebraic property: for small variations of shape around an average, they accommodate *every* conventional shape variable of the Rudolf Martin style – "small" variations in *every* ratio of interlandmark distances, *every* angle (or its sine or cosine, except near $\pm 90°$ or $0°$ and $\pm 180°$, respectively), and *every* index that combines these in further algebraic expressions. By "accommodate" we mean there is some linear combination of the shape coordinates that, in the limit of small shape variation, correlates perfectly ($r \cong 1.0$) with the distance, ratio, or index specified. This is just another **theorem**; for a more careful statement with proof, see Bookstein (1991). We will see an application of this property in Section 5.6.6.

Seemingly "just by wishing," then, we have arrived at the variable values whose summed squared differences are the squared distances of the matrices that go into the principal-coordinates analysis (Section 5.3.2). Hence these are a good set of shape coordinates, which we call **Procrustes shape coordinates,** for representing variation within or between samples.[5]

The following, which you read first in Chapter 4, is worth repeating:

The principal coordinates are the scores corresponding to the principal component analysis of the Procrustes shape coordinates.

As already mentioned in Section 5.3, when the concern is with Procrustes form space (which is appropriate for studies where allometry is either a factor or a confound), the Procrustes shape coordinate matrix just introduced is augmented by one additional column for the logarithm (base e) of Centroid Size. In other words, size is "put back into" the Procrustes representation by appending this extra column to the Procrustes shape coordinates, not by multiplying it into those coordinates or anything like that. That multiplication doesn't yield numbers having any useful statistical properties.

For essentially historical reasons (priority of the name in Bookstein, 1991), in the application to Procrustes shape analysis, the vectors that specify the linear combinations of shape coordinates produced by the eigendecompositions of Section 4.2 are called *relative warps* or, when the computations begin with Procrustes form distance, *size-shape relative warps.* The scores are correspondingly often called *relative warp scores.*

5.4.3 Examples

5.4.3.1 Relative Warps as Principal Coordinates of Procrustes Distance: The Vilmann Data Set

The methodology just introduced works quite well when applied to a data set we have already examined several times before: the Vilmann rodent neuro-cranial octagons for which the deformable template appeared in Figure 2.41. Figure 5.47 explicitly shows the eight pairs of shape coordinates underlying this exercise for each of the 144 outlines in the complete data set. All have roughly the same apparent noise (the "thickness" of these little paths), but the

---

[5] *Warning.* These coordinates are not of full rank as a set of variables. They exactly or approximately satisfy four linear constraints (2D data), or seven (3D data), corresponding to the standardizations carried out in the course of the Procrustes fits. For two-dimensional data, the coefficients in these constraint equations are just the first four rows of the matrix J in the next section. So do not use the Procrustes shape coordinates themselves as predictors in multiple regressions, canonical correlations or canonical variates analyses, or multivariate analyses of covariance. Instead, wait for Section 5.5.2, where the partial warps are introduced, or else just don't bother with the techniques that require matrix inversion, since they really aren't of much use in highly multivariate contexts like GMM.

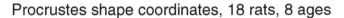

Procrustes shape coordinates, 18 rats, 8 ages

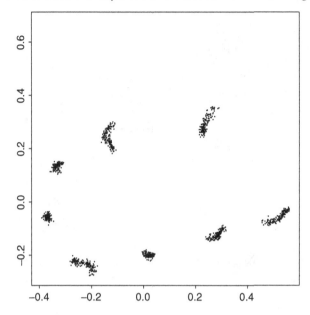

Figure 5.47 All eight Procrustes shape coordinate pairs for the complete Vilmann rodent skull shape data set.

extensions *along* the trajectory seem quite variable and also often are curved, implying that we will need at least two dimensions of explanations to account for them. (As it happens, it will take at least *four*: see Figures 5.99– 5.100.) As Figure 5.48 shows, each trajectory aligns with the age trend for the data as a whole. Individual variation around this shared trend is the subject of the traces in Figure 5.49.

The link to biological interpretation is conveyed most clearly by the diagram in Figure 5.50, which is the representation of the first two principal components by the associated patterns of joint shape coordinate displacement. The crucial associated statistical quantity is the list of squared Procrustes distance explained by the successive relative warps: these are 0.608, 0.059, 0.018, 0.012, . . . , meaning, according to Figure 4.14, that only two dimensions segregate from the noise. (The effective sample size is necessarily less than $18 \times 8 = 144$, owing to correlations of the same animal's shape across time.) As the figure indicates, the first component combines a lowering of the height of the anterior neurocranium with a substantial lengthening of the cranial base along the bottom of the diagram. This component moves monotonically along

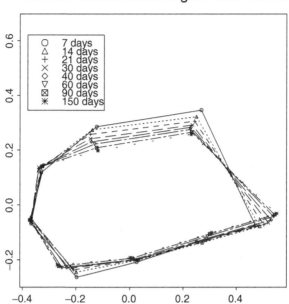

Figure 5.48 Procrustes average shapes for the Vilmann rat data age by age.

the age series in all the animals. Perpendicular to it (and also uncorrelated) is a second component that follows a U-shaped trajectory, first shearing the upper-anterior pair of landmarks (Bregma and Lambda) backward with respect to the lower-posterior pair SOS and Basion between ages 7 and 30 days, then reversing this trend between 30 days and 150.

5.4.3.2 The Same for the Human Midsagittal Cranial Data Set

We have already seen the principal coordinates for the Procrustes distances of the full Gunz data set in Figure 5.43. The further visualizations here will pertain to the subsample in the lower left panel of that figure, the analysis for the 22 specimens labeled *Homo sapiens* (including the archaic Mladeč specimen) or infant. Proceeding in parallel with the rodent example, we figure the complete original Procrustes shape coordinate scatter (Figure 5.51), and then the joint shifts in these coordinates that account for the meaningful principal components (in this example, only the first) (Figure 5.52).

Squared Procrustes distances attributable to the principal components here are 0.029, 0.014, 0.011 , ... According to Figure 4.14, only the first of these is likely to be meaningful in a sample this small. According to Figure 5.52,

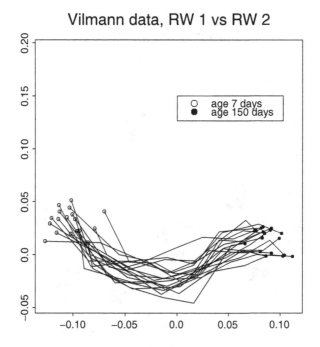

Figure 5.49 Principal coordinate trajectories for the 18 Vilmann rats separately. The axes of this plot, the first two principal components of their Procrustes shape coordinates, will be displayed as grids in Figure 5.81.

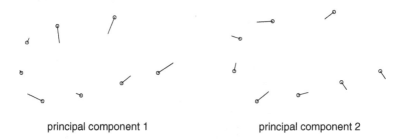

principal component 1   principal component 2

Figure 5.50 The principal coordinates of Figure 5.49 as principal components, diagrammed via the simultaneous displacements of all eight shape coordinate pairs.

this single principal component can be interpreted as a relative shortening of the segment joining Lambda to Inion without much displacement or rotation, along with a substantial anterior extension of the maxilla at left. We will see in a later figure that this pattern closely comports with the well-known pattern

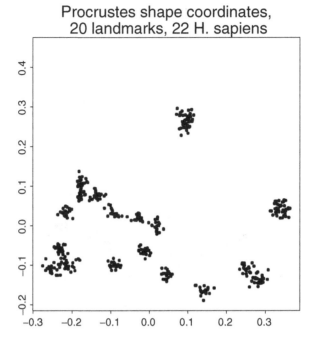

Figure 5.51 Scatter of Procrustes shape coordinates for the 20 landmarks of the midsagittal human cranial data set (Figures 5.3 and 5.43).

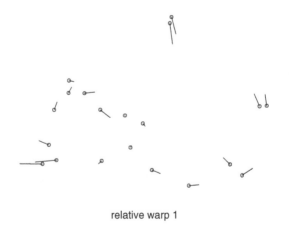

relative warp 1

Figure 5.52 Shape coordinate displacements (loadings on the first principal component) corresponding to the first principal coordinate in the lower left panel of Figure 5.43, the only apparently meaningful coordinate in this decomposition. See text.

whereby the brain more or less completes its growth long before the maxillary apparatus.

5.4.3.3 Bringing Regression Back In

The same shape coordinates that are amenable to a principal components analysis can likewise be analyzed by any other biometrically appropriate multivariate strategy. For instance, we can explicitly compute *allometry*, the effect of size on shape, by regressing the complete vector of shape coordinates on the measure of size that was partialled out in the course of the construction of the shape coordinates: the scaling factor we have called Centroid Size. If a first principal component is to be interpreted as allometry, then, as we have already explained in Section 4.2.2, it needs to substantially resemble this pattern of regressions on size. For the Vilmann rodent data, the pattern of coordinate-by-coordinate regression coefficients on Centroid Size, Figure 5.53, is a very good match to the pattern for relative warp 1 in Figure 5.50. Similarly, the regression of Figure 5.51's shape coordinates on Centroid Size, Figure 5.54, closely matches the first principal component of these 22 human midsagittal configurations.

5.4.4 The Isotropic Mardia–Dryden Distribution

Corresponding to the geometry of Figures 5.42, 5.45, 5.46 there is a statistical distribution, the **offset isotropic Gaussian distribution,** for which probability density is a function solely of Procrustes distance from the sample average. This is the distribution we have already shown in Figure 5.37 as it would appear in the digiziting space, before the GPA processing step. Formulas for this distribution, which is also called *the isotropic offset Gaussian distribution* or *the Mardia-Dryden distribution with isotropic covariance matrix*, can be found in the textbook by Dryden and Mardia. On this model, Procrustes distance is the *optimal* statistical quantity for proceeding with statistical tests such as comparisons of group mean shape or covariation of shape or form with some claimed cause or effect of form.

As far as I am aware, nobody has ever seen a real biological data set for which the isotropy of this assumption obtains. All real data have differences of variance by location or direction and local shape factors of greater or lesser scope that contradict the stark symmetry of the distribution *when stated as an empirical fact.* This is just another way of explaining why we need organismal biologists. But realism is not the reason we use Procrustes distance in a statistical context. Instead, following the principles of E. T. Jaynes (2003), we use this distribution to model our **ignorance of underlying biological processes**

rodent shape regressions on Centroid Size

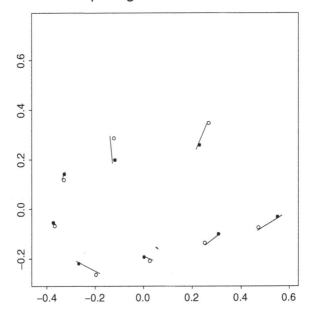

Figure 5.53 Regression coefficients for each of the Vilmann rodent landmarks expressed as the expected shift over the range of observed Centroid Size scores. Solid dots: observed average form at age 150. Open circles: observed average form at age 7. Each little line goes through the grand mean of its shape coordinates (not shown). Where these segments fail to pass through the dots, it is because of curvature in the actual trajectories of the landmark over the growth period.

prior to the data analysis. The best way of thinking about the Gaussian in this context is through the last of its characterizations in Section 2.3. The Gaussian distribution is the distribution that maximizes entropy (minimizes information, maximizes ignorance) for given mean and variance, and that desideratum, it seems to me, is the best principle to embrace if you don't have any prior quantitative knowledge according to which to modify it. (The principle is analogous to the thin-plate spline's characterization as minimizing the appearance of local shape features; see Section 5.5.1.) I know only one biometric context in which prior knowledge routinely dominates this state of earnest ignorance: structures with bilateral symmetry, to be considered in Section 5.6.7.

In these Procrustes probability distributions, noncorrelation stands for a geometric property, orthogonality. For the reader who has had some multivariate algebra, we offer the following table as the geometric decomposition of vector spaces that is tangent to the non-euclidean geometry actually

midsagittal skull shape regressions on Centroid Size, N = 22

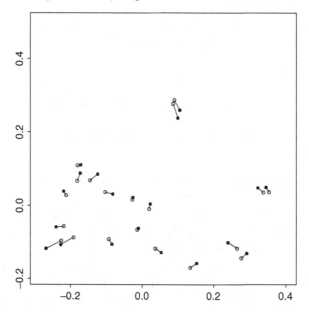

Figure 5.54 The same for the human midsagittal skull data set. Open dots: predicted shape at the smallest size (corresponding to the two-year-old child). Closed dots: at the largest size (corresponding to the Mladeč specimen). As for the rodent data set, this regression pattern closely resembles the first principal component of the same data set (Figure 5.52).

underlying all the Procrustes machinery here. *In this subsection only,* I refer to a **mean shape** μ on k landmarks $(x_1, y_1), (x_2, y_2), \ldots, (x_k, y_k)$ vectorized as $(x_1, y_1, x_2, y_2, \ldots, x_k, y_k)$ with $\Sigma x_i = \Sigma y_i = \Sigma x_i y_i = 0$, $\Sigma(x_i^2 + y_i^2) = 1$ (meaning: μ is centered, its Centroid Size is 1, and it has been rotated to principal axes horizontal and vertical). Write $\alpha = \Sigma x_i^2, \gamma = 1 - \alpha = \Sigma y_i^2$ — the central moments of the mean configuration in its principal directions — and $\delta = 1/\sqrt{k}$. Finally, set $\alpha' = \sqrt{\alpha/\gamma}$ and $\gamma' = \sqrt{\gamma/\alpha}$.

Consider the matrix J of six rows by $2k$ columns

$$
J = \begin{pmatrix}
\delta & 0 & \delta & 0 & \ldots & \delta & 0 \\
0 & \delta & 0 & \delta & \ldots & 0 & \delta \\
-y_1 & x_1 & -y_2 & x_2 & \ldots & -y_k & x_k \\
x_1 & y_1 & x_2 & y_2 & \ldots & x_k & y_k \\
\alpha' y_1 & \gamma' x_1 & \alpha' y_2 & \gamma' x_2 & \ldots & \alpha' y_k & \gamma' x_k \\
-\gamma' x_1 & \alpha' y_1 & -\gamma' x_2 & \alpha' y_2 & \ldots & -\gamma' x_k & \alpha' y_k
\end{pmatrix}
\tag{5.7}
$$

and write $J_i, i = 1, \ldots, 6$, for the ith row of J.

- J is orthonormal by rows.

For any small σ, sample configurations C of k landmark locations from the distribution $N(\mu, \sigma^2 I)$, treated as column vectors, and consider the various derived configurations

$$C^j = C - \Sigma_{i=1}^{j} J_i^t(J_i C), \quad j = 2, 3, 4, 6. \tag{5.8}$$

Because J is orthonormal, each C^i is spherically symmetric within its subspace. (The symbol C^i is read "C-super-i.")

- C^2 is centered in both even-numbered (vertical) and odd-numbered (horizontal) coordinates.
- C^3 is centered and has been rotated to a position of zero torque against μ.
- The fourth row of J scales each C to centroid size 1 (approximate, to second order in σ). (For dy small with respect to y, $(y + dy)^2 \sim y^2 + 2y \cdot dy$; y^2 is a constant, and the coefficient 2 goes away when we revert from squared Centroid Size to just plain Centroid Size, as $\sqrt{1 + \epsilon} \sim 1 + \frac{1}{2}\epsilon$ for small ϵ.) Hence C^4 is, approximately, the vector of Procrustes shape coordinates for the distribution C, written out as deviations from the sample average form.
- For small σ, because $\log(1 + \epsilon) \sim \epsilon$, C^3 is a rotation of the matrix that augments C^4 by log Centroid Size; hence it is a representation of the form space of C that was introduced at Section 5.3.4. (Remember that logs are to base e.)
- The fifth and sixth rows of J correspond to the shear and dilation terms in the uniform component of shape around μ. Hence $(J_5 C, J_6 C)$ is the uniform component of any configuration C, while C^6 is, approximately, the vector of nonaffine shape coordinates for the distribution C. The distribution C^6 has rank $2k - 6$; it is spanned by the partial warp scores, which, treated as a joint projection matrix, comprise an orthonormal basis orthogonal to J. (Two novel technical terms here, the uniform component and the partial warp scores, will be introduced in Section 5.5.)
- For an isotropic Gaussian model, the distribution of any of the C's itself remains spherical in its linearized subspace. This applies most often to the space C^4 of the usual Procrustes shape coordinates. Its particular flavor of biological meaninglessness leads to patterns having no real factors.

Translating all this back into less algebraic language: Starting from $2k$ Cartesian coordinates in 2D, we lose two dimensions of variability for centering, one for rotation and one for scaling (these last two as approximated linearly near the average form, itself rescaled to Centroid Size 1). If we stop here, after the fourth of these vectors, we get our familiar Procrustes shape coordinates. The variance *removed* at each landmark after it has been centered is proportional to its squared distance from the centroid when the configuration is at Centroid Size 1; hence the residual standard deviation at landmark r from the origin is proportional to $\sqrt{1 - r^2}$. To get to Procrustes form distance Section (5.3.4), at least in cases of limited size variability, we carry out steps 1, 2, and 3 only. For studies of integration (Section 5.6.8), we project out all six of these dimensions from each specimen.

Another approximation. The projection apparatus that drives the formalism of equation (5.7) is a least-squares procedure notated in each coordinate of the original digitization separately. For data in two dimensions we can take advantage of complex arithmetic to set down an alternate formula for a very slightly different result that is much more concise. The new formula begins in column 3 of Figure 5.42, after the two forms of interest have been centered and scaled to Centroid Size separately. Write these two configurations as two vectors $(z_1, z_2, \ldots, z_p)$ and $(w_1, w_2, \ldots, w_p)$ where the z's and the w's are all complex numbers. Then when the z-configuration and the w-configuration are almost the same, we can compute nearly the same superposition as the one at lower right in that figure by using the complex version of the least-squares machinery of line fitting we already encountered (for real numbers) in Chapter 2. The superposition of the z's over the w's is the predicted value from the regression of the w's on the z's: the set of points $C(z_1, z_2, \ldots, z_p)$, where C, the regression coefficient, is governed by essentially the same formula as in the real case, the ratio of a "covariance" to a "variance," except that for complex numbers the sums of squares and crossproducts entail taking the complex conjugate of the predictor coordinates. (This makes sense, as if you rotate the predictor clockwise by some angle, you must rotate the prediction coefficient *counterclockwise* by the same angle to get the same prediction.) In symbols, the fit of the z-configuration onto the w-configuration achieved by Figure 5.42 is very nearly

$$(w_1', w_2', \ldots, w_p') = \frac{\sum w_i \overline{z_i}}{\sum z_i \overline{z_i}} \ (z_1, z_2, \ldots, z_p). \tag{5.7a}$$

(This differs from the algorithm in Figure 5.42 only in that the prediction no longer has Centroid Size equal to 1.0; it is very slightly shrunk.) The projection residuals from the first four rows of equation (5.7) are, except for this slight shrinkage, the same as the residuals from this same regression, the values $w_i - C z_i$ with C this same coefficient, $\frac{\sum w_i \overline{z_i}}{\sum z_i \overline{z_i}}$.

Boas coordinates. I already called your attention to something odd in the explanation of Procrustes form space (Section 5.3.4). In an early step, the method there divides the original Cartesian coordinates by Centroid Size, a quantification of size in units of (say) centimeters. Later that information is restored to the data base of Procrustes coordinates, but by a different route: a logarithm, not a raw measurement, that participates as an additive component of squared "distance," not the scaling factor it originally was. These steps do not exactly cancel out, but perhaps there is a way to circumvent both of them? Yes, there is, and (in a gentle irony) it appeared in the literature more than half a century before any of the Procrustes techniques that have preceded it in this section. This is the method of the American anthropologist Franz Boas (1905), who standardized landmark configurations for position and orientation but *not* for scale. Alternatively, they are the Procrustes shape coordinates scaled back *up* by the factor of Centroid Size that we divided out to get Procrustes distance.

The diagrams generated by these novel coordinates sometimes permit a more "biological" metaphor of growth as displacement in systems where growth is truly a biological factor of the variation under study. Compare, for instance, the two versions of our familiar Vilmann rodent neurocranial growth data displayed in Figure 5.55. At upper left is the analysis of Procrustes shape coordinates we have already seen in Figures 5.47 through 5.49. The diagram shows, for instance, the relative elongation of the cranial base with respect to the calvarial roof that will turn out to be the dominant nonuniform feature of this data set. But for a system that actually grows by interstitial deposition, the figure at upper right is more suggestive of those underlying histological mechanisms. In this figure, size change is actually integrated into the description. We "see" landmarks along the cranial base "pushed apart" by increase of length of the segments separating them. Also, we "see," without having explicitly measured these things, that this directional increase is matched neither by the vertical extensions also shown nor by the horizontal respacing along the calvarial roof. Thus *for systems that are growing interstitially,* and only those, these coordinates might be preferred for generating hypotheses or explanations. At the same time, the "center" of the figure has no biological reality, nor has the appearance of centrifugality (growth away from the center). Note also how the Boas coordinates, but not the Procrustes coordinates, sometimes imitate the separation between the age-7 scatter and those at all older ages from the principal coordinates analysis of the same data in Procrustes form space (Figure 5.44).

The word "see" and the dynamic phrase "pushed apart" in the preceding paragraph are in scare quotes because your eye evolved to infer such patterns even when they are not real. This is the aspect of visual processing known

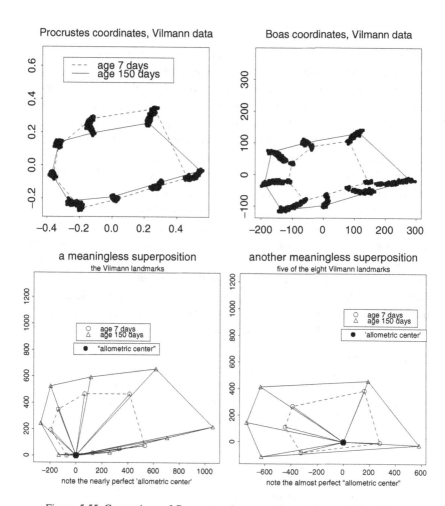

Figure 5.55 Comparison of Procrustes shape coordinates (upper left) to Boas coordinates (upper right) for the Vilmann rodent neurocranial octagons. The lines trace the averages at ages 7 days (dashed) or 150 days (solid). (bottom left, right) The scientist's eye is unskilled at detecting artifacts in superpositions like these. Here we "see" a pattern of radial displacement of the Vilmann landmarks away from an "allometric center" that depends mainly on the list of landmarks selected.

as *optical flow*, which is very useful in computer graphics and the gaming industry. A related percept is the suggestion of an "allometric center" in the figure, a point near the middle from which all the landmarks appear to be "growing away." Fortunately, there are theorems about the construction of such patterns. Unfortunately, the theorems imply that for most pairs of configurations of five landmarks one can construct a few such points (not by the centering algorithm of Section 5.4, of course) with respect to which the landmarks appear to be growing radially no matter what the biology of those landmarks actually is. In the lower row of Figure 5.55, where each panel corresponds to a minimum variance for the angles between pairs of homologous landmarks out of the putative "centers," the analyses cannot both be correct, but certainly they can both be wrong (see Bookstein, 1983, or Moss and Skalak, 1983). The problem here is similar to the problem of pattern misperception in random walk, Section 2.6.2.

It may be possible to pass from this level of informal observation to a formal multivariate method for the modeling of allometry that continues to circumvent the scaling step of the standard Procrustes construction (see Felsenstein and Bookstein, 2016). At the same time, because all the interpretation has to proceed in terms of separations between adjacent landmark pairs, the multivariate statistics of the coordinates themselves are not particularly informative *except* in the context of that same allometric hypothesis. An alternative approach for the analysis of how nearby landmarks deviate with respect to their neighbors is the analysis of integration vis-à-vis selfsimilarity in landmark configurations; I turn to this new method in Section 5.6.8.

> The matrix J is an explicit function of the mean shape μ at which it is evaluated. Different mean shapes correspond to different construals of all of the dimensions here, even the uniform component in rows 5 and 6. For a rigorous exploration of how these matrices shift under shifts of the underlying mean configuration, see Bookstein (2009c).

5.4.5 Covariance Distance

Section 4.3.5 noted an alternate interpretation of equation (4.47), one approximation to twice the logarithm of the Wishart probability distribution for covariance matrices. The sum of the squares of the logarithms of the relative eigenvalues is the natural squared distance for relating any pair of covariance matrices whether or not one is an identity matrix. Explicitly, this is

$$d^2(\Sigma_1, \Sigma_2) \equiv \sum_{j=1}^{p} \log^2 \lambda_j, \tag{5.9}$$

where p is the count of measured variables making up the matrices Σ_1 and Σ_2 of their covariances under contrasting conditions (different ages or different species, for instance) and the λ's are the relative eigenvalues, extremal ratios of variance of linear combinations between the two covariance structures, as in Figure 4.25. The formula requires only that neither matrix has any zero eigenvalues. However, the shape coordinate construction demands four zero eigenvalues (two for translation, one each for rotation and for scaling), and so an adjustment is required before it can be applied in this context. Mitteroecker and Bookstein (2009) straightforwardly suggested that shape coordinate covariance matrices be reduced not only to the dimensionality $2k-4$ of the nonvanishing shape coordinate space itself but well beyond that, all the way down to the dimension of the "meaningful part" of these covariance structures, by deletion of *all* dimensions of sufficiently small eigenvalue from the pooled within-group covariance matrix of the combined samples as a whole.[6] The result is ad hoc, no longer model-based, but produces very interesting ordinations wherever they can be shown to be stable when the count of preserved principal components is varied a bit.

For the Vilmann shape coordinate data, we computed covariances of the Procrustes shape coordinates (a total of 16), reduced to the subspace of from three to six dominant principal components (for robustness), and produced the analysis at lower left in Figure 5.56 by the distance formula and thereafter the principal coordinate analysis explained above. **Finding:** analyses are stable for counts of relative warps of 4, 5, or 6. (We will see in Figure 5.99 that four is the number of separate developmental processes combined in these growth series.) The covariance structure of this growth process makes a turn of nearly $180°$ around the time of weaning. The closer investigation in Figure 5.85 will show that the phenomenon involves a canalization (decrease in variance) of the vertical component of the uniform transformation of this shape between ages 7 and 30 days, and then a corresponding reinflation of this component of individual difference between 40 and 150 days. An explanation might proceed via the associated changes in craniofacial function, specifically action of the muscles of mastication. There is an extended discussion of this and other examples in Bookstein and Mitteroecker (2014). But the technique should not be pushed too far, where "too far" has an actual quantitative meaning: see the extended critique of this same example in Bookstein (2017a).

5.4.6 GPA Subtleties, Some Standard, Some New

This section might just as well have been entitled "Problems with Procrustes Analysis." In the three decades that the GMM community has been

---

[6] The technique generalizes Bernhard Flury's (1988) technique of *common principal components analysis*, which models all pairs of correspondingly numbered eigenvectors as parallel, so that each of the terms λ_i reduces to the ratio of corresponding eigenvalues of the matrices separately. The approach here allows those eigenvectors to rotate also, and thus embraces more geometric degrees of freedom.

keeping 3 relative warps

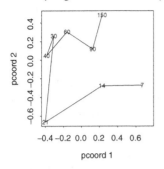

keeping 4 relative warps

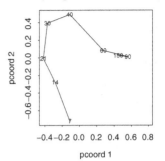

keeping 5 relative warps

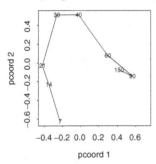

keeping 6 relative warps

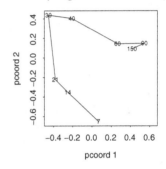

Figure 5.56 The first two principal coordinates for shape covariance distance among the Vilmann neurocranial octagons at eight ages. The four panels exploit 3, 4, 5, or 6 relative warps of the full data set. Evidently analyses of 4, 5, or 6 dimensions are fully consistent; it was (the one for five dimensions that was published in Mitteroecker and Bookstein 2009).

systematically relying on generalized Procrustes analysis, several of its predictable subtleties have come to light. In an earlier draft of this section I called them "fallacies," but that word doesn't really apply when the mathematics is working precisely as advertised. As Shakespeare might have put it, the fault, dear reader, is not in our formulas, but in ourselves. This section reviews an assortment of these predictable inconveniences, some of which can seriously interfere with an ostensibly persuasive summary narrative. I have treated many of these themes in greater detail in Bookstein (2016b).

Trade-off of noise against distance from the centroid. As noted in Section 5.4.4, for data generated as circular Gaussians around a mean, the GPA is approximately the same as a projection out of four dimensions that are

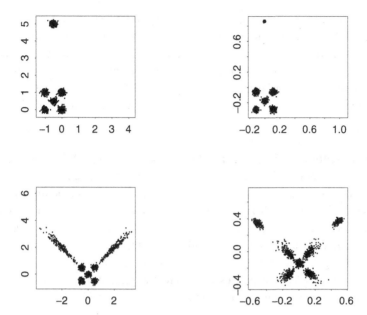

Figure 5.57 Interactions of GPA with overall landmark spacing. Both rows show simulations of 200 instances. Left column, original locations of the simulated landmarks; right column, locations after GPA. Upper row: landmark-specific variation may appear to have been "reassigned" by the GPA computation. Lower row: size allometry likewise may be "reassigned" as shape patterns (but is recoverable from the principal coordinate representation).

functions of the mean form only. The residual from these four projections is still a circular Gaussian coordinate pair with a radius proportional to $\sqrt{1 - r^2}$, where r is the distance from the centroid as scaled to a net Centroid Size of 1.0.

It follows that if one landmark is much more distant from the centroid than all the others, the output of the GPA computation will reassign nearly all of its variation to the other landmarks instead. This is demonstrated in the upper row of Figure 5.57. As a simple extension, if there are *two* landmarks at a relatively larger distance (for instance, Lambda and Inion on the anthropoid skull), the GPA fit drastically shrinks the variance of the segment between them in the course of its own least-squares operations. In a simulation of *this* pathology (Figure 5.57, lower row), the variation at the two farthest landmarks is strongly noncircular. In reducing that variability, the GPA has induced a complementary but quite fictitious noncircularity in four of the five landmarks that were originally characterized by circularity of noise. The principal coordinate of the configuration (there is only one that is meaningful) remain valid, as does the image of the corresponding relative warp: in shape terms, the size effect is on the ratio between the size of the X of landmarks and its relative displacement from the upper one or two. You should never attempt to "read" landmark-specific patterns of variance and covariance from a shape coordinate plot, as the effects of the superposition step (here, the GPA) per se are so difficult to intuit.

Misrepresentation of Procrustes distance after a GPA. When two forms are each superimposed by the Procrustes procedure on the same distant grand mean, their relation to each other can be arbitrarily biased in the direction of greater sum of squares. The effect is driven by the dependence of the formula for relative rotation, third row of the J-matrix (equation 5.7), on the details of the average form used in the formulation of J. Demonstrated in Figure 5.58, it is, once again, counterintuitive. The fit to the "grand mean" paralellogram has rotated these two rectangles by different angles, even though their own Procrustes superposition requires no relative rotation at all.

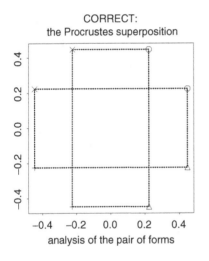
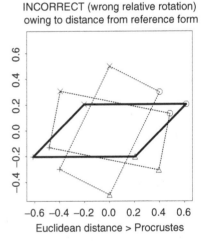

Figure 5.58 Two rectangular forms superimposed on one another by their pairwise Procrustes fit (left) and also compared after superposition on a quite different parallelopiped (right) standing for an inconveniently dissimilar sample average form (thick line). When two forms are quite disparate from the remainder of a sample of shapes in this way, the Procrustes distance between them can be arbitrarily exaggerated in the GPA fit, and, with it, the relative leverage of the pair in the principal coordinates plots and their relative separation there.

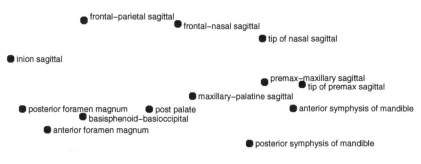

Figure 5.59 Average locations of 13 midsagittal landmarks for the 55-skull sample described in the text. This GPA mean form drives the real instance in Figure 5.60 of the problem sketched for an abstract quadrilateral in Figure 5.58.

Let me exemplify this concern via an extract from a reanalysis of a carefully collected data set published in Marcus et al. (2000), and used here with the kind permission of Erika Hingst-Zaher. As originally published by Marcus et al., the data set concerns 35 landmark points (13 midsagittal – see the listing included in this book's online resource – along with 22 from the right side) taken from solid skulls and mandibles of 57 specimens from 23 of the 27 "orders of living mammals" recognized at the time, omitting four orders for reasons given in the original publication. (As the original authors explained, "A representative sample of skull shapes were included from some orders exhibiting a greater diversity in skull shape.") From this list of 57 I deleted the cetacean owing to the extremely variant position of the nostril, which would have destroyed the GMM analysis just as in Figure 5.57, and also the representative hyena, owing to a missing datum. Digitization was by Les Marcus using a MicroScribe (a technology standard at the time) for his selections from the storerooms of the American Museum of Natural History.

The average of the full sample of 55 midsagittal 13-gons (Figure 5.59) does not much resemble the anthropoid Bauplan familiar from our courses in human biology and evolution. This disproportion between the anthropoids and the rest of the clade, highlighted in the lower left panel of Figure 5.60, is sufficient to launch the malpositioning problem detailed in the upper right panel there. The GPA has indeed overestimated the dissimilarity between *Homo* and *Gorilla* and subtly shifted its general anatomical location toward the upper posterior border of the skull.

The difference here is consequential. The lower row of Figure 5.60 shows, at left, the first two dimensions of the contrasts along this phylogeny as a

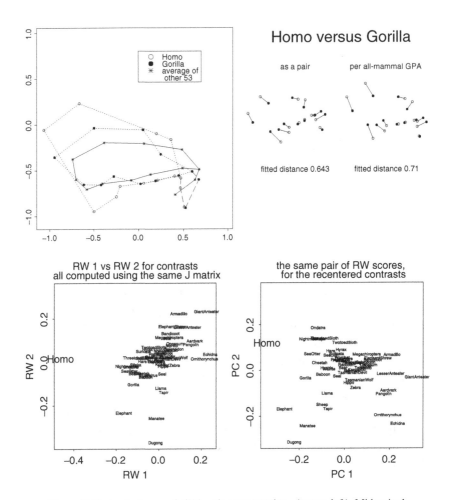

Figure 5.60 An instance of GPA misrepresentation. (upper left) Midsagittal landmark configurations from the all-mammal data set of Marcus et al. (2000), for *Homo*, *Gorilla*, and the average of the 53 other specimens. (upper right) The relation between *Homo* and *Gorilla* is overestimated in the pooled GPA and its leverage in the principal coordinates and relative warps plots is overweighted by the GPA's convention of referring to "the wrong average." The effect is made even worse in the context of phylogenetic contrasts adjusted for divergence time (which is very short for this particular pair of genera). (lower row) Implications of this problem in Figure 5.60 for the calibration of morphometrics against the consensus phylogeny of the mammals. See text.

scatterplot of their GPA principal coordinates. The point for our genus, its name printed in a larger font, is isolated outside the convex hull of the rest of this distribution, to which it is only weakly tethered by the relation to its nearest neighbor. The figure also includes the corresponding scatterplot for the recentered method recommended in this subsection.[7] (But in fact a data set of this range is well beyond the scope for which any of the approximations we have made in the course of Sections 5.2, 5.3, and 5.4 should be expected to apply routinely.)

The failure to recenter has had a drastic effect on the conventional contrast-based scatterplot from left to right. This instability is an innate failing of the principal component method itself when faced with a true synapomorphy such as our neurocranial form.[8] All the details of the positions of *Gorilla* and *Homo* have changed with respect to this central tendency – but *Homo* is, after all, the genus of greatest interest to us in the course of analyzing data sets like this one. For further discussion of this artifact, see Bookstein (2016b). When a multivariate analysis is as sensitive to details of assumptions as this one turns out to be, no "conclusions" of any kind can be trusted without a strenuous effort to survey the full range of feasible analyses. This caution applies with particular strength in high-dimensional analyses reported via their first two or three principal components – best, perhaps, *never* to trust such analyses at all unless the PCs can be rotated to align with factors of form already known to be real, as in Figure 5.82. This degree of conscientiousness is found only rarely, alas, in the actual text of published articles using principal components of contrasts. For more on this example, including the phylogeny of the mammals on which it is relying, please consult Bookstein (2016b).

---

[7] Both computations began with Felsenstein's method of contrasts of the 1980s, as reviewed in his textbook of 2004, applied to the vector space of all 26 shape coordinates of this 13-landmark configuration after a maximum-likelihood adjustment to the conventional GPA that will be described elsewhere (Felsenstein and Bookstein, 2016). The fossil record for charismatic megafauna is too spotty for us to reliably quantify how long the periods of neutral drift have lasted, versus either directional or stabilizing selection, on any of the branches of the mammalian consensus phylogeny used here. Therefore, the contrast vectors cannot reliably be corrected for elapsed time. The resulting computation is equivalent to a principal components analysis of the pairwise discrepancies between the unweighted average shapes of the two poles of each of the Felsenstein contrasts.

[8] Canonical correlations of the left and the right pair of axes in the figure are 0.998 and 0.833. The direction of least stability is the vertical in the scatter at right; even with *Homo* omitted, the canonical correlation in this direction is only 0.898.

Of course there are corresponding "subtleties" in the two-point registrations too. Advice for avoiding those was already explicit in my monograph of 1991: use relatively long baselines, with the relatively lowest coefficients of variation of length, and, wherever possible, aligned with the principal axes of the uniform component of the shape change under study and passing close to the centroid of the mean configuration as a whole. Perhaps it is an advantage that shape coordinates to a two-point baseline do not conduce to principal components analysis of "shape" per se – principal components to different baselines can be substantially different, and there is no single formula for principal coordinates (i.e., no shape distance) to which they are dual. Their application is typically to issues of group mean difference or shape regressions, not to ordinations.

Additional hidden interactions between Procrustes analysis and the principal components of their shape coordinates. The following two identities are obvious:

$$\text{cov}(x, y) = \text{var}\left(\frac{x+y}{2}\right) - \text{var}\left(\frac{x-y}{2}\right),$$

$$\text{cov}(x, y) = \frac{1}{2}\left(4\,\text{var}\left(\frac{x+y}{2}\right) - \text{var}(x) - \text{var}(y)\right).$$

Panel (a) of Figure 5.61 reminds us of the usual definition of covariance as the average of a centered crossproduct (equation 2.8), while panel (b) rearranges this according to the first identity above as the difference of two variances at $45°$ to the original xy axes. When the x and y in question are the two shape coordinates of a single landmark, as in panel (c), these two variances can be thought of as the variances of a new pair of coordinates rotated from the original system by the same $45°$.

But principal components analysis of Procrustes shape coordinates does not involve only the covariances of the two coordinates of the same landmark, but also the covariances of pairs of x-coordinates and pairs of y-coordinates for different landmarks and pairs x_i, y_j of one x-coordinate with the y-coordinate of another locus. There the implications of panel (b), when drawn out geometrically, are unexpectedly far-reaching. Suppose, for instance, that the two x-coordinates in question lie at opposite ends of a diameter of the form. Then the Procrustes registration, by trying to standardize the centroid at $(0, 0)$, has the effect of intentionally minimizing the variance of their *average*. By the second identity above, as embedded in panel (e), it follows that shape

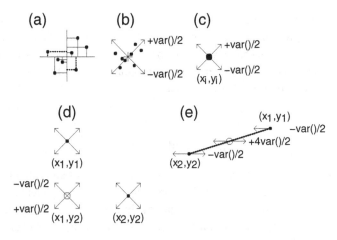

Figure 5.61 Procrustes registrations have interesting effects on covariances. (a) By definition – recall Figure 2.5 – $\mathrm{cov}(x, y)$ is the average area of rectangles like these. Dots: (x, y) pairs. Dotted lines: negative areas. (b) Equivalent quantity: the difference between two directional variances after a rotation. The terms $\mathrm{var}(x \pm y)/2$ in the first equation below are the same as half the variances of $(x \pm y)/\sqrt{2}$ in the figure; these are the rotations of the original x and y axes by $45°$. (c) When x and y are Cartesian coordinates of the same landmark, these directional variances are coordinate variances as well, in the direction of the rotated axes. (d) But the covariance of the x-coordinate of one point with the y-coordinate of a second point involves the variances of the terms $x_1 \pm y_2$. When the original landmarks lie at approximately a $90°$ angle with respect to the centroid, these variances are strongly affected by the rotational aspect of a Procrustes registration. (e) Likewise, the covariance of a pair of x coordinates or a pair of y-coordinates is affected by the translational aspect of a Procrustes registration, which tries to minimize their average (the term $\mathrm{var}(\frac{x+y}{2})$ in the second formula above).

coordinates of landmarks situated at opposite ends of a diameter of the form will tend to covary negatively in the direction of that diameter; hence the pair will typically appear as a contrast on whatever principal component they load on. Similarly, from panel (d) it follows that for landmarks at roughly $90°$ from one another out of the centroid, depending on where the centroid is, the covariance of either the *difference* between one x and the other y or their *sum* will be attenuated by the Procrustes registration, while the variance of the corresponding sum or difference, respectively, will be aggrandized; hence principal components tend to shift pairs of landmarks at $90°$ away from the centroid in a direction opposite to the shift of pairs at $90°$ in the other direction. But this is the same phenomenon as in panel (e) except now applying to pairs of landmarks instead of singletons. Neither of these contrastive phenomena has anything to do with biological processes, of course; they are mere artifacts of the Procrustes procedure. For further discussion on this point see Bookstein (2016b, appendix 2).

Summary of Section 5.4

- John Gower's *generalized Procrustes analysis* is a robust algorithm for the *Procrustes average shape* of the data sets one typically encounters in organismal biology – the shape that has the least sum of squared Procrustes distances to the specimens of most samples you will actually encounter in practice.
- The same algorithm gives you *Procrustes shape coordinates* "for free" – the vector representation of the shapes in a high-dimensional but graphically very congenial multivariate space to which the maneuvers of Chapter 4 apply elegantly.
- In this context two of the analyses of Section 4.2 yield the same result: the principal components of the Procrustes shape coordinates are at the same time the principal coordinates of their Procrustes distances. This is not true for other shape coordinate systems such as Bookstein coordinates.
- Both strengths and weaknesses of the Procrustes approach become clearer when an approximation is set down algebraically: projecting out four dimensions from the digitizing space (for Procrustes shape coordinates) or six dimensions (for the space of nonuniform transformations) in the vicinity of an average form.
- The covariance distance technique of Chapter 4 applies to shape coordinates in ways that align with aspects of the current literature of evolutionary biology through terms such as canalization or evolvability. These are inherently matrix-based properties.
- Limits on the scope of all these techniques arise both from problems with the template, such as maldistributions of landmarks, and problems of excess variation in one's sample of specimens. There are also several counterintuitive interactions between the Procrustes registration procedure and the details of the shape coordinate covariance patterns when passed to subsequent multivariate maneuvers such as principal components analysis.

5.5 Thin-Plate Splines

The fourth major theme of this syllabus, complementing landmark selection (Section 5.1), uniform tensors (Section 5.2), and Procrustes procedures (Sections 5.3–5.4), is a praxis for making the geometry of all these multivariate patterns explicitly visible in the picture plane (or space) of the typical form. In his classic *On Growth and Form* (1917), D'Arcy Thompson showed how diagrams of deformations could sometimes lead the biologist to insights into form, but left no instructions about how such diagrams could be objectively produced (Bookstein, 1978). (See my discussion of D'Arcy Thompson at the end of Section 5.1.4.) The morphometric breakthrough – routine, reproducible generation of anatomy-based analytic graphics – was made possible by a relatively esoteric advance in interpolation theory. The thin-plate spline interpolant we use for shapes was originally developed a few years earlier by applied mathematicians as an interpolant for surfaces over scattered points at which its height was somehow fixed by data or by animations. Indeed the thin-plate spline is an interpolation function, one that is linear in those "heights" and that minimizes a global figure of energy. It is crucial for our purposes, although not for that original application, that that global figure, usually called *bending energy*, is a quadratic form in the vector of "heights." The following mathematical development was first published in Bookstein (1989), an exegesis that has been cited more than 2300 times.

5.5.1 The Basic Formula

From mathematical physics we borrow the idealized equation of a thin metal plate infinite in extent, infinitely thin, and uniform in its properties, displaced by small distances perpendicular to its rest position at a finite number of distinct points in a world without gravity. Let U be the function $U(r) = r^2 \log r$, and let $P_i = (x_i, y_i)$, $i = 1, \ldots, k$, be k points in the plane. Writing $U_{ij} = U(P_i - P_j)$, build up matrices

$$K = \begin{pmatrix} 0 & U_{12} & \ldots & U_{1k} \\ U_{21} & 0 & \ldots & U_{2k} \\ \vdots & \vdots & \ddots & \vdots \\ U_{k1} & U_{k2} & \ldots & 0, \end{pmatrix} \quad Q = \begin{pmatrix} 1 & x_1 & y_1 \\ 1 & x_2 & y_2 \\ \vdots & \vdots & \vdots \\ 1 & x_k & y_k \end{pmatrix}, \tag{5.10}$$

and

$$L = \begin{pmatrix} K & Q \\ Q^t & O \end{pmatrix}, \ (k+3) \times (k+3), \tag{5.11}$$

where O is a 3×3 matrix of zeros. Write $H = (h_1 \ldots h_k\, 0\, 0\, 0)^t$ and set $W = \left(w_1 \ldots w_k\, a_0\, a_x\, a_y\right)^t = L^{-1}H$. Then the thin-plate spline $f(P)$ having heights (values) h_i at points $P_i = (x_i, y_i)$, $i = 1, \ldots, k$, is the function

$$f(P) = \sum_{i=1}^{k} w_i U(P - P_i) + a_0 + a_x x + a_y y. \tag{5.12}$$

This function $f(P)$ has three crucial properties:

1. $f(P_i) = h_i$, all i: f interpolates the heights h_i at the landmarks P_i.
2. The function f has minimum **bending energy** of all functions that interpolate the heights h_i in that way: the minimum of

$$\iint_{\mathbf{R}^2} \left(\left(\frac{\partial^2 f}{\partial x^2}\right)^2 + 2\left(\frac{\partial^2 f}{\partial x \partial y}\right)^2 + \left(\frac{\partial^2 f}{\partial y^2}\right)^2 \right) \tag{5.13}$$

   where the integral is taken over the entire picture plane.
3. The value of this bending energy is

$$\frac{1}{8\pi} W^t K W = \frac{1}{8\pi} W^t \cdot H = \frac{1}{8\pi} H_k^t L_k^{-1} H_k, \tag{5.14}$$

   where L_k^{-1}, the *bending energy matrix*, is the $k \times k$ upper left submatrix of L^{-1}, and H_k is the initial k-vector of H, the vector of k heights.

In the application to two-dimensional landmark data, we compute two of these splined surfaces, one (f_x) in which the vector H of heights is loaded with the x-coordinate of the landmarks in a second form, another (f_y) for the y-coordinate. Then the first of these spline functions supplies the interpolated x-coordinate of the map we seek, and the second the interpolated y-coordinate. It is easy to show (see Bookstein, 1989) that we get the same map regardless of how we place the (x, y) coordinate axes on the picture. For any such coordinate system, the resulting map $(f_x(P), f_y(P))$ is now a deformation of one picture plane onto the other that maps landmarks onto their homologues and has the minimum bending energy of any such interpolant. In this context one may think of the bending energy as *localization*, the extent to which the affine derivative of the interpolant varies from location to location, a variation assessed in the large according to equation (5.13). Out of all the maps that correctly pair the matching landmark locations, this particular spline is the map having the least possible amount of "local information" in this sense. The affine part of the map is now an ordinary shear, which, in the metaphor of the lofted plate, can be thought of as the shadow of the original gridded plate after it has been only tilted and rescaled but not bent.

Because $W = L^{-1}H$ in the preceding formalism, the spline is linear in the coordinates H of the right-hand form. In the application to the Procrustes construction for shape, the x- and y-coordinates we are using are actually displacements of shape coordinates after the Procrustes fit of the previous section. When the starting form of the spline is the sample average shape, then we have extended the linear machinery of shape space in $2k - 4$ dimensions to a system of exactly equivalent diagrams in two dimensions. For work in form space, we restore Centroid Size to the drawing by scaling the grid appropriately (as the exponentiation of the log of size, which is how CS entered the multivariate analysis). The relation of any specimen shape to the average and the relation of any two shapes (such as group means) that are both near the average are thereby shown as deformations the coefficients of which are linear in the shape coordinates. In this way Cartesian grids deforming the average shape have been directly incorporated into the biometric framework, a formally linear function space of nonlinear maps. We arrive thereby at a coordinate-free visualization of pairwise comparisons, shape coordinate singular vectors, or *any* pair of vectors of Cartesian coordinates. Because the spline is linear in the coordinates of the target form, furthermore, we can extrapolate it until its features are readable, or even reverse its sign; practical applications of this possibility are explored in Section 5.6.3.

5.5.1.1 Didactic Examples

The thin-plate spline interpolation formalism is an immensely powerful, even seductive visualization. To become familiar with its behavior there is no substitute for free play on the computer screen. The next two figures present a series of these.

Figure 5.62 introduces the icon by relating its form in three dimensions (the metal plate metaphor) to its form in two. The upper row shows one commonly encountered shape, which will turn out in Section 5.5.4 to be the sole partial warp (Section 5.5.2) of an exactly square four-landmark configuration. At left it is shown as the (exaggerated) deformation of a plate that begins square but is deformed by lifting at the ends of one diagonal. The rest of this row indicates the equivalent change when viewed as an in-plane deformation (which is no longer possible as physics), first when the square is upright, next when it is oriented at 45° to the grid. These are the same shape change, and one must learn to recognize that fact independent of the grid orientation.

In the second row is a standard reconfiguration feature for a different starting configuration, now the pattern with five landmarks that is usually called a *quincunx* (an analogy Galton exploited in naming his assemblage of

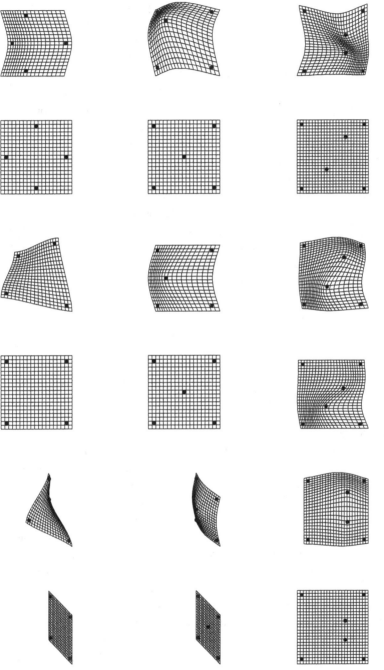

Figure 5.62 Commonly encountered features of thin-plate splines in two dimensions. Each example comprises two configurations, a starting form at left and a target form at its right. See text.

a lot of them in Figure 2.11). The transformation we are interested in here, the higher-energy partial warp of the quincunx (again see Section 5.5.2), is the shape change that shifts the central landmark while leaving the other four alone. Its appearance in three dimensions is that of a hillock, the sort of feature a hiker would either climb, for a view, or walk around, on the path to some more beautiful spot. The row continues with two in-plate examples, one where the shift of the central landmark is along a side of the square and the other where it is along a diagonal.

The general thin-plate spline (an example appears in the bottom row) is the sum of transformations for the x-coordinate and the y-coordinate separately. From left to right are shown (i) a pedagogically helpful starting form, (ii) the x-deformation only, (iii) the y-deformation only, (iv) the intended plane transformation, composite of the x- and the y-shifts together, (v) the same shape now used as a new starting configuration, and (vi) the thin-plate spline back from this target to the original starting form, a grid that represents the inverse shape change but that is not quite the inverse of the grid in (iv) as an actual map.

These were all intentionally controlled changes of landmark configuration. One can come to understand the transformation to real data by replacing these target forms with random shifts of starting forms that are somewhat richer (13 or 16 landmarks, not just six). Figure 5.63 presents an assortment of *these* corresponding to the two different probabilistic models for shape variation introduced already in Section 5.3. In the upper row are six examples of a Procrustes transformation of moderate amplitude: changes of location distributed as circular Gaussians independently at every landmark. These transformations do not conduce to coherent biological explanations. By comparison, the remaining two rows of the figure show transformations designed as in Figure 5.39, offering discrete features over a spectrum of discrete scales. Grids like these *do* seem consistent with potential biological explanations. They have the same flavor as those we shall be producing in Section 5.6 that arise from our two running examples.

The thin-plate spline is far more helpful than anyone could have expected prior to its promulgation (by Bookstein, 1989, borrowing it from the literature of computer graphics in which it had been installed a few years before). It may be that minimizing bending energy may actually be a principle of biomathematical design, or it may be that our visual systems, which are so attuned to navigating over a landscape, are appropriately processing the gradients and other inhomogeneities that are communicated here.

It is important not to attribute any truth claims to this geometry. Biological form does not deform as a thin plate in four or six dimensions, and the spline needs to be replaced by an appropriate biophysical operator whenever

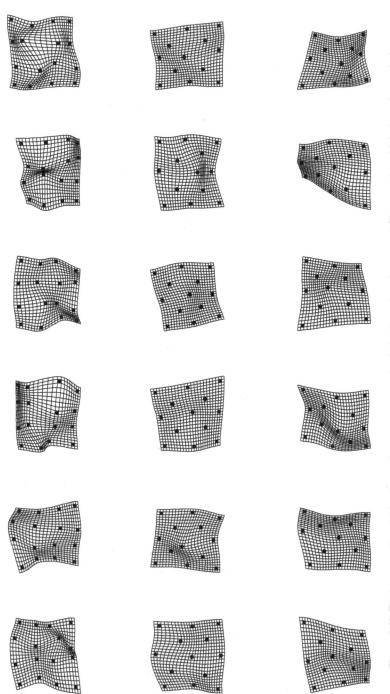

Figure 5.63 Further examples of thin-plate splines, now presented only in plane view. (upper row) Six examples with independent variation at every landmark, as in Figure 5.37. (center row) Six examples with self-similar features of the same amplitude, as in Figure 5.40. (lower row) The same for a larger setting of the feature amplitude parameter (compare any two columns of Figure 5.41).

real deformations are under the control of that operator in the application at hand. This means, in particular, that the thin-plate spline is not suited for diagramming real deformations, as of bone under strain, that are actually elastic. Its energy term has no component that is proportional to the square of displacement, which is the standard formulation of energy for analyses of in-plane material bending (part of elasticity theory). For processes like those, the thin-plate spline is minimizing the wrong quantity. (See Bookstein, 2013a.) The spline's bending energy expresses *inhomogeneities* of strain, not strain itself – these are the squared *second* derivatives, not the first derivatives, that appear in the identity (5.13) for this energy term. But most comparisons in the course of organismal biology are across specimens or over long intervals of time and hence are not amenable to these better-informed biophysical models. For comparisons of this nonphysical sort, the spline is as good a graphic as we have, and more symmetrical in its algebra than schemes like finite-element analysis that require the form to be divided up into cells prior to the description.

In 3D, the kernel function U of equation (5.10) is $|r|$, not $r^2 \log r$, the matrix Q has one more column for the z-coordinates of the landmarks in the target form, the integral has six terms instead of three and is over $\mathbf{R}^3$ (all space) instead of $\mathbf{R}^2$ (just a plane), and the constant in the bending energy equation has a minus sign. The corresponding algorithms are built into packages such as William Green's `Edgewarp` or the EVAN Toolkit designed by Fred Bookstein, Gerhard Weber, Roger Phillips, Paul O'Higgins, and William Green and released by the EVAN Society, Vienna, in 2010. This software will also fit templates on combinations of landmarks and semilandmarks as described in Section 5.5.4.

5.5.2 Bending Energy and Its Principal and Partial Warps

We passed quickly over an expression earlier, at equations (5.13–5.14):

$$\iint_{\mathbf{R}^2} \left(\left(\frac{\partial^2 f}{\partial x^2} \right)^2 + 2 \left(\frac{\partial^2 f}{\partial x \partial y} \right)^2 + \left(\frac{\partial^2 f}{\partial y^2} \right)^2 \right) = \qquad (5.13)$$

$$\frac{1}{8\pi} W^t K W = \frac{1}{8\pi} W^t \cdot H = \frac{1}{8\pi} H_k^t L_k^{-1} H_k, \qquad (5.14)$$

where f is the thin-plate interpolant for one coordinate at a time, and L and K are the matrices used in the production of the spline formula as defined near those equations. We identified this quantity, in either of its formulations, with a notion of *bending energy* of the corresponding thin-plate. If this were a real physical plate, that integral would indeed *be* proportional to the energy needed to change its shape by displacements perpendicular to its original flat configuration.

But even in this metaphorical reinterpretation, the formula in (5.14), now summed over both Cartesian coordinates, continues to have a meaning, this time a biological one. The quantities being integrated in equation (5.13) are the squared second derivatives of the grid deformation. They are zero if and only if the deformation is a uniform shear, a perfectly linear map, and so they calibrate the extent to which a grid *has* any features that differ from point to point – any features that can be localized. The larger this double integral, the more information there is that differs from point to point of the map, and thus the greater the possible biometrical yield of a closer inspection.

That closer inspection is made possible by the re-expression of the integral of equation (5.13) as the quadratic form L_k^{-1} in equation (5.14). It is possible to show (see Bookstein, 1991) that this form has three eigenvalues that are 0, corresponding to the three terms $a_0 + a_1 x + a_1 y$ at the right in equation (5.12), and that the other $p - 3$ eigenvalues (where p is the count of landmarks) come in rising order of the bending seen in a joint landmark displacement whose coefficients sum in square to 1.0. In the context of a map with two coordinates x and y, the bending energy is just the sum of the components for the two axes of the target form separately. (The matrix L in the formula, however, incorporates both axes in computing the distance functions r describing the starting form.)

In the same way that a Fourier analysis decomposes all the variation of any periodic function into multiples of terms $\cos n\theta$ and $\sin n\theta$, a sum of geometrically orthogonal terms, so the eigenvectors of this matrix L_k^{-1} decompose the variation of any pattern of displacements in one direction into a sum of a constant, a linear part, and a series of likewise geometrically orthogonal terms with greater and greater specific bending. Written out as an equation, this is

$$L_k^{-1} = WDW'. \qquad (5.15)$$

Here D is a diagonal matrix of $p - 3$ *specific bending energies*, bending (equation 5.14) per unit magnitude of net Procrustes displacement, and each column of W is the corresponding pair of dimensions (one for shifts in the x-direction, one for y). These patterns are geometrically orthogonal, meaning that the bending energy of the sum of any two of them is the sum of the bending energies of the components separately.

These $p - 3$ patterns, the columns of U corresponding to the entries of the diagonal matrix D that are greater than zero, are called the *principal warps* of the landmark configuration that provided the entries for the matrices K, Q, and

L of equations (5.10–5.11). In applications to biometric samples, their formulas depend on the mean landmark configuration only, not its variability. When they are evaluated for transformations from the mean to each individual specimen of a sample of two-dimensional data, they now have two components, one for x, one for y. Here they are called the *partial warps*, and their coefficients are the *partial warp scores*. In terms of the matrix J introduced in Section 5.4.4, these $2(k-3)$ scores form a basis for the dimensions of shape space not spanned by the rows of J. The zero eigenvalue itself matches rows 5 and 6 of J, the uniform subspace (of transformations that do not bend anything); the first four rows are zeroed by the Procrustes construction.

Let us examine these constructions for a few instructive cases. We begin (Figure 5.64) with the scenario of four starting landmarks in the form of a square. With the landmarks numbered clockwise from any starting point, the matrix L_k^{-1} of equation (5.14) is proportional to $\begin{pmatrix} 1 & -1 & 1 & -1 \\ -1 & 1 & -1 & 1 \\ 1 & -1 & 1 & -1 \\ -1 & 1 & -1 & 1 \end{pmatrix}$. This matrix has three zero eigenvalues versus only one that is nonzero. The nonzero

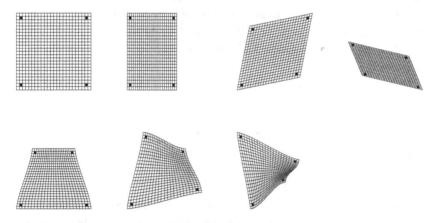

Figure 5.64 The uniform term and the single partial warp for a starting square. Upper row, left to right: the starting configuration; the first component of the uniform term for changes around this starting configuration – equal and opposite rotations of the main diagonal; the second component, shear along any convenient axis; a general uniform transformation, sum of one multiple of each component. Lower row: the single nonuniform partial warp of this four-landmark configuration, in a variety of orientations: left, square to trapezoid; center, square to kite; right, arbitrary linear combination of those two. Hidden in each form in this row is a perfect plus sign right in the middle of the grid, owing to the symmetries of the situation.

eigenvector lies along $(1, -1, 1, -1)$, which, in this numbering scheme, is just the transformation that moves both of the landmarks of one diagonal by some vector with respect to both of the landmarks of the other diagonal. The uniform term corresponds to the span of the zero eigenvalues; they turn out to involve two geometric dimensions of somewhat different appearance. One of the uniform dimensions, corresponding to row 6 of the J-matrix (equation 5.7), stretches the average scene vertically while reducing it horizontally by exactly the factor needed to leave Centroid Size unchanged; the other, corresponding to row 5 of J, shears the configuration along an axis that, for convenience, is taken horizontally in the Procrustes coordinate system. An arbitrary uniform transformation, such as the exemplar at upper right, is the sum of one of each of these, a combination often called "partial warp 0." The figure also shows three instances of the *other* partial warp, the one that involves bending, in the lower row. One is a horizontal component, one a diagonal component, and one an arbitrary combination.

The symmetries of the starting form in Figure 5.64 do not apply in general, of course. Figure 5.65 shows four multiples each (east, north, west, and south) of the same amplitude for the unique principal warp arising from each of the six random quadrilaterals displayed (along with the corresponding starting grid) in the top row. There are strong family resemblances along the cells of this display: except when some pair of the initial landmarks is unusually close together, most of the instances look approximately like bent bars or else like trapezoids.

Now restore the symmetry of Figure 5.64, but at the same time add a fifth landmark right at the center of the square, Figure 5.66. Now the matrix L_k^{-1} is

$$\text{proportional to } \begin{pmatrix} 2 & -1 & 2 & -1 & -2 \\ -1 & 2 & -1 & 2 & -2 \\ 2 & -1 & 2 & -1 & -2 \\ -1 & 2 & -1 & 2 & -2 \\ -2 & -2 & -2 & -2 & 8 \end{pmatrix}, \text{ with two nonzero eigenvalues}$$

(along with three zeroes). The larger of these two eigenvalues has eigenvector along $(-1, -1, -1, -1, 4)$ — this is just a shift of the middle landmark with respect to all the others. It is drawn in the bottom row of the figure. The smaller nonzero eigenvalue, drawn in the middle row, has eigenvector along $(1, -1, 1, -1, 0)$, meaning that the new landmark (the fifth entry) is not actually involved. This is the same partial warp as the one we already saw in Figure 5.64.

Having mastered these prototypes, you may be willing to accept the analysis in Figure 5.67, which is of an arbitrary scatter of seven landmarks. As in Figure 5.65, there is no symmetry remaining, and the four nonzero eigenvalues

·

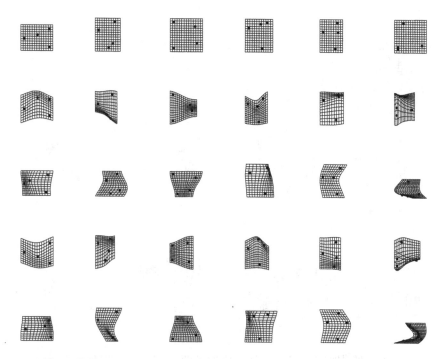

Figure 5.65 The four cardinal partial warps (displacements easterly, northerly, westerly, or southerly) for six different random quadrilaterals (top row). Pages like this encompass nearly every configuration likely to be encountered in practice for the largest-scale nonuniform aspects of deformations arising from almost any mean landmark configuration.

of the four nontrivial partial warps are likewise arbitrary: 0.180, 0.457, 1.243, and 1.684. The corresponding partial warps are now shown in the *columns* of Figure 5.67. The upper row is for a horizontal component (you can tell because all the horizontal grid lines are straight), the middle row for a vertical component (now all the vertical grid lines are straight), and the lower row for the arbitrary combination that I computed as the opposite of the sum of the first two. Notice that in one orientation the partial warp of largest scale (lowest specific bending energy), second row of column 1, closely resembles the first nonuniform partial warp we will shortly see for the Vilmann rodent skull data. In fact, this form of a bent beam or its 90° rotation the in-line growth gradient (including square-to-trapezoid and square-to-kite deformations as a special case) arises as the first partial warp of just about any average landmark configuration. It is only the later, more bent (more localized) partial warps that show obvious effects of the mean landmark configuration – here, the close spacing between selected adjacent pairs.

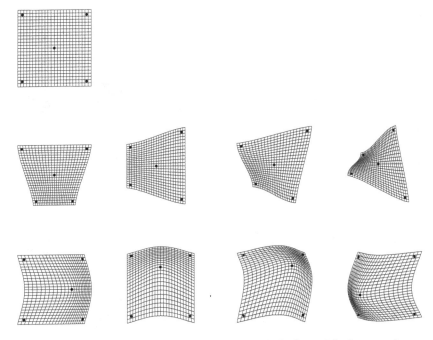

Figure 5.66 The same for a starting configuration in the form of the five-spot of a die (upper left). Middle row, left to right: the less bent partial warp, oriented horizontally, then vertically, then diagonally; then an arbitrary combination. This warp is geometrically identical to that for the square (Figure 5.64). Bottom row: the other partial warp, of highest specific bending energy. Left to right: oriented horizontally, vertically, diagonally, and then arbitrarily.

5.5.3 The Uniform Component

The partial warps just introduced span all of the curving that is part of any shape change when represented by these least-bent spline grids. But some comparisons, even growth comparisons, may be spatially so homogeneous that no mention of curving is necessary. A convenient example can be drawn from the rodent neurocranial octagon data set that has served to demonstrate many analytic suggestions in earlier sections. Figure 5.68 parcellates this octagon into six triangles and displays the principal strains of each one separately triangle by triangle before and after age 14 days. From left to right in the upper panel, these are ratios of growth rates of 1.095, 1.091, 1.117, 1.127, 1.125, and 1.100. The axes for five of these six triangles are nearly parallel (indeed almost collinear in the diagram); only the triangle at farthest left is different.

By contrast, in the transformation of shape from the 14-day average to the average at 150 days (lower panel), there is no such commonality between

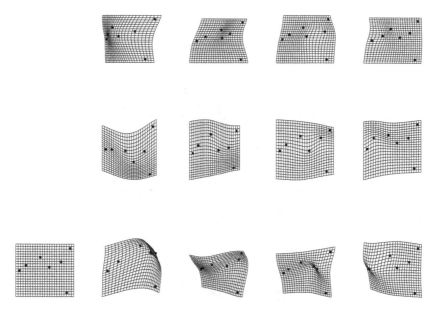

Figure 5.67 The same for an arbitrary mean form of seven landmarks, lower left. Columns are the four partial warps in order of increasing bending energy. Rows, top to bottom: a horizontal multiple, a vertical multiple, and the negative of the sum of the two.

tensors from neighboring triangles. Growth extension along the cranial base (the bottom border of the drawing) is essentially horizontal, while along the top border its directionality is quite different. Any summary in terms of a single descriptor of shear would be misleading. (We will see in Section 5.6.8 that four terms are required for a biologically interpretable description over the full temporal span of this data set.)

We can intuit the same contrast from the fully detailed thin-plate splines for the same comparisons (Figure 5.69). Above left is the spline from the 7-day average to the 14-day average. It does indeed look nearly uniform, with grid lines all nearly straight; the eye finds it quite plausibly represented by its uniform component, which arises as rows 5 and 6 of the J-matrix (Section 5.4.4). Here that component of the decomposition exhausts 83% of the full Procrustes signal. The average subsequent growth trajectory, at lower left in the same figure, is heterogeneous, with curving grid lines throughout. Its uniform component represents only 53% of the total squared Procrustes dissimilarity, and so is much less likely to be meaningful.

The uniform components at the right in Figure 5.69 can be thought of as shape-coordinate summaries of the multiple triangles from Figure 5.68.

tensors, Vilmann octagons, age 7 to 14 days

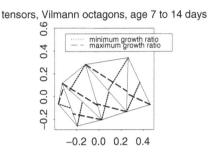

tensors, Vilmann octagons, age 14 to 150 days

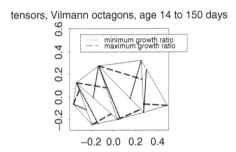

Figure 5.68 Average growth of Vilmann's rodent neurocranial octagons over two age ranges. (above) From age 7 days to 14. Except for the occipital triangle at farthest left, these tensors are nearly parallel, suggesting the usefulness of one common description in terms of directions of greatest and least rate of growth. Directions of principal strain are shown as transects through landmarks after the fashion of Figure 5.25, except that we code the polarity of the strain (greater than, or less than, the ratio of change along the baseline) by the texture of the corresponding line. (below) The same for growth from 14 to 150 days of age. Triangles with edges along the upper border have different principal axes from those with edges along the lower border; no uniform description will be effective here, even though the signal appears to be more than half uniform (in terms of shape subspace projections).

Because they are uniform transformations, as in Section 5.2 each of these can be analyzed as the shape change of "one big triangle"; Figure 5.70 shows the principal axes and the strains along them for the earliest growth period (7 to 14 days), where this component is dominant. At right is the same computation after the landmark Opisthion, which is nonconforming with the uniform transform to its anterior, is omitted. Notice that the directionality of the summary analysis is somewhat enhanced (from $1.247/1.139 = 1.095$ to $1.259/1.129 = 1.115$) when this posteriormost compartment of the octagon is deleted.

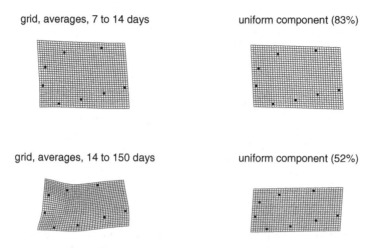

grid, averages, 7 to 14 days   uniform component (83%)

grid, averages, 14 to 150 days   uniform component (52%)

Figure 5.69 Growth changes as shown by thin-plate spline grids (left) and their uniform components (right).

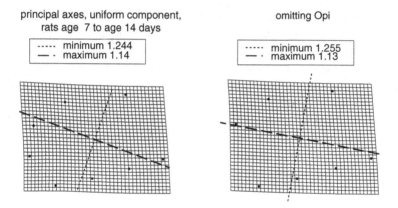

principal axes, uniform component,   omitting Opi
rats age 7 to age 14 days

```
----- minimum 1.244
— · maximum 1.14
```

```
----- minimum 1.255
— · maximum 1.13
```

Figure 5.70 The uniform component for 7-to-14-day growth as an amalgamation of all the tensors in Figure 5.68. (left) For all eight landmarks. There is an anisotropy (directionality) of about 9% along with a net size change of about 19%. (right) Omitting the landmark at Opisthion (which is nonconforming according to Figure 5.67) raises the anisotropy above 11%.

5.5.4 Semilandmarks

It is time to explain the additional dots in Figure 5.3 beyond the landmark coordinates. They represent a feedback from the thin-plate spline to the notion of landmarks with which we began: a way of using the spline to establish point correspondences when the properly biological information is partly lacking.

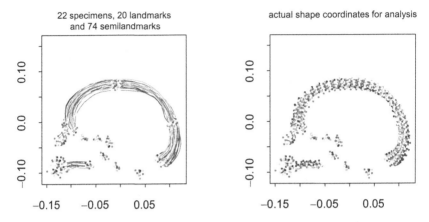

22 specimens, 20 landmarks   actual shape coordinates for analysis
and 74 semilandmarks

Figure 5.71 Semilandmarks represent curves in a scene for purposes of a shape
coordinate analysis. Each specimen is in a randomly selected color (see online
version of the figure) or gray level. After Weber and Bookstein, 2011.

Figure 5.71 shows the rest of the raw data for the forms in Figure 5.51:
curves connecting some pairs of the landmarks from the earlier analysis along
outlines of the sections made by the imaging plane within the original CT
volumes. These total five: a long arc subdividing the outer vault, another for
the inner vault, an arc along the palate, and very short segments between Alv
and ANS and between Rhi and Gla. The curves are made up of a total of
74 *semilandmarks*. Semilandmarks are points that minimize bending energy
(in the sense of the thin-plate spline; equation (5.14)) for deviations from the
average while remaining bound to the curves on which they were originally
digitized. There is a general formula driving the computations here,

$$T = -(U^t Q U)^{-1} U^t Q Y_0. \tag{5.16}$$

In most expositions, even primary peer-reviewed articles, this appears as a
naked dictum, a formula without any proof, without even any attempt to make
it seem comprehensible. But it *is* comprehensible, and this section will attempt
to place it in an appropriate pedagogical context.

   Like the thin-plate spline itself, this formalism, first introduced in Bookstein (1997) and applied to data for the first time in Bookstein et al. (1999), has
proved far more useful than anyone expected when it was originally published.
Thinking only in terms of the biomathematics of "shape measurement," we
have radically altered the ground metaphor by extending the list of ignored
variables well past the stereotyped "position, orientation, and scale" of the

Procrustes methods to incorporate the full range of possible *relabelings* of points on curves as well. (For an even more general approach to this problem of correspondence between curves, see Zhang et al., 2015.) Over in the organized system we are studying, the biological form that is growing, evolving, or just getting on with the business of living, the semilandmarks bridge the biomathematics of the Procrustes method, which deals with isolated points incapable of bounding biological extents, to the languages of morphogenesis and biomechanics, which have always dealt with bounded regions and the corresponding integrals of physiology or force generation that arise there. It is quite a surprise that the addition of one single additional geometric operation so enormously expands the visual information resources available to the systems biologist who would retrieve as much information as feasible from these ubiquitous images of organized form.

5.5.4.1 Sliding One Single Landmark

The method of semilandmarks rests on the following fundamental algebraic fact. Suppose you have two configurations of k landmarks in any two relative positions. The thin-plate spline from one to the other has some bending energy. If you add a new landmark, a $(k + 1)^{st}$ landmark, to the starting form, and place it down on the target form at exactly the point that the spline map on the first k landmarks would put it, then there is no change in the bending energy of the new $(k + 1)$-landmark spline. If, thereafter, you move this new $(k + 1)^{st}$ landmark in the target form, then the bending energy of the spline that takes it to any new position is proportional to the square of the distance of the new position from the original position that this landmark was assigned by the spline on the first k. The proportionality constant is a complicated function of the positions of all $k+1$ landmarks in the starting form: high if the new $(k+1)^{st}$ point is near any of the other k, and lower if it is far from all of them. For the sketch of a proof, see Bookstein and Green (1993).

We apply this fact to geometrize the problem of placing that new landmark somewhere on some *line* in the picture: it translates into the straightforward task of finding the closest approach of a line to a fixed point not on it. In Figure 5.72, suppose that the location where the spline on the original k landmarks, whatever their configuration, puts the new landmark is $(0,0)$ in this coordinate system, that this new landmark had actually been located at the point $(c, 0)$ (where $c < 0$ in the figure as drawn), and that it is free to slide on the line making an angle θ with the x-axis, as shown. (In reality it will be sliding on a curve, not a line, but if the original location was a reasonably good guess, the line approximation will do. One can always iterate the algorithm

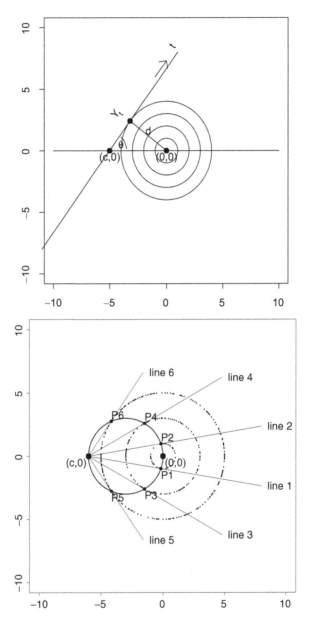

Figure 5.72 Geometry for one single semilandmark restricted to a line. (top) Sliding on a line to the foot of the perpendicular from the spline's rest position. (bottom) The locus of all possible resolutions of the sliding of a single semilandmark. As the line of support varies in all directions through the digitized point $(c, 0)$, the semilandmark traces a circle on the segment connecting the digitized location and the rest location as diameter.

after projecting the line down to match the observed boundary curve or surface and repeating everything.)

We write the points on this line as $Y_t = (c, 0) + t(\cos\theta, \sin\theta)$, where t is an unknown adjustment parameter we have to estimate, and, because bending energy for one point at a time is circular, we are looking for the value of t at which the point Y_t is closest to the rest point $(0, 0)$. That is the point for which the distance d between the line of Y_t's and $(0, 0)$ is minimum. The square of the distance d is $d^2 = (c + t\cos\theta)^2 + (t\sin\theta)^2$, and the derivative of this with respect to t is $2\cos\theta(c+t\cos\theta)+2\sin\theta(t\sin\theta) = 2c\cos\theta+2t$, which we set to zero. (Remember that $\cos^2 + \sin^2 = 1$.) Solving for t, we get $t = -c\cos\theta$ and hence

$$Y_t = (c, 0) - c\cos\theta(\cos\theta, \sin\theta) = c(1 - \cos^2\theta, -\sin\theta\cos\theta)$$
$$= -c\sin\theta(-\sin\theta, \cos\theta), \tag{5.17}$$

a point in the direction $\theta + 90°$ out of $(0, 0)$ at signed distance $-c\sin\theta$ in that direction.

As θ rotates, the line through $(c, 0)$ in its direction rotates too, and the result of the basic sliding geometry in Figure 5.72 is to locate Y_t where the constraint line is tangent to the appropriate circle in each case: the one centered on $(0, 0)$, the landmark's rest position, and having radius $-c\sin\theta$. To be tangent to such a circle is to be perpendicular to the radius through the touching point, which makes the triangle on $(0, 0)$, $(c, 0)$, and the touching point a right triangle with hypotenuse from $(c, 0)$ to $(0, 0)$. By a theorem of Euclid, this locus (all the touching points that are generated as θ varies while $Y^0 = (c, 0)$ stays the same) is a circle on the segment from $(c, 0)$ to $(0, 0)$ as diameter, as shown in the right-hand panel of Figure 5.72.

This is formula (5.16) for the case of $T = t$, a vector with only one element. In Vienna's Department of Anthropology, the rule was that nobody can get a degree based on analysis of a data set involving semilandmarks who can't reproduce this specific derivation, verbatim, at the time of the General Exam.

5.5.4.2 Sliding Any Number of Coordinates

Suppose now that more than one landmark is sliding at the same time. We can imagine the following (horrible) algorithm: pick one landmark, slide it; pick the next one, slide it to a configuration adjusted to the slid position of the first one; pick a third, slide it to a position taking into account the post-slide positions of the first two; ...; slide the last landmark given the already-slid positions of the all the others; go back and slide the first one again; then the second; ...; and loop until points aren't moving any more. This would actually work – it would eventually arrive as closely as you want to the correct minimum of total bending energy – but it would take a ridiculous amount of computing time, perhaps years.

The formula $T = -(U^t Q U)^{-1} U^t Q Y_0$ is a shortcut that computes this minimum value without the iteration, by sliding on all landmarks at once to arrive at the (unique) position of tangency $U^t Q(Y^0 + UT) = 0$ to some ellipsoidal hypercylinder of constant bending energy $Y^t Q Y$. The formalism is now of many sliding points instead of just one, so what was distance from $(0,0)$ is now bending energy $Y^t Q Y$ (for some bending energy matrix Q) over the set of target forms $Y = Y^0 + UT$ where Y^0 stands for the starting form in a notation where a form is not a matrix of landmark numbers by Cartesian coordinates but instead a single vector: not

$$Y^0 = \begin{pmatrix} x_1 & y_1 \\ x_2 & y_2 \\ \cdot & \cdot \\ \cdot & \cdot \\ x_k & y_k \end{pmatrix} \quad \text{or} \quad Y^0 = \begin{pmatrix} x_1 & y_1 & z_1 \\ x_2 & y_2 & z_2 \\ \cdot & \cdot & \cdot \\ \cdot & \cdot & \cdot \\ x_k & y_k & z_k \end{pmatrix}$$

but

$$Y^0 = (x_1\, x_2\, \cdots\, x_k\, y_1\, y_2\, \cdots\, y_k)^t \text{ or}$$
$$Y_0 = (x_1\, x_2\, \cdots\, x_k\, y_1\, y_2\, \cdots\, y_k\, z_1\, z_2\, \cdots\, z_k)^t. \tag{5.18}$$

UT needs to be a vector conformable with Y^0 (meaning: capable of being added to Y^0 — having the same shape), and T has one entry per sliding landmark, so U must be a matrix of $2k$ or $3k$ rows by one column for each landmark that is going to slide, a total count, say, of j of them. The first column of U talks about the effect of sliding the first landmark, so it probably has entries only in positions 1 and $k + 1$, which together specify the x- and y-coordinates of that first landmark (for 3D data, there is an entry in position $2k + 1$, for z_1, as well). The second column of U probably has entries only in the second and $(k + 2)^{nd}$ positions, as it is responsible mostly for x_2 and y_2 (but for 3D also position $2k + 2$ associated with coordinate z_2); and so on.

In this notation, $Y = Y^0 + UT$ is the configuration of all the semiland-marks *after* sliding, and we want to know how far to slide each one. Each semilandmark slides by its own parameter t_i times the unit vector $(U_{i,i}, U_{i+k,i})$ or $(U_{i,i}, U_{i+k,i}, U_{i+2k,i})$ that gives us the direction it's sliding in 2D or 3D. (The letter U comes from the word "unit" – in one version of this algorithm, the U are direction cosines [cosines of angles with the two or three Cartesian axes], the squares of which total 1.0.)

To work in the same spirit as for the circle, we need to use the statisticians' notation of a derivative with respect to a vector parameter like T. This means the vector is made up of the derivatives with respect to every single entry of T. The derivatives need all to be zero at the same time. The semilandmarks must slide to the points $Y^0 + UT$ at which

$$\tfrac{d}{dT}(Y^0 + UT)^t Q(Y^0 + UT) = 2U^t Q(Y^0 + UT) = 0. \tag{5.19}$$

That last 0 was a *vector*, a list of one zero derivative for each sliding parameter t_i in T. So this is really a set of j equations, one for each sliding parameter, even though each equation involves all the sliding parameters simultaneously. As we have already seen for the similar optimization task that arises in multiple regression, the matrix equation can be verified one slot at a time just by exhaustive enumeration and collection of terms.

But we can solve this equation for T: $U^t QUT$ must equal $-U^t QY^0$, so the sliding parameter vector T we seek is, again,

$$T = -(U^t QU)^{-1} U^t QY^0. \tag{5.16}$$

This is the "magic formula" that puts all the sliding landmarks into their appropriate places at the same time.

For the circle, Figure 5.72, we had $Y^0 = \begin{pmatrix} c \\ 0 \end{pmatrix}$, $Q = \begin{pmatrix} 1 & 0 \\ 0 & 1 \end{pmatrix}$, i.e.,

$(x\ y)Q\begin{pmatrix} x \\ y \end{pmatrix} = x^2 + y^2$, $U = \begin{pmatrix} \cos\theta \\ \sin\theta \end{pmatrix}$, and so $U^t QU = \cos^2\theta + \sin^2\theta = 1$,

and thus $T = t_1 = -(U^t QU)^{-1} U^t QY_0 = -(\cos\theta, \sin\theta) \cdot (c, 0) = -c\cos\theta$, which is the correct result.

The interpretation of the formula $T = -(U^t QU)^{-1} U^t QY^0$ flows likewise from the previous version $U^t Q(Y^0 + UT) = 0$. However many elements the vector T has, this is the statement of the same geometry that we immediately understood in Figure 5.72 when it applied to one sliding landmark at a time. The equation $U^t Q(Y^0 + UT) = 0$ states that at the point $Y^0 + UT$ at which we have arrived after the sliding, none of the allowable changes (shifts of the sliding parameters T applied to the point locations via the geometry coded in U) have any effect on the bending energy (for small changes – the concept is of the *gradient* of bending energy, its deviations near the optimum). That $U^t Q(Y^0 + UT) = 0$ means that at the right T the whole space of all possible slidings is tangent to the ellipsoidal hypercylinder representing the locus of constant bending energy (quite a mouthful; just think "circle"), and *that* means that we must have arrived at the global minimum we were seeking.

This single formula $T = -(U^t QU)^{-1} U^t QY^0$ applies to the curving data of the left side in Figure 5.71 to convert each form from its previous 20-landmark representation to the new 94-point configuration shown on the right. (In the electronic version of this book, each form is in a different, randomly selected color.) In this way we have brought in much of the rest of the information in each image: not the information having to do with gray levels or colors or textures, but at least the information pertaining to the locations of boundary structures and curves that display the interactions of form with function much more evocatively than landmarks can. If these were all proper landmarks, shape space would take up $2 \cdot 94 - 4 = 184$ dimensions. By virtue of the sliding, the effective dimensionality of these shapes is only $(2 \cdot 20 - 4) + 74 = 110$.

Once they have been located by this algebra, semilandmarks are treated in exactly the same way as landmarks are for all the manipulations of the morphometric synthesis. An analogous formula for vectors U in 3D permits us to estimate the one free coordinate of a point restricted to a space curve (the literature calls this a *curve semilandmark,* that is, a point sliding on the linear approximation to a curve), or the two free coordinates of a point clamped to a patch of surface (the *surface semilandmark* sliding on a tangent plane to a surface). Should greater accuracy be required, the resulting semilandmark can be "projected back down" onto the curve or surface in question and the procedure repeated. For a great deal more on such sliding semilandmarks, including more specific formulas for the 3D case, see Mitteroecker and Gunz (2009). Continuing in this vein, *both* of the coordinates of a point in 2D, or *all three* coordinates in 3D, might be estimated at the same time (in which case the metaphor of "sliding" is no longer apposite). Such situations respond to the classic problem of *missing data* in this domain of geometric morphometrics. There is a good discussion comparing this approach to a popular alternative, regression estimation, in Gunz et al. (2009). The same technology is invoked silently in the production of the "dancing grids" of the human motion example (Figure 5.83).

The display in Figure 5.71 has considerable graphical density and a slightly different superposition than that for the landmark points only. But the statistical summary diagrams of the sample of 22 specimens are not much affected – all those additional points have not actually added much information to our understanding of the system under study here. The upper left panel in Figure 5.73 plots the first two principal coordinates (relative warp scores). What we get is close to the plot in Figure 5.43, and similarly for form space (lower left), versus the previous ordination on landmarks only (lower right). At upper right in Figure 5.73 is the grid for the first principal coordinate, the horizontal axis in the plot to its left. It closely resembles the one we will see in Figure 5.80 based on the 20 landmarks only. This is often the case for analyses of data in either 2D or 3D, and should be taken as quite

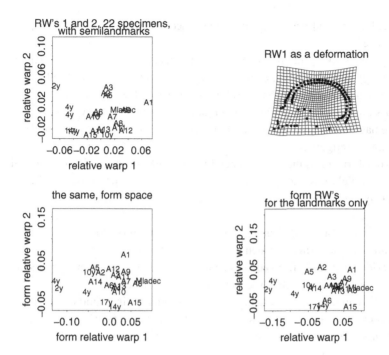

Figure 5.73 The addition of semilandmarks does not much alter our SVD-based descriptors. Upper left: first two principal coordinates of shape for the data in Figure 5.71. Upper right: the first principal coordinate as a thin-plate spline. Lower left: principal coordinates of form. Lower right: the same for just the 20 landmark points. Specimen labels are as in Figure 5.43.

reassuring. For instance, in terms of raw Procrustes distances, the two versions of those distances share $(0.976)^2$ of their summed squared variation around 0. The classic comparative anatomists did pretty well at placing the tips of their calipers on points that, taken as a collection, extracted most of the information needed for at least a qualitative understanding of the vagaries of form in the taxa they were studying. What we are using the semilandmarks to visualize here may have been in the mind of the expert all along. In the presence of enough point landmarks, they add a great deal of verisimilitude but evidently not much actual information.

Summary of Section 5.5

- The *thin-plate spline* is a robust and very broadly applicable formula that converts any pair of landmark configurations, in two or three dimensions, into a transformation grid whose formula is consistent

with linear multivariate analyses in the accompanying Procrustes shape
space.

- The particular grid produced by the thin-plate spline has the least *bending
  energy* (integral over the entire picture of the sum of squares of all the
  second derivatives of the map) for any mapping that interpolates the
  assigned pairing of landmark configurations. This bending energy is,
  remarkably, a quadratic form in the coordinates of the landmarks of the
  target configuration.
- Transformations that have no bending are *uniform shears* that map all pairs
  of parallel lines into other such pairs. Uniform transformations can be
  analyzed by the same tensor machinery that we applied to triangles in
  Section 5.2.
- Eigenanalysis of the bending-energy matrix thus provides a natural set of
  directions in terms of which to decompose the nonuniform part (the
  residual space C^6 from equation 5.8) of any single transformation or sample
  of transformations observed in the course of a data analysis.
- Information from curves and surfaces can often be incorporated in the
  Procrustes family of analyses by way of the *semilandmarks* that minimize
  bending energy of assigned matches in the presence of a mean landmark
  configuration.

5.6 Finishing the Main Examples, Along with Some New Ones

The thin-plate spline has become the de facto standard visualization linking the
arithmetic of the GMM data set to the full range of biological speculations it
might support about processes that caused the shape changes, that covary with
them, or that follow from them.

We have now introduced all the pieces of the analysis we are recommending; it is time to put them together. A **geometric morphometric [GMM]
analysis** is a choice of a Procrustes distance (shape-only or size-and-shape), a
list of landmark locations (including semilandmarks from curves or surfaces),
a scatterplot of Procrustes shape coordinates, another scatter of principal
coordinates labeled or colored by everything else you know in advance
from textbooks, specimen labels, or other measurements, and some thin-
plate splines visualizing the interesting vectors that apply to the Procrustes
coordinates as they emerge from principal coordinate [principal component]
analysis, analysis of groups or any other labeling variable, or PLS analysis
against nonmorphometric quantities, like function ecotype, or state of health,

that happen to be correlated with form. We're looking for clusters, clouds, submanifolds, trends, or outliers in the ordinations produced by the pattern engine, and at the same time we're also looking for spatially coherent patterns and scales in the deformation grids.

This section incorporates more diagrams than would fit into any publication or thesis. My purpose is to show all the figures you *might* wish to construct, even if most of them would be examined by only one person (the Ph.D. candidate, the data analyst). It is good practice to produce these splines repeatedly and generously whenever a narrative based on features of an observed shape phenomenon needs reporting: any between-group contrast of interest, each of the first few relative warps, and any within-group vector such as the regression grid of a shape on some predictor. Here follow examples of all these forms of usage in the context of our two main running examples, the Vilmann rodent neurocranial data and the Gunz et al. human midsagittal skull data. Other examples will also make an appearance from time to time. I sort the applications into eight convenient types: splines for data screening, splines for group differences, splines for relative warps, splines for partial warps, splines for shape regressions, splines for Partial Least Squares, splines for asymmetry, and splines for the visualization of integration.

5.6.1 Splines for Data Screening

One simple use for the splines in the course of any data analysis comes right at the beginning. At that time it serves to visualize the relationship of each individual specimen to the grand mean. Here is an easy context for detecting errors in the order of digitizing and individual forms, like the two *Pan* in Figure 5.74, that do not much resemble any of the others in the sample. These are two of the seven forms that were removed from this little data set in the course of settling on the lower left panel of Figure 5.43.

5.6.2 Splines for Pairwise Contrasts of Specimens or Group Mean Differences

We saw one of these at the very beginning of this chapter: the example for two "groups" of one image each that was shown in Figure 5.2. Many studies culminate in corresponding comparisons of two or more group average images. In our study of the human skulls, we can approximate the effect of age by averaging the infants and the adults separately (as we already did in the course of computing Figure 5.34) and computing the deformation grid that relates

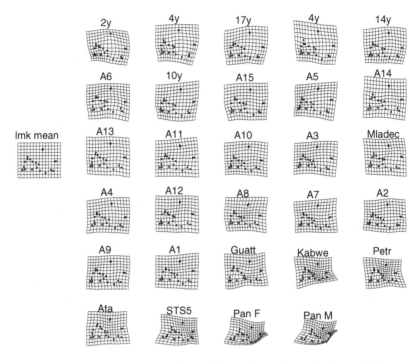

Figure 5.74 Grids for each of the original 29 specimens in Figure 5.43 as deformations of their grand mean shape (left margin), drawn in ascending order of their first principal coordinate (the abscissa in Figure 5.43). The display is a useful adjunct to that earlier figure in detecting specimens that arguably do not belong in the sample. The chimpanzees and STS5 are obviously inconsistent with the rest of the sample, while the four Neanderthal specimens seem to share a different, equally outlying feature (the sharp gradient of the grid's apparent compression across the anterior cranial base). A: adult modern *Homo sapiens*.

the two averages (Figure 5.75). There are two directions of comparison; the choice here (younger to older) is obvious. The formalism here allows us to extrapolate any observed transformation by any multiple just by extrapolating the landmark-by-landmark shift vectors. Figure 5.76 shows this for a simple example, the doubling of the changes from Figure 5.75. We will see in Figure 5.79 that this simple trick affords a much more powerful approach to selecting and reporting discrete features of shape change.

In our study of the growing rat skulls, we can compare any two ages. The comparison of adjacent ages, in particular, serves as a good "snapshot" of the growth trend imagined as the derivative of the time course. In Figure 5.77 these are shown extrapolated by a factor of 5 for legibility.

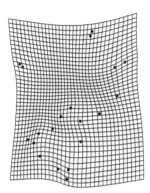
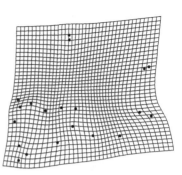

Figure 5.75 Grids for the comparison of average infant and adult 20-gons, in two orientations differing by about 45°.

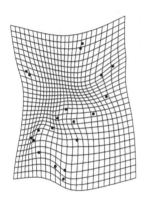
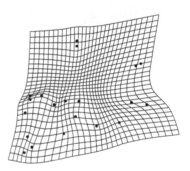

Figure 5.76 Extrapolation of the grids in Figure 5.75 by a factor of 2, illustrating the visual nonlinearity of these linear extrapolations. See text.

5.6.3 Splines for Regressions

In Section 5.4.3 we learned how to draw a regression of shape on any predictor by explicitly diagramming its effects on every shape coordinate at the same time. To these coordinated shifts correspond a thin-plate spline grid of their own, which has proved an effective diagram for a variety of regressions and analyses of covariance in many applications. Here is an example paralleling our earlier work on the effects of age on the 20 human skull landmarks. Figure 5.78 is a regression covering the full observed range of Centroid Size, from small to large (left) or from large to small (right).

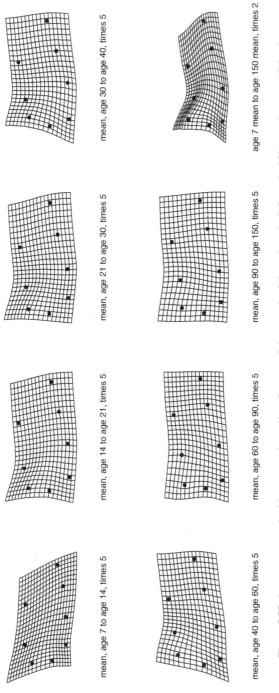

mean, age 7 to age 14, times 5   mean, age 14 to age 21, times 5   mean, age 21 to age 30, times 5   mean, age 30 to age 40, times 5

mean, age 40 to age 60, times 5   mean, age 60 to age 90, times 5   mean, age 90 to age 150, times 5   age 7 mean to age 150 mean, times 2

Figure 5.77 An assortment of grids representing salient features of the growth of the rodent skull from the Vilmann data set. (all but lower right) Grids for the transformation for each age-specific mean shape to the next, extrapolated fivefold. We can see clearly the monotone trends in extension of the cranial base and in diminution of relative height. We also see the reversal of the trend along principal coordinate 2, the relative shear of upper-anterior and lower-posterior quadrants, from before to after age 30 days. (lower right) Net change, age 7 days to 150, times 2. There is a clear large-scale change here over which is superimposed a local phenomenon at the upper posterior. See Section 5.6.8. The grid at upper left here is a fivefold extrapolation of the grid at upper left in Figure 5.69.

452

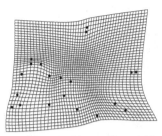 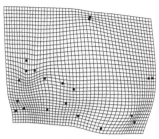

regression toward larger Centroid Size   regression toward smaller Centroid Size

Figure 5.78 Grids for the regression of shape on Centroid Size shown in Figure 5.44. Compare Figure 5.75, the contrast of two averages by age group.

Creases. An earlier proposal for the detection of separate features works by carefully tuning the extrapolation of a regression until it breaks down at precisely one locus. This will be where the local directional derivative of the mapping in a unique direction is either a global maximum or a global minimum (Bookstein, 2000 or Bookstein, 2004). Creases have proved a very effective way to organize the search for discrete foci of shape processes. The same computation applies to any group comparison: considered as a regression of shape coordinates on group number, the grid that is α times the observed difference is linearized as the deformation from S to $S + \alpha(T - S)$, where S is the starting form, T is the target, and both are taken as average Procrustes shape coordinates.

By this manual exploration, or by the algorithm published in Bookstein (2000), we find (Figure 5.79) a degree of extrapolation (namely, a factor of 2.4 times the change from average subadult to average adult) that folds the growth grid all along an extended path, the so-called *hafting zone* where the neurocranium is said to attach to the splanchnocranium rather as the head of an axe attaches to its handle. Growth is slower in the hafting zone than to either side. This is the extrapolation graphed in the left-hand grid. In the other direction, we can run the regression backward in time until tissue begins to disappear. At an extrapolation to -1.5 times the subadult-to-adult change, the thickness of the calvarial bone goes to zero more or less simultaneously in all the intervals where it is entailed in these landmarks. This suggests the presence of some joint regulatory process (which also might be managing the extension of the palatal bone at lower left).

5.6.4 Splines for Relative Warps

The method of splines seems particularly suited for visualization of the relative warps, as their computational purpose of aggregating and smoothing changes

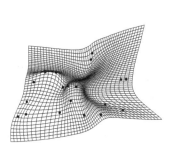
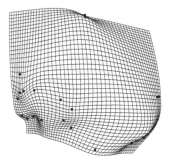

for 2.4 times the range of CS   for −1.5 times the range of CS

Figure 5.79 Calibrated extrapolations of the skull regression on Centroid Size, applied to the average subadult form. (left) Extrapolated by 2.4 times the actual shape difference from subadult to adult average form. One clearly sees the hafting zone. (right) Extrapolated in the direction of juvenility by 1.5 times the observed shape change from subadult to adult. The thickness of the bony skull falls to an extrapolated value of zero (along with localized shrinkage of the upper palate).

of landmark position closely aligns with the spline's emphasis on minimizing local variations of the first derivative. Figure 5.80 presents the grids for the two principal coordinates of the 22 skulls we have been discussing all along. Even though we are skeptical of the reality of the second of these components (recall Section 5.4.3.2), it is worthwhile to visualize it anyway, in order to see if it might correspond to some separable process (here, a local increase in maxillary height). Figure 5.81 shows the same visualizations for our 18 growing rats. The first of these relative warps aligns strikingly well with the overall growth gradient in this data set from youngest to oldest. The second, which tracks the reversal of the horizontal component of these Bookstein coordinate shifts between the first and second phases of this growth process (Figure 5.33), is strikingly close to a uniform shear.

This has not been our first encounter with grids for relative warps. They already appeared in the margins of Figure 3.49 in Section 3.6, where they sketched the dimensions of the infant corpus callosum that were most diag-nostic of prenatal alcohol effects according to the quadratic discrimination there. There these grids were actually relative eigenvectors ("relative relative" warps).

An example without landmarks. Domjanić et al. (2013) analyzed a data set of 166 soft-tissue representations from the human foot surface under normal load about two millimeters above a support plane. The 166 specimens

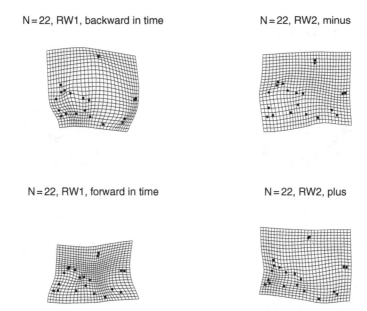

Figure 5.80 The two relative warps for the human skull data set. (left) An arbitrary multiple of RW1 and its inverse. (right) The same for RW2. RW1 is the familiar heterochrony of brain–face growth timing; RW2, if it is real (which I doubt), deals mainly with the vertical height of the maxilla.

arose from left and right feet of 83 mostly Croatian women. A reanalysis (Bookstein and Domjanić, 2015) extracted a subset of 79 of the 83 footprint pairs and, for just the outline of the sole, applied the sliding procedure reviewed in Section 5.5.4 against the sample average 36-gon. (The resulting coordinates are listed in a data set included in this book's online resource http://www.cambridge.org/9781107190948.) The computation was in the usual Procrustes framework, but the display here uses Bookstein coordinates standardized to foot length (shoe size). The first relative warp of this structure, in the top row of Figure 5.82, proved very suggestive, involving as it does not only a narrowing of the observable arch width (in effect, a raising of the arch in the third dimension) but also a reshaping of the posterior aspect of the ball of the foot. The reason this is suggestive is that these two features, the narrowing and the ball reshaping, are the two classic measures of the footprint that have appeared in the literature of the human arch since the 1920s (Figure 5.82, upper left). In fact, after two wild scores are removed, this first relative warp correlates 0.94 with a weighted difference of those two standard measures, the arch ratio (in hundredths) minus 1.3 times the arch angle

RW1, forward in time   RW2, early trend

RW1, backward in time   RW2, late trend

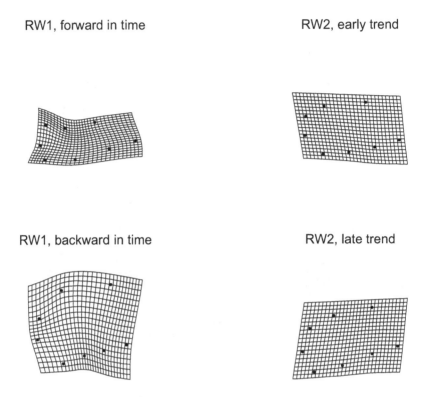

Figure 5.81 The same display for the growing rodent skulls. Left column, relative warp 1: above, approximately the same as the contrast of average forms at the youngest and oldest ages; below, the inverse transformation, such as might be used by a caricaturist trying to convey rodent babyhood (think Mickey Mouse). Right column, relative warp 2, the nearly uniform shear superimposed over the change in the first column, which reverses between halves of the full growth trajectory as scattered in Figure 5.84.

(in degrees). This actually stands for a common factor, as those two indices are negatively correlated ($r = -0.52$). Similarly, the second relative warp (same figure, bottom row) correlates better than 0.8 with the *sum* of the same two terms, arch ratio and arch angle, with the same weights, 1.0 and 1.3. In this way our contemporary relative warp analysis confirmed the insights of the podia-trists/anthrometricians of nearly 100 years ago, who had guessed at the salience of these two angles mainly as a matter of clinical judgment. That this paper was thereby a confirmation, not a refutation, of the classical approach rendered it nearly unpublishable in a variety of conventional peer-reviewed journals.

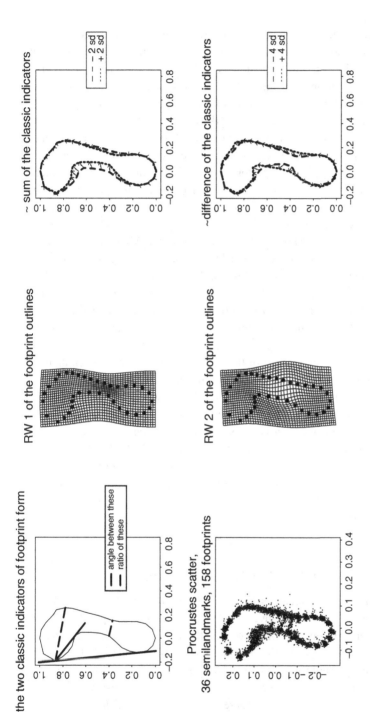

Figure 5.82 First and second relative warps of a 36-semilandmark representation of 158 footprints (right and reflected left feet of 79 young women), standardized to foot length (a surrogate for shoe size). (above left) The two standard measures whose sum and difference these two relative warps stand for. The arch angle is the angle between the solid lines; the arch ratio, the ratio of the dashed lines (ball diameter in the denominator). (below left) Shape coordinate scatter of the slipped landmarks for the sample. (center column) Visualizations of RW1 and RW2 by thin-plate spline. (right column) Visualization by two-point shape coordinate displacement, more clearly indicating the relationship of this computed dimension to the standard measures. After Bookstein and Domjanić, 2015.

457

Grids superimposed over the original imagery. The last little vignette figure in Chapter 1 is a single frame from a modern dance routine rendered as the video superposition of transformation grids based on the classic da Vinci drawing "Vitruvian Man." One day in 1997, Peter Sparling, Professor of Dance at the University of Michigan, donned a skintight costume with bright spots pasted over his joints to serve as landmarks and created a six-minute dance routine. From every sixtieth frame of the video of this dance (i.e., one image every two seconds) William D. K. Green and I located the landmark points and used them to drive a grid itself "performing" the same dance via interpolation of these key frames. The new sequence was presented in synchrony with Sparling's reenactment of the original as part of a collective performance "Seven Enigmas," also involving the work of art professor James Cogswell, that was presented at the Power Center in Ann Arbor, Michigan, that same year. In 2015, as part of the exhibition Das Wissen der Dinge (The Science of Things) at the Naturhistorische Museum, Vienna, Austria, Green extended this software to superimpose the grid over the original freezeframed videos that I had hand-digitized back in 1997. (Today, of course, the landmarks would be LEDs, not fabric, and their tracking would be automatic, using technology whose principal market is the sports sciences.) These grids are evocative in a manner uncannily parallel to that of the original dance sequence even though incommensurate in both physics and form – for instance, the grid has corners, whereas the dancer himself did not. Figure 5.83 displays a selection of my favorite freezeframes from this video series. The composites were created and the animation managed in Green's program package edgewarp; other software that superimposes grids over imagery includes the EVAN Toolbox out of Vienna and also Paul O'Higgins's pioneering package morphologika. This particular rendering tactic, while of enormous potential cognitive and aesthetic power, alas falls outside the scope of this book; I limit myself to this single remarkably suggestive example.

5.6.5 Splines for Partial Warps

Given the hints we have already seen about the interplay between the uniform component and the second relative warp of those rat skulls, it proves helpful to inspect more closely the time courses for these largest few geometric components. Figure 5.84 shows all of the scores for all animals at all ages. The pattern in the uniform component is striking, and conforms closely to what we already noted in Figure 5.49 for the Procrustes distance analysis of the configuration as a whole. There can also be seen a linear trend in

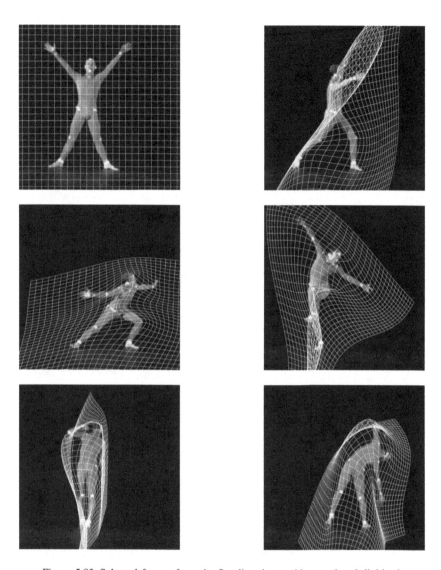

Figure 5.83 Selected frames from the Sparling dance videotaped and digitized in 1997 and superimposed over their corresponding transformation grids in 2015. The starting grid, reprinted at the end of the series for convenience, is a representation of da Vinci's well-known "Vitruvian Man." Landmarks occluded by flesh and thereby inaccessible to video digitizing were treated as "missing data" and assigned the locations corresponding to the spline from the Vitruvian pose to the positions of the visible landmarks frame by frame. The image of Prof. Sparling is used by permission.

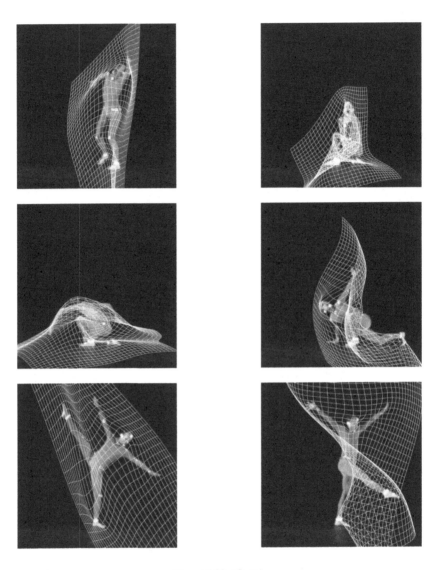

Figure 5.83 *(Cont.)*

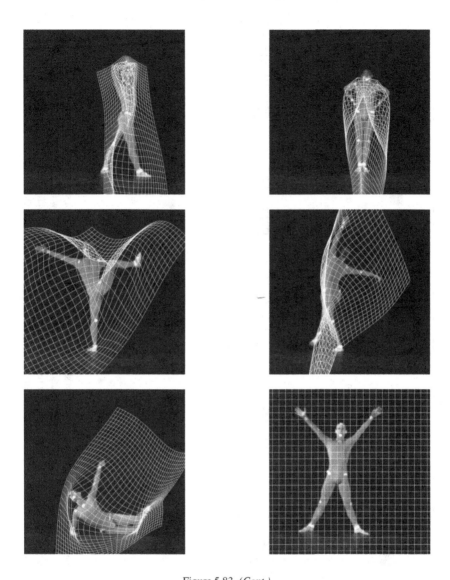

Figure 5.83 *(Cont.)*

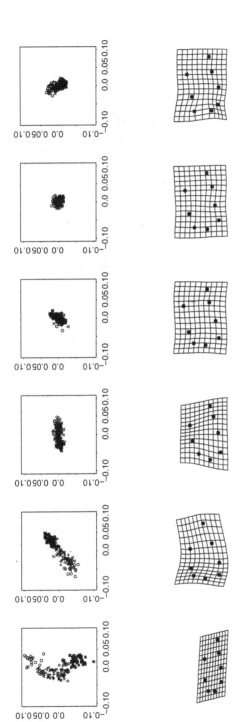

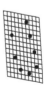

Figure 5.84 The six partial warps for the 8-landmark Vilmann rodent skull data set. Upper row: scatterplots of scores, all to the same Procrustes scale. Middle row, all but far left: grids of the corresponding deformations around the mean shape. Middle row far left: the uniform term (partial warp 0), for the change from age 7 days to age 30 days, combining reduction in height with a shear backward. Below it is the corresponding uniform term for change from age 30 days to age 150 days, combining a comparable height reduction with the opposite shear.

the largest-scale nonuniform warp that we did not notice before and, finally, a possible local feature emerging at the smallest scale. Under each of these scatters except that for the uniform term is plotted the partial warp along the axis of greatest variability. The one for PW1 looks remarkably like the first relative warp itself except that the uniform component (reduction of relative height) is gone. Both capture the relative overgrowth of the cranial base with respect to the upper margin of the calva. The last partial warp seems to reflect a phenomenon local to the IPP that is nevertheless patent in many of the mean comparisons already shown as grids in Figure 5.77. Under the uniform term (far left column) we show the mean differences from age 7 days to age 30 days (above) and age 30 days to age 150 days (below), to indicate the extent to which these changes agree in diminution of the vertical but are opposed concerning the shear of upper border versus lower.

Figure 5.85 confirms all these observations by examining the trajectories for these first three partial warps individually. Notice, in the lower left panel, the distinctive deficit in variance of the uniform term for the 30-day-olds vis-à-vis their variances at either end of these growth series. The U-shaped trace of this variance term over the growth period is responsible for the reversal in the corresponding plot of principal coordinates of these covariance structures (Figure 5.56). Note also the absence of curvature in the other two partial warps shown here: the 30-day averages lie along the lines connecting the 7-day to the 150-day averages. (In the contemporary sciences of mathematical imaging this is called the *geodesic question* – do actual temporal processes align with this geometric analogue to straight lines? For a real example of a dynamic situation where this collinearity is certainly *not* the case, see the analysis of human smiles in Figure 5.101) Figure 5.99 and 5.100 will summarize the features in Figure 5.85 along with the intermediate partial warps in a different rhetoric, *integration*, that likewise involves a contrast with the behavior of the warp of smallest scale, PW5.

5.6.6 Splines for Partial Least Squares

As the PLS computations of Section 4.2.3 result in linear combinations of the underlying variables of either measurement block, when that block consists of shape coordinates, this same splining tool can be used to represent it as a grid at "either end" of the PLS covariance extracted. A good example is Figure 5.86, which is an enhancement of a statistical scatter first published without the grids in Bookstein et al. (2002a). The data set for this analysis is the same one I used in connection with the quadratic discrimination in Figure 3.43. The shape representation here comprises one landmark only (the sharp corner

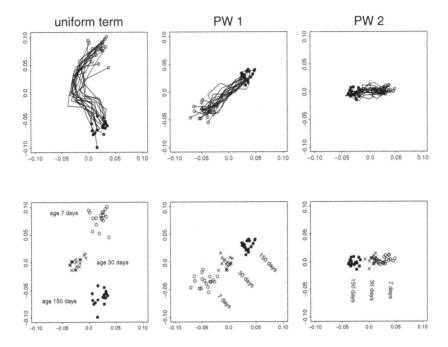

Figure 5.85 Trajectories on the uniform term and the first two partial warps for the 18 rodents separately. Above, at all eight ages; below, a clearer display for ages 7 days, 30 days, and 150 days only. Note the monotonicity of the vertical component of the uniform term, both coordinates of partial warp 1, and the single meaningful component of partial warp 2, together with reversal of the shear (horizontal) component of the uniform term.

called Rostrum) along with 39 semilandmarks computed with respect to a template as reviewed in Section 5.5.4. There is a correlation of 0.81 between a profile of neuropsychological test scores (one end connoting executive function problems, the other end motor problems) and an easily interpreted pattern combining shearing and thinning of the corpus callosum. This geometric pattern is far easier to draw than to verbalize, hence the role of those little grids along the horizontal axis. Numbers printed on the plot are the patients' measured IQ scores; evidently neither of these dimensions is associated with IQ within these fetal-alcohol-affected subsamples either separately or pooled.

That was an analysis matching a shape coordinate space to a block of scalar measures. The same SVD-driven computation applies for computing dimensions of relatively great covariance between one shape coordinate space and another. To demonstrate this option, Figure 5.87 returns to the 22-specimen, 20-landmark human midsagittal data set. Purely for the purposes

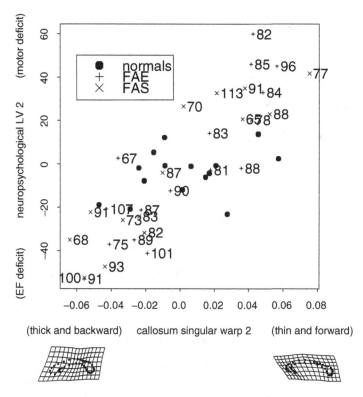

Figure 5.86 Example of a spline used to visualize a partial least-squares finding. Here, as in Figure 3.47, the grids actually comprise part of the figure axis labeling, not the main data display. In keeping with the advice at the end of Section 4.2.4, these behavioral measures have all been converted to z-scores before the SVD computation. (The shape coordinates are already in a common unit, the Procrustes unit.) Numbers near 100 are IQ scores. After Bookstein et al., 2002a.

of this demonstration, I divided it arbitrarily into a "neural" component and a "facial" component as shown in the upper left panel of the figure. These components do not overlap, but they do not comprise all the landmarks, either. A PLS analysis of the two shape coordinate spaces indicated there results in one dominant pair of latent variables correlating about 0.74 and accounting for 63% of the summed squared covariances of the ten shape coordinates of the face compartments against the twelve shape coordinates of the brain compartments. (The deficiency of rank of these Procrustes shape spaces separately – four zeroed dimensions each – has no effect on the reporting of the larger singular values. Recall that PLS is robust against projection into Procrustes space or any other data subspace.) The upper center panel shows

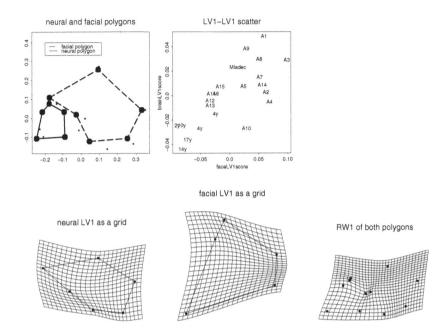

Figure 5.87 Partial Least Squares analysis of one shape space against another. Upper left: a "facial" polygon and a "neural" polygon from the 20-landmark configuration we have used in earlier demonstrations. Upper center: scatter of the first pair of PLS latent variables, with specimens identified as in the legend of Figure 5.43. The positioning of the children and adolescents with respect to each other and the adults is not entirely satisfactory. Lower left and center: grids for the first neural and facial latent variables. Lower right: the first dimension from an analysis of the same 11 landmarks by relative warps. This grid taps a different aspect of the shape covariance structure than the PLS analysis does. Notice that the hafting zone is a common boundary between the anatomical components; some of the resulting correlation must therefore be artifact.

the scatter of the scores corresponding to this first pair of LV's (equation 4.25). At lower left is a multiple of the neural LV from this analysis, drawn as a grid transformation of the average form; at lower center, the same for the facial component. This pair of grids is strongly consistent with the fused analysis in the panel at lower right, the first relative warp of the pooled list of 11 landmark points (versus the full complement of 20 for the analysis of Figure 5.43). This first relative warp accounts for only 33% of the Procrustes shape variance of its 11-landmark configuration, and so the PLS of the neural "half" against the facial "half" clearly is a more efficient descriptor of whatever morphogenetic processes they are presumed to have in common. This is partly because the transformation we are investigating has one component that is a strong gradient across the posterocraniad dimension of this plane, which is very efficiently captured by the relation between its two extremes, and partly because the "hafting zone" in between them, which is quite complicated in its geometric gradients, has been omitted from the PLS analysis.

Knowledge of other factors can supersede a pro-forma PLS. The uniform component we reviewed in Section 5.5.3 is not only a simplification (no bending) of a deformation grid but also an explanatory hypothesis of its own: the hypothesis of a homogeneous shape effect corresponding to a uniform common cause, perhaps a biomechanical one. Other hypotheses can be built atop a GMM analysis in a similar biomechanically nuanced way that is explained in some detail in Bookstein (2015c). In the context of the analysis of the 22 human midline cranial landmark configurations that we just used for the PLS demonstration, suppose we want to consider one of the standard explanations of hominization, the possible selection process for a shift in the face size – brain size ratio. (The bigger the brain, the smaller the teeth need to be, once food can be cooked; see Wrangham, 2010.) The PLS analysis in Figure 5.87 involves two polygons that overlap along part of the border of each, the hafting zone; hence some of the PLS correlation reported here must be artifact. An analysis would be more persuasive that extracted entirely separate measures from the same pooled analysis. .

We can do this, as long as each module measure has the same dimensions of cm/cm, from the pooled analysis. Figure 5.88 shows the geometry by which this goes forward. For measures that are functions of interlandmark distances only, it can be shown that the only row of the matrix J that needs to be considered is its fourth row, the size adjustment row. For our sublist of 11 landmarks the entries of this row can be diagrammed in the vectors of the upper left panel in the figure. The measures theory suggests for the interpretation of the PLS (upper right panel) are, first, the length of the maxilla (the separation of two landmarks toward the left, drawn in solid line) and, second, the centroid size of the rear part of the brain, the part not bounded by the hafting zone (the centrifugal pattern in dashed line in the same panel).

The clever step in this application of the GMM toolkit is the projection of these vectors down into the Procrustes shape space. At lower left we see, in the solid lines, an adjustment of the upper maxillary landmarks toward the centroid (to a small extent) in compensation of the increase in Centroid Size consequence on the moving of the leftmost landmark further left. Similarly, to make hindbrain size change a proper Procrustes index, its loadings must be adjusted for the consequent size change as shown by the dashed lines here.

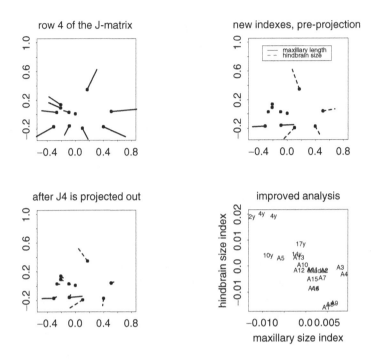

Figure 5.88 Improving on PLS by remembering your functional anatomy. (upper left) Map of the fourth row of the J-matrix, the only dimension requiring projection in this example. Landmark CaO, canalis opticus, is indistinguishable from the centroid of this little configuration, and so its coefficients in the fourth row of J are too small to be visible. (upper right) The two extents that the text suggests for superseding the PLS analysis. Solid bars, differentials of a maxillary length measure; dashed segments, differentials of hindbrain size (row 4 of its own J-matrix). (lower left) The same after projecting out the fourth row of J. (lower right) A scatterplot of the resulting pair of indices correlates 0.813, considerably better than the PLS first latent variable pair. Note the separation of the three infants with deciduous dentition and the much more satisfactory placement of the three adolescents in a position intermediate between the infants and the adults.

Notice, for instance, how the change of hindbrain size toward its posterior end actually changes Centroid Size at nearly the same rate, and so the Procrustes representation of such a change must concentrate on the shift of the anterior pair of landmarks of this quadrilateral: the pair move forward together but diverge in the vertical coordinate of this change. The resulting pair of indices, a proper linear combination of Procrustes shape coordinates, correlate -0.813, as shown in the final figure panel. (Comparing this to the correlation of 0.74 in Figure 5.87 confirms that PLS is not in the business of maximizing correlation.)

Because both of these indices are functions of the Procrustes superposition, the appropriate reference value for this correlation is not the conventional 0.0 of the packages, but instead the correlation one would observe from the offset isotropic (Mardia–Dryden) distribution on the same average shape. From simulations, this reference correlation is about -0.24. Transforming both to Fisher's z's, equation (3.19), the difference between them is about 2.75 times its standard error for independent samples of size 22. So the correlation of -0.813 we just constructed is no artifact of Procrustes fitting but instead a potentially real aspect of the regulation of human skull growth.

The analysis in Figure 5.88 is better than the one in Figure 5.87 in many ways. One is that the report deals not with linear combinations of ten or twelve shape coordinates, but with ordinary extents, lengths or areal moments, which are much easier to incorporate in linear models of the type we reviewed in Chapters 2 and 3. Another is that the deformation grid itself, with all its visual complexity, is no longer a necessary part of the narrative. (Extents are much easier to put into words than deformations are.) Now that PLS has computed this pair, we are permitted to substitute the obvious scalar for the corresponding pattern. A third advantage is the circumvention of what would otherwise be a severe artifact, the overlap of the boundaries of our "modules" along the cranial base. Fourth, we have found a novel hint in the new scatterplot, namely a separation of the infants from the older children as well as the adults of the sample. In a larger sample of humans, that would suggest that the maxilla grows to some extent in response to the eruption of the permanent dentition. But that investigation would require an entirely different kind of sample, with more children who were followed longitudinally and surely some additional landmarks on the mandible. The grand longitudinal growth studies at Michigan and Denver might easily support such an analysis combining tooth size measures with GMM of bony landmarks. I argue elsewhere (Bookstein, 2015c) that analyses of this type should supersede relative warps in any morphometric exploration of the biomechanical aspects of skeletal form.

5.6.7 Bilateral Symmetry and Asymmetry

There is at least one common research context where properties of the average shape are no longer a "nuisance variable," but rather a substantial concern of the scientist working with shape coordinates. This is the study of a *bilaterally symmetric* structure such as the vertebrate body. In this context, the Procrustes method offers a modification of all the standard SVD-based approaches that applies directly to the comparison at issue. For rigid objects that have both a left side and a right side, the formal model involves a set of landmarks most of

in the laboratory, perhaps   in shape space

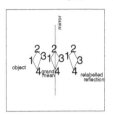

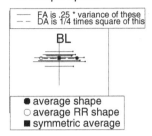

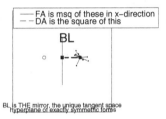

Figure 5.89 Procrustes construction of bilateral symmetry. FA, fluctuating asymmetry; DA, directional asymmetry; BL, the plane of perfect bilateral symmetry; RR, reflected relabeling.

which are paired – left eye corner, right eye corner – along with a possible list of unpaired points up a nominal "midline" or "midplane."

Typical approaches (e.g., Palmer and Strobeck, 1986) would measure the two sides of the form separately, or else measure distances from the paired landmarks separately to some approximate midline. In the Procrustes approach, we instead measure the distance of the entire form from its own mirror image. Because of the independence from rotation that characterizes Procrustes distance, this measurement is independent of any specific choice of a midplane for the reflection. It is, instead, reflection in the Procrustes geometry itself (Figure 5.89): reflection in the hyperplane of all possible perfectly symmetric shapes with the same counts of paired and unpaired landmarks. As part of the mirroring procedure, we have to renumber the landmarks so that left and right sides are restored; this is the reason for the term "relabeled reflection" in the figure, along with its acronym RR.

As the figure's upper left panel indicates, the average of a form and its own relabeled reflection is a perfectly symmetrical form, from which the original form has a Procrustes distance (which is half its distance from its own relabeled reflection). A sample of forms yields a sample of these relabeled reflections, a

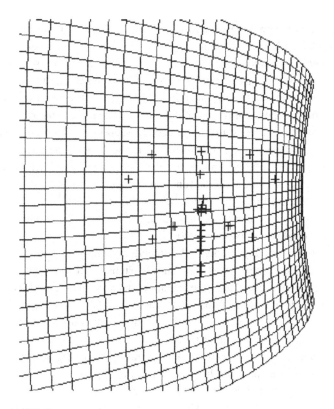

Figure 5.90 Representation (by quadratic-kernel thin-plate spline) of the component of human craniofacial asymmetry for bilateral difference in the uniform component. The actual left-right asymmetry of these data (anteroposterior cephalograms of good-looking human children) has been magnified tenfold here for visibility.

sample average, and a sample average of the averages; this is the point plotted at the solid square in either right-hand panel of the figure. Mardia et al. (2000) and Schaefer et al. (2006) show how to extract quantities standing for the various standard quantifications of asymmetry (fluctuating, directional, total) from a scheme like this – it reduces to an ordinary analysis of variance, and Bookstein and Mardia (2003) show how the descriptors we have adopted can be used to visualize *types of asymmetry.* These include differences in size or shape of the left and right halves with respect to one another, differences of their positions with respect to the midline, rotation of the unpaired structures with respect to the mirroring line between the sides, and unflatness of the midline.

Figure 5.90, from Bookstein (2004), shows one of these components for another classic craniofacial data set, the "Broadbent–Bolton standards" for craniofacial growth in three dimensions. This is a sample of about 30 Cleveland children selected for the pleasantness of their appearance (i.e., not a definable sample of any population), who were imaged by head x-rays in two directions, permitting a 3D reconstruction of some of the characteristic points from Figure 5.16. Analysis here is of a frontally projected view. The thin-plate spline pictured is the deformation of the true average form to its own relabeled reflection, but it is not the spline introduced in Section 5.5. That spline is linear at infinity, and to see how the sides differ at large scale, we want instead a spline that is quadratic at infinity. This is arranged by replacing the kernel function $|r|$ of the standard spline with the function $|r^3|$ and augmenting the bordering matrix Q in the formulas of Section 5.5 by the products $x^2, xy, \ldots, z^2$ of the Cartesian coordinates as well as their actual values. (For the mathematics that allows us to do this, see Wahba, 1990.)

In the display of Figure 5.90, the intended focus is not on the average landmark locations themselves (the little + signs — if you look hard, you can see all the pairs, and also the unpaired stack along the midline) but on the largest-scale features of the grid. The left side of the figure is larger than the right side everywhere, and the dilation is directional: it has become wider faster than it is becoming taller. As a result, the cusp where the spline dwindles to a zero derivative is aligned vertically (at the right margin) rather than horizontally, as it would have been had the opposite gradient applied to the raw data. The left-right difference has been exaggerated by a factor of ten so that this feature of the grid will appear near enough to the data to be printed at the same scale.

For another application of a Procrustes-like symmetrization, for a template comprising one closed curve without any landmarks at all, see Bookstein and Ward (2013). In that application, bilateral asymmetry is considered mere developmental noise, to be removed from the biometric analysis on explicitly functional grounds.

Symmetrization. In addition to computing these sums of squares for asymmetry, it is often useful to examine the symmetrized form itself, the form around which these sums of squares have been taken. That computation is likewise a straightforward Procrustes calculation that can be followed in the panels of Figure 5.91. At upper left, courtesy of Dr. Sonja Windhager of the University of Vienna, is a typical organismal form of 71 (semi)landmarks that is "nominally" bilaterally symmetric, meaning that it is a combination of *unpaired* or *midline* landmarks, such as #20 or #46, along with *paired bilateral landmarks or semilandmarks* such as (#37, #55). Assume that this nominal mirroring plane is nearly vertical in your Procrustes plot. Then

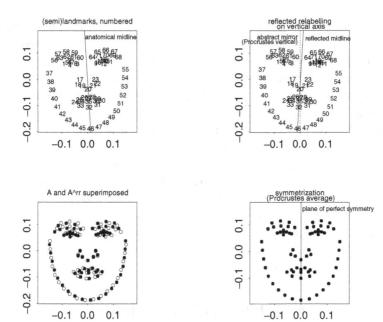

Figure 5.91 Symmetrization of a bilaterally labeled form. (upper left) A Procrustes average form, nominally but not geometrically symmetric. The anatomical midline lies askew and the other landmarks are not placed precisely symmetrically with respect to it. (upper right) The *reflected relabeling* – all *x*-coordinates have their signs reversed and then the new left-side landmarks are renumbered according to the old left side numbers, and conversely. (lower left) Superposition of the original and mirrored forms. (lower right) The Procrustes average of this pair has perfect mirror symmetry around the Procrustes vertical.

produce a new form, the *reflected relabeling*, by reversing the sign of every *x*-coordinate of the original form (point 37 goes from $(-0.1496, .0232)$ to $(0.1496, .0232)$, for instance) and then, as before, switching the numbers between the sides (so that this new point becomes #56 instead). This operation involves the specification of that *mirroring list*, which, in one program package language, looks like mirroring<-c(11:9, 12, 15:13, 16, 3:1, 4, 7:5, 8, 23:17, 30:24, 33:31, 36:34, 55:37, 68:64, 71:69, 60:56, 63:61), meaning that points 1, 2, 3, 4, 5, 6, 7, 8 reflect to points 11, 10, 9, 12, 15, 14, 13, and 16, *and vice versa*, 9 through 16 reflecting to 3, 2, 1, 4, 7, 6, 5, 8. Midline points, like #20 here, correspond to their own mirroring. For instance, points 17, 18, 19, 20, 21, 22, 23 mirror to 23, 22, 21, 20, 19, 18, 17, respectively, so point #20 does not change its number.

In the superposition of these two forms (lower left panel), the summed squared distances between corresponding points (neighboring pairs of solid and open dots) is four times the sum of squares for asymmetry at lower right in Figure 5.89. Whether or not that quantity is of interest, we can take the Procrustes average of the two forms here following the scheme of Figure 5.89. They have the same Centroid Size, and the rotation step of GPA guarantees that the actual choice of the mirroring plane for the *x*-coordinate change is irrelevant. So the final result (lower right) is a precisely symmetrical form, with midline precisely straight and precisely vertical as shown.

There is another variant of this calculation, the version that Mardia et al. (2000) call *object asymmetry*. In this setting, there are two different forms involved, for instance, a left hand and a right hand, and the asymmetry computation is just the ordinary group difference of the two subgroups after one or the other has been reflected (as by changing the sign of every *x*-coordinate after digitizing). In that setting, also, one produces a symmetrized form by averaging the two organs, left and right, of the same organism, along with the mirroring of these averages.

5.6.8 "Modularity" and "Integration"

This section summarizes an argument set out at considerable length, with additional examples, in Bookstein (2015b, 2016b).

The discussion of bilateral symmetry in the preceding section is connected to a powerful generalization offering more ways in which the large-scale pattern analysis of a landmark configuration can be organized in its geometry. (In some sense the halves of a bilaterally symmetric scene must be regarded as modules, and certainly bilateral symmetry enforces an integration at very large scale.) Chapter 2 already showed you one good example of this interpretation, an example a hundred years old: the Sewall Wright analysis of the correlations among six length measures on 276 chickens. The structure of this data set proved hierarchical (Figure 2.31, equation 2.21), with wings predicting legs better than either predicted skulls and either proximal measurement predicting its own distal measure better than the other proximal one. Olson and Miller (1958) built this sort of observation into a classic book-length argument about the magnitudes of correlations among positively correlated variables.

Unfortunately, that reasoning does not transfer over into the domain of GMM. The difficulty is that shape coordinates do not behave like the "extents" that Wright, Olson, and Miller were studying; growth does not make shape coordinates bigger. They sum exactly to zero in four different ways (the first four rows of the *J*-matrix, Section 5.4), and so they cannot possibly all correlate positively, the way Wright's chicken length measures did.

Instead, what we mean by an integrated pattern of shape variation must be rooted in spatial aspects of the pattern claim. A uniform shear is integrated across every little patch of tissue in our map – the shape change is, literally, the same everywhere. A perfectly symmetric organismal form is *also* perfectly integrated *in the same abstract sense* – there are exact equalities governing the relation of distinct parts of the form. The difference is not one of decimal values but a matter of counting: perfect bilateral symmetry among $2k + m$ landmarks involves $2k + m$ exact equalities, where k is the count of paired landmarks and m the count of unpaired, and perfect uniformity among l landmarks involves $2l - 6$ exact equalities, namely the zeroing of all the nontrivial partial warp scores from Section 5.5.2. Either situation can be perfectly integrated, but the perfection of the pattern is different in the two cases. Importantly, while bilateral integration does involve "modules" (the left and the right sides, separately), the uniform transformation example does not. The words "modularity" and "integration" not only are not opposites but actually have nothing important to do with each other.

With this in mind, page back to Figure 5.84, a summary of the partial warp analysis for the Vilmann neurocranial octagons. Notice, now, that the visual extents of the plots in the top row there – in effect, the variances of the successive partial warps – fall steadily from left to right except for the very last column. Instead of numbering these warps, we may characterize them by their own spatial scale, in the form of their specific bending energy (their eigenvalue from the analysis that produced them, equation 5.15).

The log-log plot of this scheme (Figure 5.92), is very suggestive. What is important is not that the regression line shown slopes downward – this will be true of every data set the biologist ever encounters – but that its slope is steeper than -1. A calculation that explicitly separates out digitizing noise from biological variability (Bookstein, 2015b) suggests that this slope is even steeper, with an estimated value of -2.2.

The slope threshold of -1 is important because it corresponds to the phenomenon of *selfsimilarity,* shape variation at the same scale for every small quadrilateral regardless of position, orientation, or scale. Such models correspond to the organismal biologist's trained strategy of searching for phenomena to be explained, or for their explanations, at every geometric scale a data set can offer, from the full image of the organism down to the smallest variations of organ outlines that can be discerned in an image. The model of Figure 5.39 is not consistent with this strategy, but there is a closely related model that is. Figure 5.93 shows realizations of both of them on the same starting configuration. As Procrustes shape scatters they appear quite similar, but the covariance structures hidden here are strikingly different, as shown in

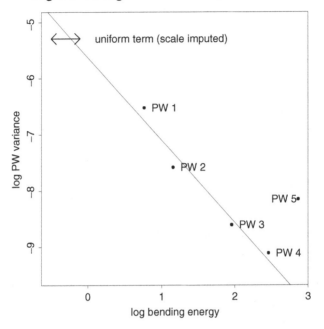

Figure 5.92 Log bending energy against log partial warp variance for the Vilmann neurocranial octagons. The points for partial warps 1 through 4 lie close to a straight line. The uniform component does not have a log bending energy; it has been placed on the graph by hand at an estimated location corresponding to the variance of its vertical component. The downward-slanting line is the regression of log PW on log BE for the first four partial warps, slope −1.47.

Figure 5.94. For the distribution of shapes at the left, the variance on every partial warp is the same, up to sampling noise; but at the right, variance drops as the inverse of bending energy. There is a hint of this, but only a hint, in Figure 5.93: the apparent dominance of variance at the corners over variance at the mid-edges and the center, which dominate, in turn, the variance at the other four landmarks. What is meant by selfsimilarity is clearest, perhaps, from the comparisons across the rows in Figure 5.95. The upper row shows how in the offset isotropic Gaussian (Mardia–Dryden) distribution, with variance the same at every landmark prior to the Procrustes arithmetic, the nonuniform component of shape variation rises as the landmark subconfiguration becomes smaller. But in the selfsimilar model of the lower row, the extent of shape variance is the same for every scale of a possibly informative feature. This latter is much more compatible with biological styles of investigation and explanation. The grids in Figure 5.96 are samples from this distribution. If we

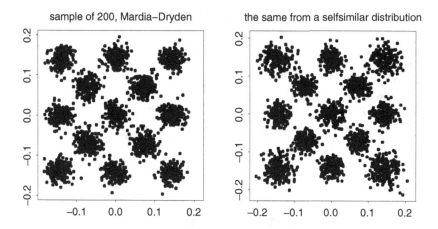

Figure 5.93 Procrustes shape coordinate scatters for two different models of variation around the same average form. Left, the model of independent variation, Figure 5.39. Right, the selfsimilar model of Bookstein, 2015b.

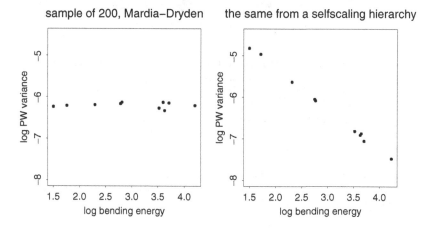

Figure 5.94 Log partial warp variance by log bending energy for the two models in the previous figure. Left, the model of independent variation: the variance of each partial warp is about the same. Right, the selfsimilar model: partial warp variance is proportional to the reciprocal of bending energy. Note the twofold and fourfold degeneracies (up to sampling noise) induced by the symmetries of the mean 13-point design.

did not know in advance that they were just random samples, each one would suggest a suitable report narrative.

The data for Figures 5.93 through 5.96 were simulated per equation (8) of Bookstein (2015b):

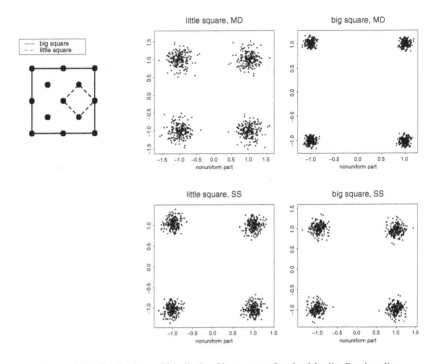

Figure 5.95 Confirming selfsimilarity. Upper row: for the Mardia–Dryden distribution: the nonuniform shape standard deviations of a large square (right) are $1/\sqrt{8}$ that of a small square (left). Lower row: in a selfsimilar distribution, the nonuniform shape variability of these two squares is the same. In all panels, the scatters of the four landmarks are completely redundant (identity along diagonals, perfect multiplication by -1 between them), in keeping with the geometry of the partial warp in question in Figure 5.64. Inset: situation of the two squares upon the mean of the scatters in Figure 5.93. They differ not only in scale but also in position (relative to the centroid) and orientation. It is remarkable that any such selfsimilar distribution should exist. SS: the selfsimilar distribution. MD: the isotropic Mardia–Dryden distribution.

$$defl = Pmean + \sum_{l=1}^{k-3} \sqrt{\frac{E_1}{E_l}} (W_l \cdot Pdist) W_l \qquad (5.20)$$

where *Pmean* is the Procrustes mean shape of the simulated sample, *Pdist* the corresponding distribution of Procrustes shape coordinates case by case, the E's are the nonzero bending energies of its $k - 3 = 10$ partial warps W_l, $l = 1, \ldots, 10$, and the quantities $W_l \cdot Pdist$, taken as complex numbers, are the corresponding 10 partial warp scores. In words, one begins by sampling from an isotropic Mardia-Dryden distribution (GPA of 13-gons analogous to

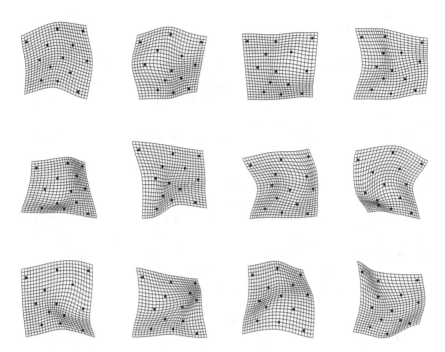

Figure 5.96 Twelve samples from the selfsimilar distribution on a 13-gon. These are far more conducive to the possibility of biological explanations than analogous samples from an isotropic offset Gaussian distribution as in Figure 5.38.

Figure 5.37), rotates to the basis of their partial warps (ignoring the uniform component), deflates each nonuniform partial warp by the square root of its specific bending energy, and finally sums up all the components after that deflation.

To these displays corresponds a new language for discussions of integration and modularity that accommodates the presumptive similarity of displacements of adjacent landmarks in a biologically sensible way. **It is always inappropriate to submit these patterns to "significance tests."** I am strongly opposed to the current fashion for "testing" for integration or modularity by permuting displacements over landmark numbers somehow. Integration is a *biometrical* hypothesis, not a statistical one. It requires biological modeling that embraces all of the auxiliary information available in the measurement design. To show that a data set is integrated, one shouldn't be testing a "null" hypothesis of "non-integration" – such a null is incompatible with life. Instead one needs to model the integration by some explicit geometry, such as symmetry, a uniform term or (the example below) a growth gradient. Fit the model; interpret the fit. The idea of a "null model" for integration is as absurd as the idea of the Procrustes shape distribution as a descriptor of reality. It is not, as we have seen; it serves only as a descriptor of ignorance. Likewise, permutation tests have no role to play in this domain. Our job is to say what we mean by integration, not what we mean by disintegration, given that we are absolutely, positively guaranteed not to see it (inasmuch as the organisms we study are or were alive).

This is important enough to be worth repeating in its own offset paragraph.

Permutation tests against biologically meaningless null hypotheses (e.g., random associations among landmark locations, or random partitions between candidate modules) have no useful role to play in the study of morphological integration whether over evolution or over development. Instead one must fit actual, geometrically specific models of integrated shape change, then assess their parameters against various theoretical specifications. Neither evolution nor development ever permutes landmark numbers around their average locations.

What would be a suitable augmentation of the language of integration that has already been demonstrated in this chapter, a language that includes uniform terms but also bilateral symmetry, each with its own quantitative rhetoric? I suggest a next entry for this directory that is borrowed from a source nearly as old as biometrics itself, Julian Huxley's *Problems of Relative Growth* of 1932 (the book that launched the concept of allometry via its differential-geometric interpretation). A proper GMM approach to integration in the context of growth (which is, after all, the setting in which we are most often concerned to understand it) should center on the appropriate generalization for space of Huxley's notions in the time domain. Following a suggestion in my 1991 monograph, this could very well be the classic setting of the *growth-gradient,* the next degree of geometric parametrization of spatial trends beyond the uniform component that we have already strenuously exercised here. (In fact, the term "at infinity" of the second-order thin-plate spline demonstrated in Figure 5.90 is actually an example of such a growth gradient: its formula is quadratic in all two or all three spatial coordinates.)

To describe integration along these lines, a modification of the J-matrix (Section 5.4) is helpful. Add six rows that specify the three quadratic terms of x, y-dependence (x^2, xy, y^2) for shifts in the two target coordinates (horizontal and vertical) separately. And don't forget to project out the first six rows, of course – we want only the *new* information that was not already there in the Procrustes fit and the uniform term. When all this is done and tidied up, we learn that one single growth-gradient (Figure 5.97), accounts for 89% of all the nonuniform variability in the Vilmann data set. This progressive

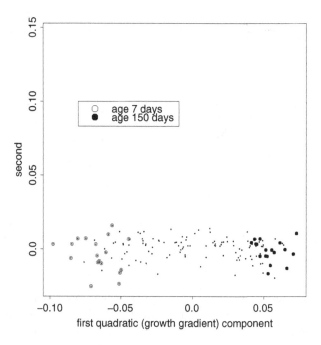

Figure 5.97 Scatter of the first two dimensions of the quadratic (second-order)
subspace, of dimension 6, for the Vilmann data. Clearly the first component is the
one that will carry our notion of integration here.

gradient manages to embrace nearly all of the nonlinearity in the previous
plot of the first two principal coordinates (Figure 5.84), and it runs quite
equably in time from the youngest animals (at the left) to the oldest (at the
right).

Figure 5.98 shows, at the left, the corresponding grid diagram for this
single dimension of integrated growth gradient, and, to its right, the analogous
computation from the standard Procrustes toolkit, the principal component of
the residuals of the shape coordinate configurations after projecting out from
each its own uniform term. The resemblance between these grids is startling
but not perfect. There is a clear shape feature at the upper left of the actual
nonaffine principal component that is not captured by the principal growth-
gradient. The residual from this smooth gradient looks just like the twist
between IPP and Lambda that we already saw in Figure 5.84. This last partial
warp thereby becomes the diagram for the least integrated part of our octagon.
If there is any "module" to be detected in these data, it is there: a locale that
maximally deviates from predictability by the best-predicting global gradient.
The complete interpretation of this growth sequence, eight landmarks over
eight ages, is laid out in Figure 5.99.

Vilmann data set, N = 144
first (and only) quadratic component

Vilmann data set,
first nonaffine relative warp

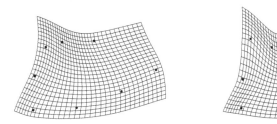

Figure 5.98 The principal component of our growth-gradients is similar to but not identical with the principal component of the actual residual from the uniform term of these shape changes.

We thereby learn a great deal more about how the growth of these 18 rodent neural skulls was organized. That knowledge is not based on permutation tests, but arises from a close consideration of what it would *mean* for a midsagittal configuration to be integrated vs. decomposing into multiple separate features. A two-segment uniform process, a single integrated process, and a localized module together account for 93% of all the shape variation in the data (versus 94% for the sum of the first four eigenvalues of the relative warps, which try to maximize "explained" variance without actually explaining anything). This is a far more nuanced description of this growth process than anything available to Olson and Miller's methods for extent measures. It is also much more informative than either of the separate breakdowns of Section 5.5, the breakdown by relative warps or the breakdown by partial warps. That is because it is the biologist who is asking the questions now, using the installed knowledge base of the *way* morphogenetic processes are integrated (which is not remotely the same as the way that kinetic networks are integrated, or genomes, or bilateral structures). If there is to be a methodology for modularity and integration as descriptions of morphometric phenomena, then the parameters of the methodology need to be the parameters of the underlying biological explanations, not the parameters of their Procrustes covariance matrices, which, as we have seen, offer no meaningful biological interpretability at all. Integration is not about the *fact* of correlated shape coordinates but the *manner* of that correlation. It is to be described, not "tested." After all, if an organism were not integrated, it would certainly be dead: that is what "disintegrated" implies.

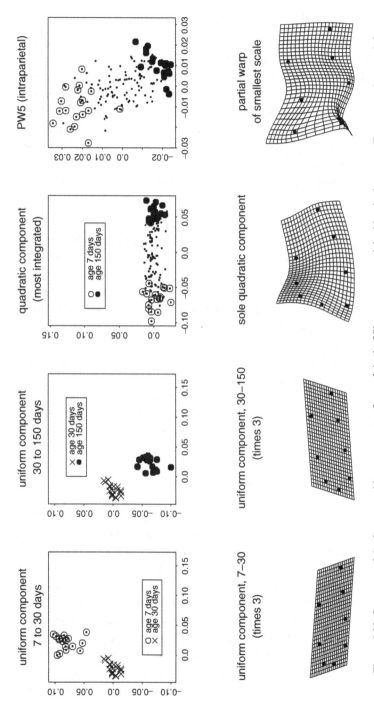

Figure 5.99 Summary of the four separable components of growth in the Vilmann neurocranial midsagittal octagon. From top to bottom, left to right, these are the two phases of uniform shear (posterocranial early, anterocranial late), the unique integrated dimension of large-scale change (the nonuniform growth gradient), and the focal divergence between landmarks IPP and Opi.

5.6.9 Two Recent Extensions

The analysis in Figure 5.99 broke the symmetries of the standard Procrustes/
PCA approach by explicit injection of biological insight: selection of particular
subspaces in which to pursue single-factor component analysis, or selection
of specific partial warps for biological interpretation. Two recent extensions
in this spirit modify the principal component approach more radically. Both
discard the underlying Procrustes metric in favor of new multivariate pattern
analyses much more aligned with the biological knowledge base that motivated
the experimental or comparative study in the first place. The examples in this
final section construe this assignment – the subordination of multivariate
arithmetic to biological understanding – in somewhat opposite ways.

5.6.9.1 Varimax Factor Rotation of Residualized Partial Warps

This approach, introduced in Bookstein (2017b), embraces a very old tactic
from the adjacent discipline of psychometrics, whereby a suitable principal
component analysis is followed by a separate geometric operation, *rotation*.
What results can often more closely approach the so-called *simple structure*
whereby most loadings of most variables on most dimensions are small enough
to be ignored over the course of subsequent explanations. (This class of
methods, collectively known as *factor analysis*, was reviewed very thoroughly,
though without applications like this one, in Reyment and Jöreskog 1991.)
But there is a further trick involved: the variables sent for rotation are not
the Procrustes shape coordinates, nor even the partial warp scores (which
are already a rotation), but a new set of variables representing these warp
scores after each is rescaled to its *residual* from a regression like the one
in Figure 5.92. The resulting analysis, restricted to the nonuniform (i.e.,
localizable) aspects of the shape variation or shape change under study,
no longer makes any reference to Procrustes distance. For this particular
assignment, the rotation of residualized partial warp scores, I recommended the
varimax method of Kaiser (1958). (The name is a portmanteau word: the sum
of the **vari**ances of the squares of the rotated factor loadings is **max**imized.)
Varimax rotation is among the approaches discussed in Reyment and Jöreskog.

Applied to the neurocranial octagons of the instant example (Figure 5.99),
the new technique leaves columns 1 and 2 unaltered, but supplements column
3, there interpreted as a single growth-gradient, by an additional component of
the nonaffine space for a particular reproportioning of the body of the sphenoid.
Also, the analysis splits the rightmost column of Figure 5.99, the unique pattern
corresponding to the last partial warp, into two components, one for its vertical
aspects and the other for its horizontal aspects. The resulting set of six patterns

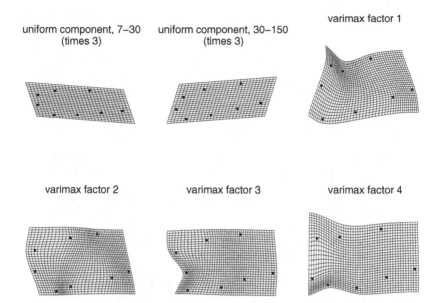

Figure 5.100 Enhancing Figure 5.99 by varimax rotation of residualized partial warp scores (Bookstein, 2017b). The rotation greatly simplifies the geometric structure of the multivariate pattern analyses, easing the translation into biological explanations. Upper left, center: the two factors of the uniform term, unaffected by the residualized varimax rotation. Upper right: a slightly modified version of the "general factor," still close to the first Procrustes principal component of the nonaffine subspace. Lower left: factor for the relative expansion of the middle segment of the cranial base, the separation of spheno-ethmoid synchondrosis from intersphenoidal synchondrosis (see Figure 2.41). Lower center, right: horizontal and vertical aspects of local remodeling across the foramen magnum (basion to opisthion).

is diagrammed in Figure 5.100. See Bookstein (2017b) for a deep critique of the standard methods of principal component analysis when applied to shape coordinates from growth studies, for a thorough explication and justification of the varimax method itself (along with two versions of the crucial software fragment), and for much more insight into this example.

5.6.9.2 A Dynamic Analysis at the Largest Two Scales

By contrast with the preceding exegesis, my final example of a modified multivariate analysis emphasizes only the two symmetric partial warp components of largest scale. These are shown in the top row of Figure 5.101 for a decagon of data corresponding to changes in shape of a soft-tissue configuration, the human lip outline, as observed over 28 smiles: 14 for subjects trained to

The integrated part of   ... comprises this pattern (1y)   ... along with this pattern (uy)
smile dynamics ...   (~ action of zygomaticus major) .   (~ action of orbicularis oris).

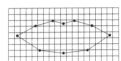
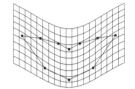
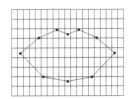

Figure 5.101 Aspects of the dynamic smile analysis, Section 5.6.9.2. Top row: the mean decagon (left) and the two factors that suffice for an explanation by familiar muscle actions: the contraction of zygomaticus major, corresponding to the vertical component 1y of partial warp 1 (center), and the relaxation of orbicularis oris, corresponding to the vertical component *uy* of the uniform term. Landmarks and semilandmarks, clockwise from left: (1) right cheilion, (2) midpoint between 1 and 3, (3) right christa philtri, (4) labiale superius, (5) left christa philtri, (6) midpoint between 5 and 7, (7) left cheilion, (8) midpoint between 7 and 9, (9) labiale inferius, (10) midpoint between 9 and 1. Middle row: scatterplots of absolute values of all the partial warp loadings for the 28 experimental dynamical sequences (open-lips and closed-lips smiles for the 14 subjects). ×, loadings for the vertical component of the uniform term; +, loadings for the vertical component of the first partial warp; ○, the other 196 loadings. FAC12: the closed-lips smile, muscle action 12 of the Facial Action Coding system (action of zygomaticus major only). FAC1225: the open-lips smile, muscle actions 12 and 25 of the Facial Action Coding system (zygomaticus contraction and orbicularis relaxation combined). Bottom row: dynamics of all 28 experimental smiles between rest and the configuration of maximum expression, registered on that rest position. The two smile conditions show comparable shifts of PW1 but opposite shifts of the uniform term. Note, however, the relative homogeneity of the FAC12 smiles in contrast to the substantial heterogeneity of the FAC1225 smiles. Filled black circle: common registration for all 28 rest configurations. Open circles: the configurations of maximum smile expression for each of the 28 smiles. (After Bookstein, Khambay, et al., 2017.)

produce a closed-lips smile, the other 14 for the same subjects now instructed to produce an open-lips smile, all while leaving the mandible fixed (and hence the teeth in occlusion). The six landmarks and four semilandmarks, listed in the figure caption, are the obvious ones for this cartoon. For details of data capture, please see Bookstein, Khambay, et al. (2017).

The top row goes on to sketch two particular partial warps for the variation around the average rest shape of this lip decagon. These two were selected because (1) in the dynamical analysis of the full sequence of video images for either type of smile, the dominant contributions to the first two relative warps were *always* these two specific partial warps, and also (2) each corresponds to the action of one single facial muscle known in advance to be responsible

abs(loadings), RW1–2, 14 FAC12 smiles   abs(loadings), RW1–2, 14 FAC1225 smiles

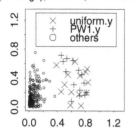 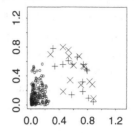

all histories, uy–1y, 14 FAC12 smiles   all histories, uy–1y, 14 FAC1225 smiles

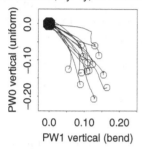 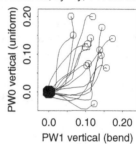

Figure 5.101 *(Cont.)*

for the smiles the subjects were instructed to produce. (Thus the design of this study ultimately traces to D'Arcy Thompson's original insight that grid diagrams like these can be used to explore "the origins of form in force.") The arithmetic justifying this simplification is laid out in the two frames of the middle row, which distinguish the loadings of the vertical uniform component uy (the $\times$ symbols) and the vertical component $1y$ of partial warp 1 (the $+$ symbols) from all 14 of the other partial warp components for each of the 14 experimental subjects (the $\circ$ symbols). When projections separate as perfectly as these do, there is no good reason not to immediately replace the 16-dimensional space of Procrustes coordinates by a single two-dimensional projection (uy by $1y$) that is consistent both with the data and with the a priori functional anatomy of the human smile.

The bottom row of the figure shows the dynamics of all 28 smiles in this projection onto the selected pair of meaningful components. It is obvious that the smiles are different – no statistician is needed for that observation, which passes the "interocular trauma test" (Edwards et al., 1963, as quoted in Bookstein, 2014:xxviii): it hits you between the eyes. But the contrast is

a little subtler than that. For action FAC12, the closed-lips smile, most of
these trajectories are similarly shaped, deviating from a linear path in shape
space to a relatively stable ending configuration by only slight curvatures
that are almost all convex-downward. By comparison, the individual shape
changes from beginning to end of the open-lips smiles vary wildly not only
in the final configuration (even though that involves an upward shift of the
uniform component in all examples except one) but in the relative tempo of
the contributions of the two components to this dynamical summary. The open
circles third and fourth from the bottom in the right panel, in particular, achieve
nearly the same final smile by quite different physiologies (in one case, an
initial segment that is entirely a zygomaticus action, followed by a segment
that is wholly orbicularis; in the other case, proportional contributions of both
muscles all along the trajectory). For an extensive discussion of this example,
together with details of the arithmetic and then the biology of this little study,
see, again, Bookstein, Khambay, et al. (2017).

Summary of Section 5.6

- Multivariate analysis (Chapter 4), Procrustes coordinates (Section 5.4), and
  the thin-plate spline visualization (Section 5.5) combine in a powerful and
  diverse collection of tools for the exploration of many different aspects of
  quantitative organismal morphology whenever morphometric landmark or
  semilandmark data are a part of the archive.
- At the very outset of a project, pages of multiple thin-plate splines, each
  specimen against an average, are useful for *data screening* and for
  motivating specific feature reports.
- Projects aimed at the discovery and presentation of contrasts among *group
  averages* benefit from the thin-plate splines that contrast these averages in
  pairs.
- Descriptions of large-scale variation often culminate in plots that combine
  the principal coordinates of a Procrustes analysis with their principal
  components, drawn as thin-plate splines contrasting one end of their range
  to the other. Often such diagrams confirm the insights that earlier
  generations of biologists incorporated in explicitly constructed shape
  indices (proportions or angles).
- The partial warps, eigenfunctions of the bending energy matrix, are a useful
  way of sorting both between-group contrasts and within-group variability
  across the range of spatial scales.
- Regressions of shape upon its determinants can be drawn by thin-plate
  spline grids of the corresponding predicted forms.

- Likewise, a partial least squares analysis of a shape space against a covarying block of measurements is often usefully diagrammed by the grids corresponding to the shape latent variables. When both blocks of variables are shape coordinates, often one can say even more, by designing specific scalar indices that simplify the grids of an exploratory PLS.
- The newly standardized methods for Procrustes analysis of bilateral symmetry produce comparisons of averages (such as the form versus its reflected relabeling) and dimensions of asymmetry that are more easily interpreted when presented as splined grids.
- The topic of *morphological integration*, currently in a state of some ferment, benefits greatly from a formalism whereby shape features are explicitly calibrated by their bending energy as the first step in their study. For this purpose the model of independent identical variation at every landmark needs to be replaced by a different model, the model of selfsimilarity, in which the variance of every partial warp is inverse to its bending energy. Growth processes often show patterns of the fall of variance with bending energy even steeper than that.
- Recent innovations in this class of methods deal with *simplifications* of morphometric reports so that they might correspond more closely to the language of biological explanation: localization of shape changes to specific foci or directions, and the matching of dynamical changes or comparisons to anatomical entities specified a priori.

5.7 Envoi

We have reached the end of the book, but it is not the end of the journey. Too much of the methodology recounted here has been *bricolage*, tinkering with existing materials from various scientific departments (anthropology, evolutionary biology, applied statistics) separately. And these materials arose in different epochs: the average date of the references to Chapters 2, 3, and 4 is about half a century earlier than citations from Section 5.2 onward. In 1977, just as I was beginning my own work on these themes, everything that is covered in Chapters 2, 3, and 4 was already known, certainly in the technical statistical literature and often over in the applied literatures of biometrics and evolutionary biology as well. Yet at that time *none* of the contents of Chapter 5 existed beyond its very first topic, the legacy of Rudolf Martin and the anthropometric tradition of the early twentieth century (which, here in my Vienna department, we still teach to the graduate students). Morphometrics was the last elementary unworked domain of statistics, the last area for which simple techniques, like the two-point coordinates, were just lying around on the ground to be stumbled over.[9] Even the tie with information theory was in place by midcentury – though information per se had been broached as a formal topic of applied mathematics only during World War II, it had already been translated into the language of linear statistics by Kullback (1959) while I was still in short pants.

Since then, linear statistical methods have stabilized – Rao's great textbook of 1973 is still a fine resource for a graduate sequence today, as is the reference by Mardia, Kent, and Bibby just a few years later – whereas morphometrics, driven by the sea-change in imaging resources, has proceeded from one "revolution" to another, digitizing tablets to graphical workstations to CCD cameras to neural nets, industrial face recognition, and personalized avatars.

We morphometric toolbuilders thereby must grapple with an enormous technoscientific lag. Quantification of the primary spatial and spatiotemporal data, all those individual surfaces and volumes, proceeds steadily faster, and likewise quantifications in genomics, proteomics, and all the other symbol-manipulating and code-manipulating branches of bioinformatics. But the *spatial matching functions* of morphometrics – that "biomathematical rhetoric of anatomical variation" and the conversion that it drives of those big piles of images into actual marked-up data bases – have developed far more slowly wherever they can be said to have developed at all. Paul Weiss's *bon mot* of 1956 – "Identical twins are much more similar than any microscopic sections from corresponding sites you can lay through either of them" – remains true and, by virtue of its multiscale paradoxes, remains a major barrier to future progress in quantification. Thus we have no updates in our catalogues of "normal human variants" beyond Anson's atlas of 1950, really – nothing that responds yet to Puget's (2012) plaintive request that we learn how to describe "what track the bullet would follow after it entered this body," meaning this *particular* body.

This is not to say that the role of morphometrics in organismal biology is standing still. Clothing design is making good use of body surface scans (a homely example was our analysis of the footprint, Figure 5.82, which actually derived from a doctoral dissertation on female footwear). There is good recent work on human movement (gait, sports, dance), on attractiveness and other projections of personality into form, on the direct assessment of emotional state

---

[9] These coordinates were like fossils in another sense as well: they had originally been published by Francis Galton in 1907, and were thereafter ignored by everyone except Karl Pearson in his role as Galton's scientific hagiographer. They were named Bookstein coordinates much later owing to Stigler's Law of Eponymy, which is that methodologies are named after the person who recognizes them *second*. Who first discovered Stigler's Law?

from facial form and motion, and on more and more lifelike cartooning and image rendering for video entertainment (what one might call "impersonation," really). There is excellent work on surface effects of birth defects, notably in connection with schizophrenia and with fetal alcohol syndrome. There is excellent work on the details of form that are directly relevant to our best current theories of particular diseases: studies of joint surfaces in connection with joint pain, studies of the optic nerve head in connection with glaucoma.

And yet whole realms of public anthropology are separating their biometry from our morphometrics at the speed of light. Svante Pääbo's work on the Neanderthals, for instance, is almost wholly bioinformatic at this time, having little use for any measures of the organism beyond its genome. In spite of excellent morphometrics from Philipp Gunz and his colleagues at the same institution (e.g., Gunz, Neubauer et al., 2010), the turn of Neanderthal science away from bones toward the surviving molecules they shelter feels to me like a step backward from Gorjanović-Kramberger's work of a hundred years earlier. For public intellectuals, the meaning of anthropometry is inseparable from "man's conception of himself," from the *philosophical* anthropology that pursues continual enlightenment about the habitus of human life over the full range of species (apparently there are five of us now? or six?) that are entitled to be called sapient humans. Nothing in the molecular sciences can make up for the information that is currently missing about the forms, the biomechanics, and the mentalities of the hominids that bore those molecules. Nowadays the "tree of life" is computed from DNA (see, e.g., Hinchliff, 2015), and the role of morphometrics is to explain (or attempt to explain) evolutionary trends and speciations whose reality is demonstrated mainly by molecular evidence, not by morphology.

Other frontiers of our subject are not so band-limited. The study of ordinary human variability needs to be brought into communication with the enormous multiscale resources of CT and MR archives across the world's medical centers. During the years that this book was in preparation, I have busied myself with a range of sharply focused methodological speculations – on the joint information theory of morphometrics and biomechanics (Bookstein, 2013a), on the properties of high-dimensional random walk as detectable from the fossil record (Bookstein, 2013b), on a pseudo-Procrustes method for symmetric outlines without any landmarks (Bookstein and Ward, 2013), on the ties between GMM and today's formal kinematics of locomotion and predation (Bookstein, 2015c) – any of which might end up expanding the scope of GMM precisely by virtue of the expanded scope of hypotheses from neighboring disciplines to which the GMM descriptors are newly required to articulate. Well before that, Kanti Mardia and I (Mardia et al., 2006) floated the new

theory of multiscale morphometrics based on models along the lines of the
right-hand panel in Figure 5.93, which evolved into the fullblown methodology
of integration in Bookstein (2015b, 2016b) sketched in Section 5.6.8. It is time
that others took up efforts like these.

There is also a sociological side to these concerns of mine. Geometric
morphometrics is not so much a branch of statistics as a tool for all the
*inter*disciplines that are emerging to take advantage of the new instrumentation
of organismal form – and that network of interdisciplines now badly requires
a rebalancing. The current synthesis reviewed in these pages used GMM tools
to complete a toolkit for the biometry of the twentieth century. For the twenty-
first, the emphasis will fall on the extension of all these approaches to respond
to new questions about development, aging, disease, and evolution of our
particularly interesting species. Yes, in order to understand the natural history
of organisms, including *Homo sapiens,* we will need to master the information
content of form and the pattern engines that deal with it. Nevertheless, we
will never be able to understand morphology just from measurements of
morphology, and certainly not if that morphometric information is limited to
surfaces alone. We need to incorporate the rest of morphological structure as
well, at both reductionist and holistic levels. This requires quantities exported
for joint pattern analyses and the inferences about biological processes that
may follow. It is not that GMM's job *is* the inferences – inferences from GMM
alone are as impoverished as inferences from genomics alone. GMM's job is to
supply the quantities that, sent on for joint pattern analyses with observations
from other channels (development, behavior, health, physiology), eventually
result in inferences useful for understanding man's place in nature and the
individual's place in the species.

Biometrics took about one hundred years to build, from the 1870s to the
late twentieth century, and that was all *after* the instruments that supplied its
data, from calipers to photogrammetry, had been perfected by the end of the
Industrial Revolution. We are just about thirty years into the construction of
this companion technology of morphometrics, but the images that are driving
this progress are still ramifying, and it is all we can do to keep up with their
representations (cf. Weber and Bookstein, 2011), even if we have no time left
to deal with issues of variation. Taken all together, I would guess that we are
about half done with the necessary foundation-building for the morphometric
technology transfers of the present century. Any future edition of this book
will need to import tools from fields other than biometrics – from genomics,
from medical imaging, and from spatiotemporal statistics, to choose only three
from the library – in order to drive its pattern engines efficiently. Here in 2018,
the morphometrics of landmark points, curves, and surfaces seems suited to

its role in these tasks. But the toolbox for the next frontier, the morphometrics of volumes, of growth and development, of textures, of the distributions of molecules and tissues, and of the effects of genes and environment on all of these, has barely been imagined. We know almost nothing about how to phrase questions that will suit methodologies that have not yet been invented. I eagerly look forward to the equivalent of Wishart distributions, shape coordinates, and thin-plate splines for these steadily more and more complex data resources. Bon voyage.

References

Allen, B., B. Curlew, and A. Popović. The space of human body shapes: Reconstruction and parameterization from range scans. ACM SIGGRAPH 2003, July 2003. ACM.

Andersen, P. K., and L. T. Skovgaard. *Regression with Linear Predictors.* New York: Springer, 2010.

Anderson, D. R. *Model Based Inference in the Life Sciences: A Primer on Evidence.* New York: Springer, 2008.

Anderson, G. W., A. Guionnet, and O. Zeitouni. *An Introduction to Random Matrices.* Cambridge: Cambridge University Press, 2010.

Anderson, T. W. Asymptotic theory for principal component analysis. *Annals of Mathematical Statistics* 4:122–148, 1963.

Anderson, T. W. *An Introduction to Multivariate Statistical Analysis.* New York: Wiley, 1984.

Anson, B. J. *An Atlas of Human Anatomy.* Philadelphia: W. B. Saunders Company, 1950. Second edition, 1963.

Arias, E. United States Life Tables, 2003. *National Vital Statistics Reports* 54:14, 2006.

Bachelier, M. L. *Théorie de la Spéculation.* Paris: Gauthier-Villard, 1900.

Ball, P. *The Self-Made Tapestry: Pattern Formation in Nature.* Oxford University Press, 1999.

Ball, P. *Patterns in Nature: Why the Natural World Looks the Way It Does.* University of Chicago Press, 2016.

Berta, A., ed. *Whales, Dolphins, and Porpoises. A Natural History and Species Guide.* University of Chicago Press, 2015.

Biegert, J. Der Formwandel des Primatenschadels. Gegenbaurs Morphologisches Jahrbuch 98:77–199, 1957.

Blackith, R. E., and R. A. Reyment. *Multivariate Morphometrics.* Academic Press, 1971.

Blalock, H. M., Jr. *Causal Inferences in Nonexperimental Research.* University of North Carolina Press, 1964.

Boas, F. The horizontal plane of the skull and the general problem of the comparison of variable forms. *Science* 21:862–863, 1905.

Bollen, K. A. *Structural Equations with Latent Variables.* Wiley-Interscience, 1989.

494

Bookstein, F. L. *The Measurement of Biological Shape and Shape Change*. Lecture Notes in Biomathematics, vol. 24. Springer-Verlag, 1978.

Bookstein, F. L. The geometry of craniofacial growth invariants. *American Journal of Orthodontics* 83:221–234, 1983.

Bookstein, F. L. Tensor biometrics for changes in cranial shape. *Annals of Human Biology* 11:413–437, 1984.

Bookstein, F. L. Principal warps: Thin-plate splines and the decomposition of deformations. *IEEE Transactions on Pattern Analysis and Machine Intelligence* 11:567–585, 1989.

Bookstein, F. L. *Morphometric Tools for Landmark Data: Geometry and Biology*. Cambridge University Press, 1991.

Bookstein, F. L., and W. D. K. Green. A feature space for edgels in images with landmarks. *Journal of Mathematical Imaging and Vision* 3:231–261, 1993.

Bookstein, F. L. Landmark methods for forms without landmarks: Localizing group differences in outline shape. *Medical Image Analysis* 1:225–243, 1997.

Bookstein, F. L., K. Schaefer, H. Prossinger, H. Seidler, M. Fieder, C. Stringer, G. Weber, J. Arsuaga, D. Slice, F. J. Rohlf, W. Recheis, A. Mariam, and L. Marcus. Comparing frontal cranial profiles in archaic and modern *Homo* by morphometric analysis. *The Anatomical Record – The New Anatomist* 257:217–224, 1999.

Bookstein, F. L. Creases as local features of deformation grids. *Medical Image Analysis* 4:93–110, 2000.

Bookstein, F. L. "Voxel-based morphometry" should never be used with imperfectly registered images. *NeuroImage* NIMG.2001.0770, 14:1454–1462, 2001.

Bookstein, F. L., P. D. Sampson, A. P. Streissguth, and P. D. Connor. Geometric morphometrics of corpus callosum and subcortical structures in the fetal-alcohol-affected brain. *Teratology* 64:4–32, 2001.

Bookstein, F. L., and W. D. K. Green. *User's Manual, EWSH3.19*. 102 pages. `ftp://brainmap.stat.washington.edu/edgewarp/manual/`, posted March 2002.

Bookstein, F. L., A. Streissguth, P. Sampson, P. Connor, and H. Barr. Corpus callosum shape and neuropsychological deficits in adult males with heavy fetal alcohol exposure. *NeuroImage* 15:233–251, 2002a.

Bookstein, F. L., P. D. Sampson, P. D. Connor, and A. P. Streissguth. The midline corpus callosum is a neuroanatomical focus of fetal alcohol damage. *The Anatomical Record – The New Anatomist* 269:162–174, 2002b.

Bookstein, F. L., P. Gunz, P. Mitteröcker, H. Prossinger, K. Schäfer, and H. Seidler. Cranial integration in *Homo*: Singular warps analysis of the midsagittal plane in ontogeny and evolution. *Journal of Human Evolution* 44:167–187, 2003.

Bookstein, F. L., and K. V. Mardia. The five components of directional asymmetry. Pp. 35–40 in R. Aykroyd et al., eds., *Stochastic Geometry, Biological Structure, and Images*. Department of Statistics, University of Leeds, 2003.

Bookstein, F. L. After landmarks. Pp. 49–71 in D. E. Slice, ed., *Modern Morphometrics in Physical Anthropology*. Kluwer Academic Publishers, New York, 2004.

Bookstein, F. L. Morphometrics and computed homology: An old theme revisited. Pp. 69–81 in N. MacLeod, ed., *Proceedings of a Symposium on Algorithmic*

Approaches to the Identification Problem in Systematics, Museum of Natural History, London, 2007.

Bookstein, F. L., P. D. Connor, J. E. Huggins, H. M. Barr, K. D. Covell, and A. P. Streissguth. Many infants prenatally exposed to high levels of alcohol show one particular anomaly of the corpus callosum. *Alcoholism: Clinical and Experimental Research* 31:868–879, 2007.

Bookstein, F. L. Measurement, explanation, and biology: Lessons from a long century. *Biological Theory* 4:6–20, 2009a.

Bookstein, F. L. How quantification persuades when it persuades. *Biological Theory* 4:132–147, 2009b.

Bookstein, F. L. For isotropic offset normal shape distributions, covariance distance is proportional to Procrustes distance. Pp. 47–51 in A. Gusnanto, K. V. Mardia, and C. Fallaize, eds., *Proceedings of the 2009 Leeds Annual Statistical Research Workshop*, University of Leeds, 2009c.

Bookstein, F. L., and A. Kowell. Bringing morphometrics into the fetal alcohol report: Statistical language for the forensic neurologist or psychiatrist. *Journal of Psychiatry and Law* 38:449–474, 2010.

Bookstein, F. L. Allometry for the twenty-first century. *Biological Theory* 7:10–25, 2013a.

Bookstein, F. L. Random walk as a null model for geometric morphometrics of fossil series. *Paleobiology* 39:52–74, 2013b.

Bookstein, F. L., and P. D. Ward. A modified Procrustes analysis for bilaterally symmetrical outlines, with an application to microevolution in *Baculites*. *Paleobiology* 39:214–234, 2013.

Bookstein, F. L. *Measuring and Reasoning: Numerical Inference in the Sciences.* Cambridge: Cambridge University Press, 2014.

Bookstein, F. L., and P. M. Mitteroecker. Comparing covariance matrices by relative eigenanalysis, with applications to organismal biology. *Evolutionary Biology* 41:336–350, 2014.

Bookstein, F. L. No quantification without qualification, and vice versa. *Biological Theory*, thematic issue on quality and quantity, doi:10.1007/s13752-015-0221-3, 10:212–227, 2015a.

Bookstein, F. L. Integration, disintegration, and self-similarity: Characterizing the scales of shape variation in landmark data. *Evolutionary Biology*, doi 10.1007/s11692–015–9317–8, 42:395–426, 2015b.

Bookstein, F. L. The relation between geometric morphometrics and functional morphology, as explored by Procrustes interpretation of individual shape measures pertinent to function. *Anatomical Record* 298:314–327, 2015c.

Bookstein, F. L. Statistics is founded on entropy, not evolutionary psychology. (Review of *Tychomancy* by M. Strevens.) *Biological Theory*, 2015d.

Bookstein, F. L., and J. Domjanić. The principal components of adult female insole shape align closely with two of its classic indicators. *PLOS ONE* DOI:10.1371/journal.pone.0133303, August 26, 2015.

Bookstein, F. L. Reconsidering "The inappropriateness of conventional cephalometrics." *The American Journal of Orthodontics and Craniofacial Orthopedics* 149:784–797, 2016a.

Bookstein, F. L. The inappropriate symmetries of multivariate statistical analysis in geometric morphometrics. *Evolutionary Biology* doi: 10.1007/s11692-016-9382-7, 43:277–313, 2016b.

Bookstein, F. L. A newly noticed formula enforces fundamental limits on geometric morphometric analysis. *Evolutionary Biology* doi:10.1007/s11692-017-9424-9, 44:524–541, 2017a.

Bookstein, F. L. A method of factor analysis for shape coordinates. *American Journal of Physical Anthropology* doi:10.1002/ajpa.23277, 164:221–245, 2017b.

Bookstein, F. L. Review of Gilroy and MacPherson, *Thieme's Anatomy Atlas*, third edition, Latin nomenclature. *Journal of Anatomy* doi:10.1111/joa.12684, 231:1019–1020, 2017c.

Bookstein, F. L., B. Khambay, J. T. Kent, and K. V. Mardia. Bridging geometric morphometrics to medical anatomy: An example from an experimental study of the human smile. Manuscript in preparation, 2017.

Brennan, S. E. Caricature generator: The dynamic exaggeration of faces by computer. *Leonardo* 18:170–178, 1985.

Bumpus, H. C. The elimination of the unfit as illustrated by the introduced sparrow, *Passer domesticus*. *Biological Lectures of Woods Hole Marine Biological Laboratory*, 209–225, 1898.

Calvin, W. H. *A Brain for All Seasons: Human Evolution and Abrupt Climate Change*. University of Chicago Press, 2002.

Campbell, D. T., and H. L. Ross. The Connecticut crackdown on speeding: Time-series data in quasi-experimental analysis. *Law and Society Review* 3:33–54, 1968.

Campbell, D. T., and J. C. Stanley. *Experimental and Quasi-Experimental Designs for Research*. Rand-McNally, 1966. Originally published in Gage, N. L., ed., *Handbook of Research on Teaching*. Rand-McNally, 1963.

Cook, D. L., M. L. Neal, F. L. Bookstein, and J. H. Gennari. Ontology of physics for biology: Representing physical dependencies as a basis for biological processes. *Journal of Biomedical Semantics* 4:41, 2013.

Cronbach, L. J. *The Dependability of Behavioral Measurements: Theory of Generalizability for Scores and Profiles*. New York: Wiley, 1972.

Daumier, H. *Masques de 1831. La Caricature* (Paris), March 8, 1832.

Delattre, A. and Fenart, R. *L'hominisation du crâne: étudiée par la méthode vestibulaire*. Éditions du Centre national de la recherche scientifique, 1960.

Desimini, J., and C. Waldheim. *Cartographic Grounds: Projecting the Landscape Imaginary*. New York: Princeton Architectural Press, 2016.

DeWitte, S. N. Mortality risk and survival in the aftermath of the medieval Black Death. *PLOS ONE* 9:e96513, 2014.

Diaconis, P., S. Holmes, and R. Montgomery. Dynamical bias in the coin toss. *SIAM Review* 49:211–235, 2007.

Domjanić, J., M. Fieder, H. Seidler, and P. M. Mitteroecker. Geometric morphometric footprint analysis of young women. *Journal of Foot and Ankle Research* 6:27–34, 2013.

Draper, N. R., and H. Smith. *Applied Regression Analysis*, 3rd ed. New York: Wiley-Interscience, 1998.

Dryden, I. V., and K. V. Mardia. *Statistical Shape Analysis*. New York: Wiley, 1998. Second edition, 2016.

Dürer, A. *Vier Bücher von menschlicher Proportion.* 1528.

Eckart, C., and G. Young. The approximation of one matrix by another of lower rank. *Psychometrika* 1:211–218, 1936.

Edwards, A. W. F. *Likelihood.* Baltimore: Johns Hopkins University Press, 1992.

Edwards, W., H. Lindman, and L. J. Savage. Bayesian statistical inference for psychological research. *Psychological Review* 70:193–242, 1963. (This essay is reprinted in the collected essays of Jimmie Savage, in Volume 1 of S. Kotz and N. L. Johnson, eds., *Breakthroughs in Statistics* [Springer, 1993], and elsewhere.)

Einstein, A. [The three immortal papers from *Annalen der Physik,* 1905.] "On a Heuristic Viewpoint Concerning the Production and Transformation of Light" [the photoelectric effect], June 9. "On the Motion of Small Particles Suspended in a Stationary Liquid, as Required by the Molecular Kinetic Theory of Heat" [Brownian motion], July 18. "On the Electrodynamics of Moving Bodies" [special relativity theory], September 26.

Elsasser, W. M. *The Chief Abstractions of Biology.* Amsterdam: North-Holland Publishing Co., 1975.

Elsasser, W. M. *Reflections on a Theory of Organisms.* Cambridge, MA: MIT Press, 1998.

Farkas, L. G. *Anthropometry of the Head and Face.* New York: Raven Press, 1994.

Feller, W. *An Introduction to Probability Theory and Its Applications,* Volume 1, second edition. New York: John Wiley and Sons, 1957.

Felsenstein, J. *Inferring Phylogenies.* Sunderland, MA: Sinauer Associates, 2004.

Felsenstein, J., and F. L. Bookstein. Morphometrics on phylogenies. Manuscript in preparation, 2018.

Finch, C. E. *The Biology of Human Longevity: Inflammation, Nutrition, and Aging in the Evolution of Lifespans.* New York: Academic Press, 2007.

Fisher, R. A. Frequency distribution of the values of the correlation coefficient in samples from an indefinitely large population. *Biometrika* 10: 507–521, 1915.

Fix, E. Distributions which lead to linear regressions. In Neyman, J., ed., *Proceedings of the Berkeley Symposium on Mathematical Statistics and Probability* 1949, pp. 79–91.

Flury, B. *Common Principal Components and Related Multivariate Models.* New York: Wiley, 1988.

Fog, D. The geometrical method in the theory of sampling. *Biometrika* 35: 46–54, 1948.

Fornell, C., and F. L. Bookstein. Two structural equation models: LISREL and PLS applied to market data. *Journal of Marketing Research* 19:440–452, 1982.

Freedman, D. A. Statistical models and shoe leather. *Sociological Methodology* 21:291–313, 1991.

Freedman, D. A. *Statistical Models: Theory and Practice,* second edition. Cambridge: Cambridge University Press, 2009.

Freedman, D. A., and H. Zeisel. From mouse to man. *Statistical Science* 3:3–56, 1988.

Galton, F. *Hereditary Genius: An Inquiry into its Laws and Consequences.* London: Macmillan, 1869.

Galton, F. [Letter to George Darwin, 1877.] In Pearson, K., *The Life, Letters, and Labours of Francis Galton.* Cambridge: Cambridge University Press, 1930, III:465–466.

Galton, F. *Natural Inheritance.* London: Macmillan, 1889.

Galton, F. Classification of portraits. *Nature* 76:617–618, 1907.

Gerard, R. W., ed. *Concepts of Biology.* Publication 560. National Academy of Sciences, 1958.

Ghosh, M., and B. K. Sinha. A simple derivation of the Wishart distribution. *The American Statistician* 56(2):100–101, 2002.

Glaeser, G. *Geometry and Its Applications in Arts, Nature and Technology.* Vienna: Springer, 2012.

Gleick, J. *The Information: A History, a Theory, a Flood.* New York: Pantheon, 2011.

Gorjanović-Kramberger, K. *Der diluviale Mensch von Krapina in Kroatien: ein Beitrag zur Paläoanthropologie.* Wiesbaden: Kreidel's Verlag, 1906.

Gower, J. C. Some distance properties of latent root and vector methods used in multivariate analysis. *Biometrika* 53:325–338, 1966.

Gower, J. C., and G. B. Dijksterhuis. *Procrustes Problems.* Oxford: Oxford University Press, 2004.

Gower, J. C., and D. J. Hand. *Biplots.* London: Chapman and Hall, 1995.

Gunz, P. M., P. M. Mitteroecker, S. Neubauer, G. W. Weber, and F. L. Bookstein. Principles for the virtual reconstruction of hominin crania. *Journal of Human Evolution* 57:48–62, 2009.

Gunz, P., S. Neubauer, B. Maureille, and J.-J. Hublin. Brain development after birth differs between Neanderthals and modern humans. *Current Biology* 20:R921–R922, 2010.

Hackshaw, A. K., M. R. Law, and N. J. Law. The accumulated evidence on lung cancer and environmental tobacco smoke. *British Medical Journal* 315:980–988, 1997.

Hallgrimsson, B. S. "Morphometrics and the middle-out approach to complex traits." Rohlf Award Lecture, http://www.youtube.com/watch?v=kwo9QnJfwn0, October 28, 2015.

Harrison, C. R., and K. M. Robinette. CAESAR: Summary statistics for the adult population (ages 18–65) of the United States of America. United States Air Force Research Laboratory, Wright-Patterson Air Force Base, 2002.

Harvey, P. H., and J. R. Krebs. Comparing brains. *Science* 249:140–146, 1990.

Hastie, T., R. Tibshirani, and J. Friedman. *The Elements of Statistical Learning: Data Mining, Inference, and Prediction,* second edition. New York: Springer, 2009.

Hellung-Larsen, P., and A. P. Andersen. Cell volume and dry weight of cultured *Tetrahymena. Journal of Cell Science* 92:319–324, 1989.

Herculano-Houzel, S. *The Human Advantage.* Cambridge, MA: MIT Press, 2016.

Herculano-Houzel, S., K. Catania, P. R. Manger, and J. H. Kaas. Mammalian brains are made of these: A dataset of the numbers and densities of neuronal and nonneuronal cells in the brains of glires, primates, scandentia, eulipotyphlans, afrotherians and artiodactyls, and their relationship with body mass. *Brain, Behavior and Evolution* 86:145–163, 2015.

Hinchliff, C. E., and 21 others. Synthesis of phylogeny and taxonomy into a comprehensive tree of life. *PNAS* 112:12764–12769, 2015.

Hogben, L. *Chance and Choice by Cardpack and Chessboard.* New York: Chanticleer Press, 1950.

Hogben, L. *Statistical Theory: The Relationship of Probability, Credibility, and Error.* New York: W. W. Norton, 1957.

Huxley, J. *Patterns of Relative Growrth*. New York: Dial Press, 1932.

Jackson, J. E. *A User's Guide to Principal Components*. New York: Wiley-Interscience, 1991.

James, W. *The Varieties of Religious Experience*. London: Longmans Green & Co., 1902.

Jardine, N. The observational and theoretical components of homology: A study based on the morphology of the dermal skull-roofs of rhipistidian fishes. *Biological Journal of the Linnaean Society* 1:327–361, 1969.

Jaynes, E. T., and G. L. Bretthorst. *Probability Theory: The Logic of Science*. Cambridge: Cambridge University Press, 2003.

Jerison, H. J. Paleoneurology and the evolution of mind. *Scientific American* 234(1): 90–101, 1976.

Kaiser, H. F. The varimax criterion for analytic rotation in factor analysis. *Psychometrika* 23:187–200, 1958.

Kampourakis, K. *Understanding Evolution*. Cambridge: Cambridge University Press, 2014.

Keay, J. *The Great Arc: The Dramatic Tale of How India Was Mapped and Everest Was Named*. New York: HarperCollins, 2000.

Kendall, D. G. Shape manifolds, Procrustean metrics and complex projective spaces. *Bulletin of the London Mathematical Society* 16:81–121, 1984.

Kendall, M. S. Comment on H. Hotelling, "New light on the correlation coefficient and its transforms." *Journal of the Royal Statistical Society, Series B*, 15:225–226, 1953.

Koch, G. S., and R. F. Link. *Statistical Analysis of Geological Data*. New York: Wiley, 1971.

Krieger, M. H. *Doing Physics: How Physicists Take Hold of the World*. Bloomington: Indiana University Press, 1992. Second edition, 2012.

Kuhn, T. S. The function of measurement in modern physical science. *ISIS* 52:161–193, 1961. Also, pp. 31–63 in Woolf, ed., 1961.

Kullback, S. *Information Theory and Statistics*. New York: Wiley, 1959.

Lande, R. Quantitative genetic anaysis of multivariate evolution, applied to brain:body size allometry. *Evolution* 33:402–416, 1979.

Law, M. R., J. K. Morris, and N. J. Wald. Environmental tobacco smoke exposure and ischaemic heart disease: An evaluation of the evidence. *British Medical Journal* 315:973-980, 1997.

Li, S. Z., and A. K. Jain, eds. *Handbook of Face Recognition*, 2nd edition. London: Springer, 2011.

Lieberson, S. *Making It Count: The Improvement of Social Research and Theory*. Berkeley: University of California Press, 1985.

Lord, F. M., and M. R. Novick. *Statistical Theories of Mental Test Scores*. Reading, MA: Addison-Wesley, 1968.

Lukacs, E. Characterization of populations by properties of suitable statistics. In Neyman, J., ed., *Proceedings of the Third Berkeley Symposium on Mathematical Statistics and Probability*, 1956, pp. II:195–214.

Mandelbrot, B. B. *The Fractalist*. New York: Pantheon, 2013.

Marcus, L. F. Traditional morphometrics. In Rohlf and Bookstein, eds., 1990, pp. 77–122.

Marcus, L. F., M. Corti, A. Loy, G. J. P. Naylor, and D. E. Slice, eds. *Advances in Morphometrics*. New York: Springer, 1996.

Marcus, L. F., E. Hingst-Zaher, and H. Zaher. Application of landmark morphometrics to skulls representing the orders of living mammals. *Hystrix* 11:27–47, 2000.

Mardia, K. V., F. L. Bookstein, and J. T. Kent. Alcohol, babies, and the death penalty: Saving lives by analysing the shape of the brain. *Significance* 10(2):12–16, 2013.

Mardia, K. V., F. L. Bookstein, and I. J. Moreton. Statistical assessment of bilateral symmetry of shapes. *Biometrika* 87:285–300, 2000.

Mardia, K. V., F. L. Bookstein, J. T. Kent, and C. R. Meyer. Intrinsic random fields and image deformations. *Journal of Mathematical Imaging and Vision* 26:59–71, 2006.

Mardia, K. V., J. T. Kent, and J. Bibby. *Multivariate Analysis*. New York: Wiley, 1979.

Mardia, K. V., and R. J. Marshall. Maximum likelihood estimation of models for residual covariance in spatial regression. *Biometrika* 71: 135–146, 1984.

Martin R. *Lehrbuch der Anthropologie in systematischer Darstellung*. Jena: Gustav Fischer, 1914. 2nd ed., three volumes, 1928.

Martin, R. D. Relative brain size and basal metabolic rate in terrestrial vertebrates. *Nature* 293:57–60, 1981.

Masoro, E. J., and S. N. Austad, eds. *Handbook of the Biology of Aging*, 7th edition. New York: Academic Press, 2010.

Medawar, P. B. The shape of the human being as a function of time. *Proc. Royal Society of London B* 132:133–141, 1944.

Medawar, P. B. Postscript. In R. D'A. Thompson, *D'Arcy Wentworth Thompson*, Oxford: Oxford University Press, 1958.

Millikan, R. A. A direct photoelectric determination of Planck's "*h*." *American Journal of Physics* 7:355–390, 1916.

Mitteroecker, P. M., and F. L. Bookstein. The ontogenetic trajectory of the phenotypic covariance matrix, with examples from craniofacial shape in rats and humans. *Evolution* 63:727–737, 2009.

Mitteroecker, P. M., and F. L. Bookstein. Linear discrimination, ordination, and the visualization of selection gradients in modern morphometrics. *Evolutionary Biology* 38:100–114, 2011.

Mitteroecker, P. M., and P. Gunz. Advances in geometric morphometrics. *Evolutionary Biology* 36:235–247, 2009.

Mitteroecker, P., P. Gunz, G. Weber, and F. L. Bookstein. Regional dissociated heterochrony in multivariate analysis. *Annals of Anatomy* 186:463–470, 2004.

Mosimann, J. E. Size allometry: Size and shape variables with characterizations of the log-normal and generalized gamma distributions. *Journal of the American Statistical Association* 65:930–945, 1970.

Moss, M. L., R. Skalak, M. Shinozuka, H. Patel, L. Moss-Salentijn, H. Vilmann, and P. Mehta. Statistical testing of an allometric centered model of craniofacial growth. *American Journal of Orthodontics* 83: 5–18, 1983.

Mosteller, F. Nonsampling errors. In D. L. Sills, ed., *International Encyclopedia of the Social Sciences*. New York: Macmillan and the Free Press, 1968, III:113–132.

Mosteller, F., and J. W. Tukey. *Data Analysis and Regression: A Second Course in Statistics.* New York: Addison-Wesley, 1977.

Moyers, R. E., and F. L. Bookstein. The inappropriateness of conventional cephalometrics. *American Journal of Orthodontics* 75:599–618, 1979.

Muirhead, R. J. *Aspects of Multivariate Statistical Theory.* New York: Wiley, 1982.

Olson, E. C., and R. L. Miller. *Morphological Integration.* Chicago: University of Chicago Press, 1958.

Ono, M., S. Kubick, and C. D. Abernethey. *Atlas of the Cerebral Sulci.* New York: Thieme, 1990.

Oxnard, C. E. *The Order of Man: A Biomathematical Anatomy of the Primates.* New Haven, CT: Yale University Press, 1984.

Oxnard, C., and P. O'Higgins. Biology clearly needs morphometrics. Does morphometrics need biology? *Biological Theory* 4:84–97, 2009.

Pakkenberg, B., and H. J. G. Gunderson. Neocortical neuron number in humans: Effect of sex and age. *Journal of Comparative Neurology* 384:312–320, 1997.

Palmer, A. R., and C. Strobeck. Fluctuating asymmetry: Measurement, analysis, patterns. *Annual Reviews of Ecology and Systematics* 17:391–421, 1986.

Paulos, J. A. *A Numerate Life: A Mathematician Explores the Vagaries of Life, His Own and Probably Yours.* Amherst, NY: Prometheus Books, 2015.

Pearson, K. *The Grammar of Science.* London: Walter Scott, 1892. 2nd ed., London: Adam and Charles Black, 1900. 3rd ed., London: Adam and Charles Black, 1911.

Pearson, K. On lines and planes of closest fit to systems of points in space. *Philosophical Magazine* Series 6, 2:559–572, 1901.

Pearson, K. On the inheritance of the mental and moral characters in man, and its comparison with the inheritance of the physical characters. *Journal of the Anthropological Institute of Great Britain and Ireland* 33:179–237, 1903.

Pearson, K. Walter Frank Raphael Weldon, 1860–1906. *Biometrika* 5:1–52, 1906.

Pearson, K., and L. N. G. Filon. Mathematical contributions to the theory of evolution. IV. On the probable errors of frequency constants and on the influence of random selection on variation and correlation. *Philosophical Transactions of the Royal Society of London A* 191:229–311, 1898.

Pearson, K., and A. Lee. On the laws of inheritance in man. I: Inheritance of physical characters. *Biometrika* 2:357–462, 1903.

Perrin, J. *Atoms,* 2nd English edition, revised. London: Constable, 1923.

Peters, R. H. *The Ecological Implications of Body Size.* Cambridge: Cambridge University Press, 1983.

Platt, J. R. Strong inference. *Science* 146:347–353, 1964.

Pólya, G. *Mathematics and Plausible Reasoning,* two volumes. Princeton, NJ: Princeton University Press, 1954.

Puget, A., J. L. V. Mejino, Jr., L. T. Detwiler, J. D. Franklin, and J. F. Brinkley. Spatial-symbolic query engine in anatomy. *Methods of Information in Medicine* 51:463–478, 2012.

Ramsay, J., and B. W. Silverman. *Functional Data Analysis,* second edition. New York: Springer, 2010.

Rao, C. R. *Linear Statistical Inference and Its Applications,* second edition. New York: John Wiley & Sons, 1973.

Rentgen, S. *Information Graphics*. Cologne: Taschen, 2012.

Reyment, R. A. *Multidimensional Palaeobiology*. Oxford: Pergamon, 1991.

Reyment, R. A., R. E. Blackith, and N. Campbell. *Multivariate Morphometrics*, second edition. New York: Academic Press, 1984.

Reyment, R. A., and K. H. Jöreskog. *Applied Factor Analysis in the Natural Sciences*. Cambridge: Cambridge University Press, 1993.

Riggs, D. S. *The Mathematical Approach to Physiological Problems: A Critical Primer.* Cambridge, MA: MIT Press, 1963.

Riolo, M. L., R. E. Moyers, J. A. McNamara Jr., and W. S. Hunter. *An Atlas of Craniofacial Growth*. Craniofacial Monograph 2, Center for Human Growth and Development, University of Michigan, 1974.

Robinette, K. M., H. Daanen, and E. Paquet. The CAESAR project: A 3-D surface anthropometry survey. In *Proceedings of the Second International Conference on 3-D Digital Imaging and Modeling*, IEEE, 1999.

Rohlf, F. J. On the use of shape spaces to compare morphometric methods. *Hystrix*, 11:9–25, 2000a.

Rohlf, F. J. Statistical power comparisons among alternative morphometric methods. *American Journal of Physical Anthropology* 111:463–478, 2000b.

Rohlf, F. J., and F. L. Bookstein, eds. *Proceedings of the Michigan Morphometrics Workshop*. Ann Arbor: University of Michigan Museums, 1990.

Rohlf, F. J., and D. E. Slice. Methods for comparison of sets of landmarks. *Systematic Zoology* 39:40–59, 1990.

Rohlf, F. J., and R. R. Sokal. *Biometry*, 4th edition. New York: W. H. Freeman, 2012.

Ross, A. A., K. Nandakumar, and A. K. Jain, eds. *Handbook of Multibiometrics*. Boston, MA: Springer, 2006.

Rosse, C. The challenges of representing anatomical spatial relations. *Methods of Information in Medicine* 51:457–462, 2012.

Rosse, C., and J. L. V. Mejino, Jr. A reference ontology for biomedical informatics: The Foundational Model of Anatomy. *Journal of Biomedical Informatics* 36:478–500, 2001.

Roth, G., and U. Dicke. Evolution of the brain and intelligence in primates. Pp. 413–430 in M. A. Hofman and D. Falk, eds. *Progress in Brain Research*, vol. 195: *Evolution of the Primate Brain: From Neuron to Behavior*. Elsevier, 2012.

Schäfer, K., T. Lauc, P, Mitteroecker, P. Gunz, and F. L. Bookstein. Dental arch asymmetry in an isolated Adriatic community. *American Journal of Physical Anthropology* 129:132–142, 2006.

Schmidt-Nielsen, K. *Scaling: Why Is Animal Size So Important?* Cambridge: Cambridge Univesrity Press, 1984.

Schoenemann, P. T. An MRI Study of the Relationship Between Human Neuroanatomy and Behavioral Ability. PhD dissertation, University of California at Berkeley, 1997.

Seber, G. A. F., and C. J. Wild. *Nonlinear Regression*. New York: Wiley-Interscience, 2003.

Secher, N.J., H. Djursing, P. K. Hansen, C. Lestrup, P. S. Eriksen, B. L. Thomsen, and N. Keiding. Estimation of fetal weight in the third trimester by ultrasound. *European Journal of Obstetrics & Gynecology and Reproductive Biology* 24:1–11, 1987.

Small, C. *The Statistical Theory of Shape*. New York: Springer 1996.

Sneath, P. H. A. Trend-surface analysis of transformation grids. *Journal of Zoology* 151:65–122, 1967.

Sokal, R. R., and P. H. A. Sneath. *Principles of Numerical Taxonomy*. San Francisco: W. H. Freeman Co., 1965.

Stigler, S. M. *The History of Statistics: The Measurement of Uncertainty before 1900*. Cambridge, MA: Harvard University Press, 1986.

Stone, M. An asymptotic equivalence of choice of model by cross-validation and Akaike's criterion. *Journal of the Royal Statistical Society* B39:44–47, 1977.

Streissguth, A. P., F. L. Bookstein, H. M. Barr, P. D. Sampson, and J. K. Young. Risk factors for adverse life outcomes in Fetal Alcohol Syndrome and Fetal Alcohol effects. *Journal of Developmental and Behavioral Pediatrics* 25:228–238, 2004.

Strevens, M. *Tychomancy: Inferring Probability from Causal Structure*. Cambridge, MA: Harvard University Press, 2013.

Stuart, A., and K. Ord. *Kendall's Advanced Theory of Statistics*. Volume 1, *Distribution Theory*. 1994 edition. London: Griffin.

Taigman, Y., M. Yang, M'A. Ranzato, and L. Wolf. DeepFace: Closing the gap to human-level performance in face verification. Pp. 1701–1708 in *2014 IEEE Conference on Computer Vision and Pattern Recognition (CVPR)*. IEEE, 2014.

Taleb, N. N. *The Black Swan*. New York: Random House, 2007.

Tanner, J. M., and P. S. W. Davies. Clinical longitudinal standards for height and height velocity for North American children. *Journal of Pediatrics* 107:317–329, 1985.

Federative International Programme on Anatomical Terminologies. *Terminologia Anatomica: International Anatomical Terminology*. Stuttgart: Thieme, 1998. Second edition, 2011.

Thompson, D'A. W. *On Growth and Form*. Cambridge: Cambridge University Press, 1917. Second, enlarged edition, 1942. Abridged edition (J. T. Bonner, ed.), 1961.

Torgerson, W. S. *Theory and Methods of Scaling*. New York: Wiley, 1958.

Tuddenham, R. D., and M. M. Snyder. Physical growth of California boys and girls from birth to eighteen years. *University of California Publications in Child Development* 1:183–228, 1954.

Wahba, G. *Spline Models for Observational Data*. Philadelphia: SIAM, 1990.

Weber, G. W., and F. L. Bookstein. *Virtual Anthropology: A Guide to a New Interdisciplinary Field*. Berlin: Springer Verlag, 2011.

Weiner, J. *The Beak of the Finch*. New York: Vintage, 1995.

Weisberg, S. *Applied Linear Regression*, third edition. New York: John Wiley & Sons, 2005.

Weiss, P. A. [Comments.] In Gerard, 1958, p. 140.

West, G. *Scale*. New York: Penguin Press, 2017.

West, G. B., J. H. Brown, and B. J. Enquist. A general model for the origin of allometric scaling laws in biology. *Science* 276:122–126, 1997.

Whittaker, E. The modern approach to Descartes' problem: The relation of the mathematical and physical sciences to philosophy. The Herbert Spencer Lecture in the University of Oxford. London: Thomas Nelson, 1948.

Wigner, E. The unreasonable effectiveness of mathematics in the natural sciences. *Communications in Pure and Applied Mathematics* 13:1–14, 1960.

Williams, R. J. *Biochemical Individuality: The Basis for the Genetotrophic Concept.* New York: John Wiley and Sons, 1956.

Wilson, E. B. *An Introduction to Scientific Research.* New York: McGraw-Hill, 1952.

Wilson, E. O. *Consilience: The Unity of Knowledge.* New York: Knopf, 1998.

Wishart, J. The generalized product moment distribution in samples from a normal multivariate population. *Biometrika* 290A:32–52, 1928.

Wright, S. General, group, and special size factors. *Genetics* 17:603–619, 1932.

Wright, S. *Evolution and the Genetics of Populations.* Volume 1, *Genetic and Biometric Foundations.* Chicago: University of Chicago Press, 1968.

Yablokov, A. V. *Variability of Mammals.* Washington, DC: Amerind, Ltd., for the Smithsonian Institution and the National Science Foundation, 1974.

Zhang, A., Q. Xie, and A. Srivastava. Elastic registration and shape analysis of functional objects. Pp. 218–235 in I. L. Dryden and J. T. Kent, eds., *Geometry-Driven Statistics.* Chichester: Wiley, 2015.

Ziman, J. *Reliable Knowledge.* Cambridge: Cambridge University Press, 1978.

Index

The following index combines people, topics, techniques, notations, acronyms, and examples. Persons are cited by last name and one or two initials. References to figures are in **boldface**. Entries pointing to footnotes go as page number followed by "n" and then footnote number, e.g., "352n2". Multiple crossreferences are separated by semicolons; within a cross-reference, a comma indicates subordination (e.g., *see* A, B means "look up B under main index term A").

Printed in the United States
by Baker & Taylor Publisher Services